Mechanistic Toxicology

Mechanistic Toxicology

The molecular basis of how chemicals disrupt biological targets

Urs A. Boelsterli
Head, HepaTox Consulting
Pfeffingen
Switzerland

and

Professor of Toxicology
Institute of Clinical Pharmacy
University of Basel
Switzerland

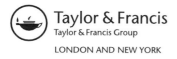
Taylor & Francis
Taylor & Francis Group

LONDON AND NEW YORK

First published 2003 by Taylor & Francis
2 Park Square, Milton Park, Abingdon, Oxon, OX14 4RN

Simultaneously published in the USA and Canada
by Taylor & Francis Inc,
270 Madison Ave, New York, NY 10016

Reprinted 2005

Taylor & Francis is an imprint of the Taylor & Francis Group

© 2003 Taylor & Francis

Typeset in 10/12pt Goudy by Graphicraft Ltd, Hong Kong
Printed and bound in Great Britain by TJ International Ltd, Padstow, Cornwall

British Library Cataloguing in Publication Data
A catalogue record for this book is available from the British Library

Library of Congress Cataloging in Publication Data
Boelsterli, Urs A., 1948-
    Mechanistic toxicology : the molecular basis of how chemicals disrupt biological
targets / Urs A. Boelsterli.
        p. cm.
    Includes bibliographical references and index.
    1. Molecular toxicology.   I. Title.

RA1220.3 .B64 2002
615.9—dc21   2002072726

ISBN 0-415-28458-9 (hbk)
ISBN 0-415-28459-7 (pbk)

Contents

Figures

Tables

Preface

This book is an introductory textbook and a gateway to the area of mechanistic toxicology. It addresses both undergraduate and graduate students in pharmaco-toxicology and environmental toxicology, but it is also intended to be a source of reference for interested readers from other disciplines. The idea for this book originated from an introductory course on 'Mechanisms underlying the toxicity of xenobiotics' taught for many years at the Swiss Federal Institute of Technology in Zurich, Switzerland. During the continued reviewing and updating of the lectures, and thanks to the feedback from students and colleagues, the contents of the book slowly crystallized into its present form.

Because this textbook highlights one particular area of toxicology (mechanisms), it can only scratch the surface of other related fields. It is, therefore, not intended to compete with the many other excellent textbooks on general toxicology nor does it provide a comprehensive documentation of toxic chemicals or organ systems affected by xenobiotics. Rather, this book focuses on the general principles that link xenobiotic-induced toxicity with molecular pathways underlying these toxic effects.

To illustrate such molecular mechanisms and pathways, many specific examples of drugs, environmental pollutants, and other chemicals were chosen. These examples are paradigms for which the underlying mechanisms are particulary well understood or for which the elucidation of a particular mechanism has been applied for human risk assessment or used as a rationale to develop therapies or antidotes. For the sake of clarity and to make a case, it was inevitable that some key points would be highlighted, thereby often neglecting the fact that the same xenobiotic may use other pathways and exert its toxicity via other mechanisms as well.

The real challenge in compiling the chapters was not so much to find examples for a given mechanism as the right selection of appropriate paradigms, given the rapidly increasing wealth of information and the exploding knowledge in molecular toxico-logy. In addition, it was often necessary to choose to omit details and make things understandable without distorting the real story. For a clear understanding of the mechanisms of toxicity, it will often be indispensable for the reader to recall briefly the biological, biochemico-molecular, or toxicological background; therefore, some of this basic background is provided in boxes in a condensed frame.

For each chapter, a concentrated selection of recent review articles or pivotal original articles is given. I thank the authors who are not specifically mentioned for understanding that not all the pertinent work could be included. This occurred due to space limitation rather than a lack of appreciation of the others' work.

I am most grateful to my teachers and peers, in particular the late Gerhard Zbinden, who convinced me (many years ago) that the elucidation of the molecular events underlying the toxicity of xenobiotics was a topical field and an exciting area of research. This has not changed over the years, and it is hoped that the reader will share in some of this excitement. I would also like to extend my thanks to all my former postdocs, graduate students, and undergraduate students who gave me feedback and pointed out gaps and better ways to communicate the toxicological science in academic classes.

Importantly, I would like to express my warmest thanks to my colleagues who critically read the chapters and provided valuable clues for improvement. Notably, I thank Dr Christopher A. Bradfield, Dr Steven D. Cohen, Dr George B. Corcoran, Dr Jürgen Drewe, Dr Hans-Pietro Eugster, Dr James P. Kehrer, Dr Anke Kretz-Rommel, Dr B. Kevin Park, Dr José E. Manautou, Dr Urs Rickenbacher, Dr Stephan Ruetz, and Dr Kendall B. Wallace for their input.

Finally, I wish to thank the members of staff of Taylor & Francis who have been involved with the publication for their professional guidance.

And last but not least I thank my family for their support, patience, and encouragement.

Chapter 1

Introduction

Contents

1.1. Why molecular mechanisms?

Mechanistic toxicology describes the processes of *how* chemicals exert their toxic effects in biological systems. Mechanistic toxicology therefore not only delineates a hazard for a particular chemical, and defines the potency of one compound in comparison with its congeners, but also aims at identifying the underlying molecular events that lead from initial exposure to the chemical to the ultimate manifestation of toxic injury in an organism.

Because these molecular events are causal and occur in a defined temporal sequence, branching out into different directions, this area of toxicology investigates and addresses a number of fundamental questions.

1 How do xenobiotics (i.e. foreign compounds, as opposed to endogenous compounds) enter an organism (or a cell), and how are they distributed and metabolized?
2 How do xenobiotics interact with target molecules?
3 How do xenobiotics exert their toxic effects at the molecular level?
4 What are the downstream biological consequences and how does the organism deal with the insult?

Sometimes the mechanisms are well investigated and understood at one level but not known at all at another level. For example, there are examples where the initial

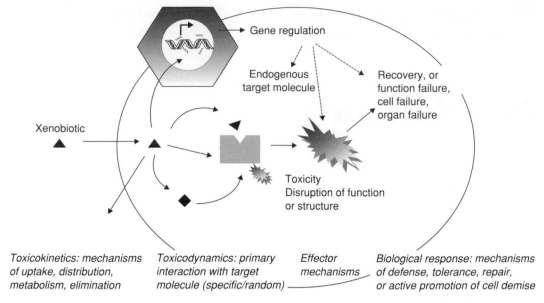

Gene regulation

Endogenous
target molecule

Recovery, or
function failure,
cell failure,
organ failure

Xenobiotic

Toxicity
Disruption of function
or structure

*Toxicokinetics: mechanisms
of uptake, distribution,
metabolism, elimination*

*Toxicodynamics: primary
interaction with target
molecule (specific/random)*

*Effector
mechanisms*

*Biological response: mechanisms
of defense, tolerance, repair,
or active promotion of cell demise*

Figure 1.1. Mechanisms of toxicity can be studied at different levels, following the sequence of events that occur during exposure to a potentially toxic compound. First, a xenobiotic is taken up into the body or by a particular organ, where it is distributed and subject to possible biotransformation, and where it is in an equilibrium with its elimination. Next, a xenobiotic or its metabolite interacts with a target molecule where it exerts a toxic effect, either through specific intermolecular recognition sites or in a less selective manner. This interaction is amplified by specific signals. Finally, the cell, organ, or body reacts with a specific response to this insult, which can be an adaptive or compensatory reaction, induction of tolerance, or repair, or it may succumb to the insult, or even actively promote cell death or organ failure. All these events can be up- or down-regulated by altered gene expression induced by the xenobiotic.

interaction of a xenobiotic with a target macromolecule in the cell is well understood at the molecular level, yet the downstream molecular events that lead to toxicity are enigmatic. Alternatively, the more distal cascades of pathophysiological events that lead to a toxic effect may be well understood, while the types of molecular interactions of a xenobiotic with an initial target are completely unknown (see Figure 1.1).

But why is the unraveling of such molecular mechanisms important, and why should we invest an enormous amount of time, financial resources, and energy in elucidating biological mechanisms that are involved in the causation of a toxic effect? There are a number of important factors that more than justify these efforts. One of the most plausible reasons for improving our detailed understanding of molecular mechanisms is the fact that a deeper understanding of such mechanisms will help us to extrapolate data better and to improve risk assessment of potentially toxic chemicals for human safety. This is true not only for pharmaceutical drugs in development but also for environmental pollutants, chemicals in the workplace, and synthetic and naturally occurring hazardous compounds in food or residues in the drinking water (see Table 1.1).

Table 1.1 Biomedical applications where a more detailed understanding of the mechanisms underlying the toxicity of a particular xenobiotic is helpful

- To improve assessment of risk to human health
- To define high-risk subgroups in human populations
- To define threshold exposure level for toxic compound including carcinogenic compounds (genotoxic versus non-genotoxic carcinogens)
- To guide and accelerate the development of safer pharmaceutical drugs
- To develop antidotes for prevention of acute intoxications and therapy for their treatment
- To develop biomarkers that monitor exposure to toxins and development of chronic toxicity
- To target and selectively kill cells or tissues (e.g. in tumor therapy)

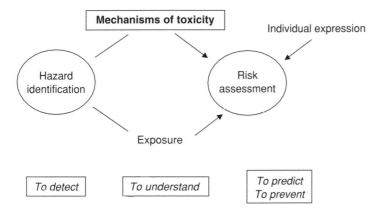

Figure 1.2. Elucidation of mechanisms of toxicity is one of the most important bridges connecting hazard detection with risk assessment for human health, ultimately leading to toxicity prediction and prevention.

A host of potentially hazardous chemicals has been detected in the past, and the number of new chemicals added to this list is steadily growing. The step from the mere detection of a toxic hazard (qualitative aspect) to the final assessment of risk in human populations (quantitative aspect) involves, however, a number of sophisticated estimations and considerations. For a chemical it is certainly not sufficient merely to set a safety margin, based on animal data or cell culture experimentation. Instead, realistic exposure data have to be taken into account. In addition, and importantly, mechanistic aspects of toxicity are increasingly used to calculate more accurately the risk for humans (see Figure 1.2).

A typical example of how biomechanistic data on the effects of xenobiotics in the body can be successfully used for interspecies extrapolation, and ultimately for the assessment of human risk, is unleaded gasoline (see Figure 1.3).

Unleaded gasoline is a complex mixture of organic chemicals to which we all are exposed to varying degrees. It has been well documented that chronic administration of unleaded gasoline to rats increases the number of tumors (tubular carcinomas) in the kidney. Interestingly, only male rats were affected, and unleaded gasoline was not carcinogenic in mice of either sex. What is the risk for humans? While exposure data are available, they alone do not further help in determining whether humans would respond to unleaded gasoline like male rats or rather like mice.

Mechanistic studies have revealed that activated substances in unleaded gasoline (e.g. *tert*-butyl alcohol) bind to a specific plasma protein, α2u-globulin, a low molecular weight protein synthesized in the liver and which functions as a protease inhibitor. This protein is filtered at the glomerulus, and a great portion of it is reabsorbed in the kidney proximal tubular cells. Normally, α2u-globulin is degraded in lysosomes. However, the chemically-altered protein is degraded more slowly by lysosomal enzymes and hence accumulates in the epithelial cells. As a consequence, the tubular epitheliar cells are lethally damaged. The continuing cycle of cell demise and regeneration greatly increases the rate of cell proliferation in the kidney, which is an established epigenetic mechanism of carcinogenesis. Because α2u-globulin is a male rat-specific protein, which is not expressed in female rats or mice or in humans, it is reasonable to conclude that the risk for unleaded gasoline to be nephrocarcinogenic in humans is small.

We tend to describe such mechanisms, especially when they are well defined, as isolated single events. Even if we appreciate the fact that several mechanisms might be involved in a toxic reaction, we often think in linear terms and see 'a mechanism' as a chain of molecular and cellular events. Although this is often helpful in order to reduce the complex picture to a simpler model that we understand better and that is amenable to experimental analysis, it is clear that nature is much more complex. Thus, mechanisms of toxicity include more than one biochemical or molecular event;

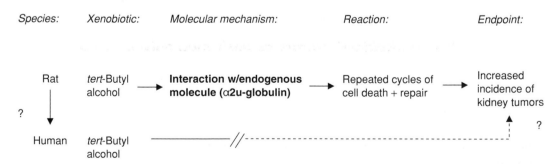

Figure 1.3. Elucidation of the mechanism of the nephrocarcinogenic potency of components of unleaded gasoline is a valuable tool in human risk assessment. As humans (unlike male rats) do not express α2u-globulin, this nephrotoxic mechanism is not relevant in humans.

there are both sequential and concurrent pathways, cascades of events, with complex feedback mechanisms involved, that create a complex network of molecular reactions. Of course, we are far from understanding these events. Nevertheless, through carefully choosing the right models and experimental approaches, we have been able to elucidate a few.

Many attempts have been made to classify mechanisms. However, the list is becoming longer and longer, and new mechanisms are added as we detect new pathways of how chemicals interact with biological targets. Such a classification is complicated by the fact that we look at these mechanisms from different angles and at different levels. Nevertheless, a few important mechanisms have been emerging as particularly relevant, and these are discussed in this book.

1.2. Toxicokinetics and toxicodynamics

Both toxicokinetic and toxicodynamic factors can greatly determine the toxicity of a xenobiotic. The term *toxicokinetics* describes the changes of the concentrations of a compound in the organism over time. These changes are mostly determined by the uptake of the compound into the organism or into a particular tissue, its body distribution, its metabolic conversion into metabolites that each again can have different kinetic behavior, and, finally, excretion of the compound. For example, selective uptake and accumulation of a particular xenobiotic in a specific tissue or cell type can lead to toxicity which does not occur in the majority of other tissues or cells (see Chapter 3). Alternatively, inhibition of the normal export of a potentially toxic metabolite from a cell may also cause toxicity.

On the other hand, the term *toxicodynamics* describes the dynamic interactions of a compound with a biological target and its downstream biological effects. For example, covalent interactions of a xenobiotic with a macromolecule of the cell, or interaction and activation of a cellular receptor can be linked with toxicity (see Chapters 9 and 12). In the vast majority of known cases and in most examples that are described below, it is only a small number of isolated steps within this toxicodynamic cascade and branching-out network which are currently known to play a causal role in the overall pathogenesis of a toxic effect. For the sake of simplicity, these isolated events are mostly dissected from their dynamic background and described as isolated pathways. This reduction to the essential steps helps one to better understand the overall mechanism and eventually to construct models.

1.2.1. Toxicokinetic factors as basic mechanisms of toxicity

In many cases, the species-selectivity or organ-specificity of a toxic effect provoked by a xenobiotic is driven by toxicokinetic factors.

Because in many instances the toxicity of a chemical is dependent on its concentration at the critical site (cell, tissue that will be damaged), and because the concentration is determined by toxicokinetic factors, abnormally high exposure level can be the cause for the toxicity. Factors that increase the exposure of a xenobiotic include enhanced absorption, decreases in the rate of metabolic degradation, inhibition of the compound's removal from a site and retention in a particular tissue compartment, repeated cycles of reabsorption and re-excretion, and overall inhibition in the excretion. Sometimes a combination of some or all of these factors can even more extensively augment the toxicity.

One example that illustrates the mechanistic role of toxicokinetic factors is a rare but serious adverse effect caused by a group of cholesterol-lowering agents, the statins.

Statins, or 3-hydroxymethyl-3-glutaryl-CoA (HMG-CoA) reductase inhibitors, are widely used therapeutics aimed at decreasing plasma cholesterol levels and thus reducing the morbidity and mortality associated with coronary heart disease. The drugs attenuate cholesterol biosynthesis in the liver by inhibiting the rate-limiting enzyme for cholesterol synthesis, HMG-CoA reductase.

Although they are generally safe drugs, a rare side effect of statins, when combined with certain other drugs, is myotoxicity, manifested as muscle fiber necrosis and fragmentation, and rhabdomyolysis, an acute fulminant and potentially fatal condition of skeletal muscle destruction, resulting in release of myoglobin. As a consequence, there is myoglobinemia and myoglobinuria with serious complications and renal failure. In 2001, the HMG-CoA reductase inhibitor, cerivastatin, was withdrawn from the market because of an unacceptably high number of such cases of rhabdomyolysis. The actual molecular mechanisms underlying statin-induced rhabdomyolysis are not known. However, current hypotheses hold that abnormally increased exposure levels might affect mitochondrial function. Indeed, statins are able to induce apoptosis in cultured rat myocytes.

Mechanisms of statin-induced myotoxicity: A number of possible causes for the increase in the concentration-versus-time area under the curve (AUC) and, hence, greater exposure of the body to statins have been considered. Among these causes, an inhibition by other compounds of the metabolic clearance of statins, which primarily proceeds by enzymatic metabolism involving cytochrome P450 (specifically, CYP3A4) (see section 4.2.1) has been suggested as the most plausible one. According to this concept, other drugs that are metabolized by the same enzyme would inhibit in a competitive manner the metabolic clearance of the statins and thus increase their half-life.

However, it has become clear that besides competitive inhibition of drug-metabolizing enzymes, another mechanism might equally contribute to the increased exposure. The rate-limiting step for elimination of the statins from the organism is their hepatic uptake and elimination into bile. This is achieved by an anion export pump (P-glycoprotein = multidrug resistance protein, MDR1) (see section 3.3.2), located at the canalicular membrane of hepatocytes, and which pumps the statin metabolites into the bile. If this pump is inhibited by another drug, then the biliary clearance is impaired. Thus, the clinical interaction of statins with other drugs is due to mechanisms at the level of toxicokinetics: impaired catalytic activity of CYP3A4 and/or (maybe even exclusively) decreased P-glycoprotein function (see Figure 1.4).

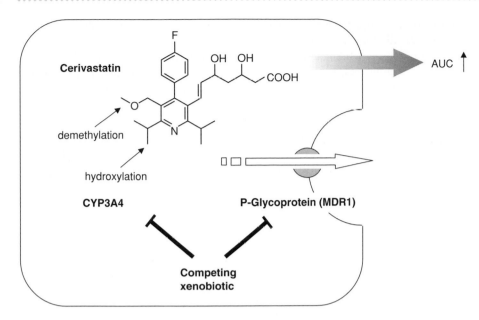

Figure 1.4. Drug–drug interactions impair the function of both the major statin-biotransforming enzyme (CYP3A4) and the canalicular export pump (MDR1), greatly decreasing the rate of excretion of cerivastatin and enhancing systemic exposure.

1.2.2. Toxicodynamic factors as basic mechanisms of toxicity

Toxicodynamic factors, i.e. interactions between a potentially toxic compound and a molecular target, may trigger functional or structural alterations in a cell and ultimately lead to a toxic effect. For example, a foreign compound (or one of its metabolites) can interact in a non-specific manner with a target macromolecule (a protein, membrane lipid, or nucleic acid), due to a combination of the chemical reactivity of the compound and its vicinity to the target molecule (see sections 5.2 and 9.1). If the extent of damage is large enough, and if the damaged target is critical and escapes possible repair mechanisms, then irreversible injury at the molecular level may ensue.

In contrast, interactions between a xenobiotic and a target molecule may be much more specific and depend on high-affinity binding sites that make the interactions very selective. This selectivity explains why only certain molecular structures, and not slightly different congeners, bind to the target molecule. It also provides a logical basis for the fact that toxicity can be restricted to certain tissues or organs, because these high-affinity binding sites to which a xenobiotic may selectively bind are abundant in these particular tissues but may be expressed at low or very low level only in non-target tissues.

Such highly specific targets are often receptors, located either on the cell surface (plasma membrane receptors) or in the cytoplasm and/or nucleus (nuclear receptors) (see Chapter 13). The xenobiotic can then either induce an agonist response or prevent the physiological ligand from binding to the receptor, thus inducing an antagonist response by inhibiting receptor function. Other high-affinity targets that specifically bind to a foreign substance (or 'pseudosubstrate') are enzymes (see Chapter 12), transmembrane transporters (carriers or ion channels) (see Chapter 14), or binding proteins that transport endogenous compounds (see Chapter 12). In many cases such interactions disrupt the physiological function of the targeted protein or protein complex and entail cell or tissue-specific toxicity.

Another type of highly specific interaction can occur when a structural moiety of a foreign molecule 'matches' with a specific target site of a macromolecule. The xenobiotic may not necessarily be reactive by itself and damage the endogenous macromolecule, but due to its high affinity and persistent binding may prevent the macromolecule, or parts of it, from interacting with other physiological molecules. By doing so, the toxic compound inhibits a vital physiological process or interferes with a regulatory step.

An example of such a reaction, at the molecular level, is the interaction of thalidomide with certain regions of DNA. By selectively binding to the promoter region of some crucial genes, this xenobiotic is able to disrupt gene activation and thus inhibits cell differentiation and growth. Importantly, this happens in an amazingly narrow tissue- and time-restricted 'window'. The interactions between this xenobiotic and a target macromolecule are the molecular basis explaining the drug's embryotoxic effects. Thalidomide has caused one of the most tragic events in the history of drug toxicology, which occurred almost half a century ago: the potential of thalidomide to induce malformations in the unborn child.

Thalidomide (Contergan®), introduced in Germany in 1956, was a popular drug used as a mild sedative and against morning sickness during pregnancy. One reason why the drug was so popular was that, for adults, it was a safe drug, and therefore the risk of abuse with overdoses of thalidomide was minimal. In the following years, an unusual increase in the number of newborns bearing malformations was seen in Germany. The major symptoms were malformations of the limbs, predominantly shortened arms (phocomelia), and sometimes completely missing arms (amelia). Later, this increase in the number of babies with limb malformations was observed in other countries too. Worldwide it is estimated that approximately 7,000–10,000 children with malformations were born in this period. It was not until 1961 that a physician suspected a possible causal link between these malformations and the use of thalidomide in pregnant women. In the same year the drug was withdrawn from the market, and since 1962 such malformations have again become quite rare.

Thalidomide is a typical compound that can exert teratogenic effects in humans. Teratogenicity (a special form of embryotoxicity) is defined as the induction of abnormalities (malformations) by exogenous compounds during the process of organogenesis. These effects are caused by an interference of the xenobiotic (or its metabolites) with morphogenetic differentiation during embryogenesis.

Why was such a catastrophe possible, and why was the drug industry not aware of the possibility that this could happen? One has to recall that in

---

those days it was generally believed that the embryo was firmly shielded away from maternal blood and that the placenta functioned as a barrier against exchanges of chemicals between the embryo/fetus and the mother. As a consequence of the thalidomide catastrophe, the US FDA issued the first guidelines for reproductive toxicology studies that had to be included in the general preclinical toxicity testing of new drugs. Nowadays, teratogenicity studies are routinely performed in the rat and rabbit. In past decades, a host of experimental studies confirmed the teratogenic effect of thalidomide in non-human primates (Figure 1.5), where similar types of toxicity could be induced to that observed in humans. In certain rabbit strains, similar malformations can also be produced. In the rat, the situation is different; as the oral bioavailability of thalidomide is poor in the rat, malformations cannot be induced by the oral route but only by adminstration of thalidomide via the intravenous route.

Almost unbelievably, and although thalidomide has been banned for many years, this drug has been revisited. As it is virtually non-toxic in adults, and as it features a number of excellent therapeutic features, it has been introduced again for certain indications. For example, thalidomide is the drug of choice to treat certain skin reactions associated with lepra. It is even used to treat

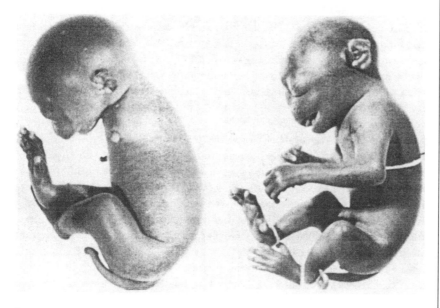

Figure 1.5. Thalidomide embryopathy in the Rhesus monkey. *Left,* 100-day old monkey after treatment of the mother with a single dose of 30 mg/kg thalidomide on day 26 of gestation; *right,* normal 100-day old fetus.
Source: Wilson, J.G. (1972) Abnormalities of intrauterine development in non-human primates, *Acta Endocrinol. Suppl.* 166; 261–292, with permission of the Society of the European Journal of Endocrinology.

AIDS, certain forms of cancer, and as an anti-rheumatic drug. Unfortunately, some new cases of thalidomide-related teratogenicity were seen in some of the countries where thalidomide has been used.

Only the rigorous efforts aimed at elucidating the mechanism underlying thalidomide embryopathy have allowed the development of drug derivatives that retain the therapeutic properties (e.g. anti-inflammatory activity, probably mediated through inhibition of TNF-α production) but eliminate the reactions that lead to teratogenic effects.

Mechanisms underlying thalidomide embryotoxicity: The critical time window during which thalidomide is able to induce these severe malformations is narrow and restricted to days 24–33 of pregnancy. This is the time period during which organogenesis occurs. In particular, this is the period in which the limb bud tissue undergoes extensive proliferation and differentiation into arms and legs, and also where ears and eyes start to differentiate. Because thalidomide was unable to induce these toxic effects before or after limb bud differentiation, it is logical to assume that the underlying mechanism must be related to a tissue-specific effect involved in this differentiation process.

A number of hypotheses have been suggested, but not all of them have proved to be relevant. For example, a number of toxicokinetic factors could be responsible for the embryo-selective effects. These include formation of toxic metabolites, or accumulation of the drug or its metabolites in embryonic tissue compartments. These factors alone cannot account for thalidomide embryopathy.

In contrast, a number of toxicodynamic factors have been suggested, and some of these isolated hypotheses have been independently confirmed. Put together, they allow for a unifying hypothesis that could help to explain the severe thalidomide effects in the developing limb buds, but also in the eyes and ears, where some abnormalities have also been observed.

It has been known for quite some time that thalidomide can intercalate into DNA. In fact, a stacked complex is formed between the flat phthalimide double ring structure and deoxyguanosine. However, this fact alone could not explain the tissue- and time-related toxicity. More recent investigations have shed more light on this. They revealed that thalidomide inhibits angiogenesis, i.e. the production of new blood vessels from preexisting micro vessels, in the embryo. Furthermore, it has been demonstrated that thalidomide inhibits the expression of specific cell adhesion molecules, the integrins, which play a pivotal role in cell growth and tissue differentiation. Finally, it has become clear that thalidomide can inhibit the action of a number of specific growth factors. But how does all this fit together?

One attractive possibility is that thalidomide interferes with mechanisms of gene expression that are involved in the regulatory pathways for integrin production and angiogenesis. It has become clear that thalidomide binds specifically to the promoter regions of genes involved in such regulatory pathways. As a consequence, gene transcription of specific integrins ($\alpha v \beta 3$ subunits) is blocked (see Figure 1.6).

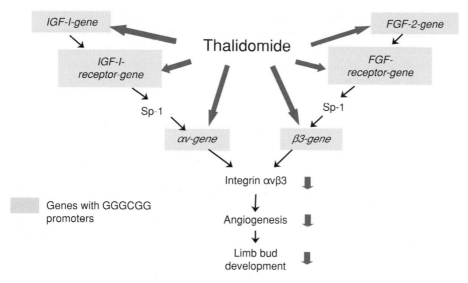

Figure 1.6. Thalidomide binds to (and blocks) the promoter region of specific genes involved in angiogenesis and limb bud development.

> **Role of growth factors and integrins in the developing limb bud.** Integrins belong to the large group of intercellular adhesion molecules and play a pivotal role in cell–cell communication and, hence, in tissue differentiation. The production of the specific integrin αvβ3, which is composed of the two subunits, αv and β3, is synergistically stimulated by the two growth factors, IGF-I (insulin-like growth factor I) and FGF-2 (fibroblast growth factor type 2). Integrin αvβ3 in turn stimulates angiogenesis and is an important factor in the developing limb buds and other embryonal structures.
>
> The transcription and subsequent production of integrin αvβ3 are regulated by a promoter-specific transcription factor, Sp1. A pivotal step in gene activation is binding of Sp1 to guanine-rich promoter regions in the genes for both αv and β3. *Thus, the normal function and accessibility of these poly-guanine sites, which also occur in the promoter regions of the genes for IGF-I and FGF-2, is crucial for gene activation.*

A further clue to the mechanism of action of thalidomide inhibition of angiogenesis and normal limb bud development came from two important observations.

1 It is known that those promoters of the genes coding for the integrin subunits αv and β3, and of those of IGF-I and FGF-2, are guanine-rich (poly-G), i.e. they possess multiple GGGCGG sequences. This is important for understanding the possible toxicodynamic drug-target molecule interactions.

2 It is also known that thalidomide exists in two racemic forms, the *S*-(−)-form and the *R*-(+)-form (and was marketed originally as a racemate). *Interestingly, it is only the S-enantiomer that is teratogenic.* It is therefore inviting to speculate that a stereospecific interaction between the thalidomide molecule and these promoter regions might occur.

Indeed, molecular models have revealed that thalidomide can intercalate into the DNA where it binds to specific poly-G sites in the promoter regions. It is only the *S*-enantiomer of the thalidomide molecule that exactly fits into the 'major groove' of the double helix and subsequently binds to poly-G; the non-teratogenic *R*-thalidomide is unable to bind, because of sterical hindrance. Thus, this stereoselective binding behavior is a plausible explanation for the differential embryotoxic potential of the two enantiomers (see Figure 1.7).

Although these novel findings provide an intriguing explanation with respect to thalidomide's molecular mechanism of disturbance of limb bud differentiation, they leave us with the unanswered question of why this occurs in such a restricted tissue-selective manner. Indeed, the reason for the 'organotropic' (affecting selective tissues of the embryo only, not the adult) effect of thalidomide is only incompletely known. It has been speculated that intercalation and binding of thalidomide to DNA have the greatest adverse effect in those regions where guanine-rich promoters of genes critically involved in limb bud development are abundant (which is the case for the integrin subunits αv and β3, and for IGF-I and FGF-2). Generally, it is only a minority of genes (<10 percent) that possess multiple GGGCGG sequences in their promoter region. In other words, >90 percent of all genes would not be affected by thalidomide. In addition, the majority of genes that do possess these poly-G regions are housekeeping genes, featuring little if any regulation and minimal transcriptional activity.

To conclude, the embryotoxicity associated with thalidomide is ultimately determined by mechanisms at the level of toxicodynamics: molecular interactions of the drug with guanine-rich promoter regions of specific genes.

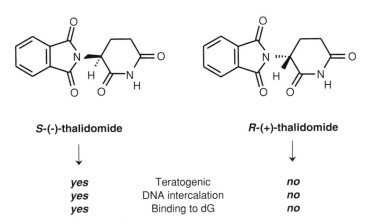

S-(-)-thalidomide		R-(+)-thalidomide
↓		↓
yes	Teratogenic	no
yes	DNA intercalation	no
yes	Binding to dG	no

Figure 1.7. The teratogenic activity of thalidomide is stereoselective.

Learning points

- Mechanisms of toxicity can be studied at different levels: (i) how a xenobiotic is taken up into the body or by a cell, and how it is metabolized and distributed (toxicokinetic factors); (ii) how a xenobiotic interacts with primary target molecules including the secondary signaling pathways and effector mechanisms (toxicodynamic factors); (iii) how a xenobiotic affects the biological response of defense, tolerance, and repair, or promotes cell damage or demise; and (iv) how a xenobiotic may alter gene expression that modulates all these factors.
- Elucidation of molecular mechanisms underlying the toxicity of a chemical compound, together with quantitative exposure data, is of paramount importance for risk assessment in humans.
- Molecular mechanisms should not be viewed as a linear sequence of events, but rather as complex networks of reactions, branching out into different directions, and subject to tight regulation.
- At the toxicokinetic level, the myotoxicity of statins can be explained by drug–drug interactions acting at both inhibition of drug-metabolizing enzymes and the drug export pump, leading to abnormally high exposure.
- At the toxicodynamic level, the embryotoxicity of thalidomide can be explained by selective binding of thalidomide to the promoter regions of genes involved in integrin transcription, thereby inhibiting angiogenesis and limb bud development.

Further reading

General reading
Gregus, Z. and Klaassen, C.D. (2001) Mechanisms of toxicity, *Casarett's and Doull's Toxicology. The Basic Science of Poisons*, 6th edition, McGraw-Hill, New York, NY, pp. 35–81.
Zbinden, G. (1992) The three eras of research in experimental toxicology, *Trends Pharmacol. Sci.* 13: 221–223.

Unleaded gasoline nephrotoxicity
Borghoff, S.J., Prescott, J.S., Janszen, D.B., Wong, B.A. and Everitt, J.I. (2001) α2u-Globulin nephropathy, renal cell proliferation, and dosimetry of inhaled *tert*-butyl alcohol in male and female F-344 rats, *Toxicol. Sci.* 61: 176–186.
Dietrich, D.R. (1995) Alpha 2u-globulin: Species- and sex-specific protein synthesis and excretion, association with chemically induced renal toxicity and neoplasia in the male rat, and relevance in human cancer risk assessment, *Rev. Biochem. Toxicol.* 11: 115–180.

Statin-induced myotoxicity
Ucar, M., Mjörndal, T. and Dahlqvist, R. (2000) HMG-CoA reductase inhibitors and myotoxicity, *Drug Safety* 22: 441–457.
Wang, E.J., Casciano, C.N., Clement, R.P. and Johnson, W.W. (2001) HMG-CoA reductase inhibitors (statins) characterized as direct inhibitors of P-glycoprotein, *Pharm. Res.* 18: 800–806.

Thalidomide embryotoxicity

Neubert, R., Nogueira, A.C. and Neubert, D. (1993) Thalidomide derivatives and the immune system. I. Changes in the pattern of integrin receptors and other surface markers on T lymphocyte subpopulations in marmoset blood. *Arch. Toxicol.* 67: 1–17.

Service, R.F. (1995) Can thalidomide be rehabilitated? *Science* 269: 1340.

Stephens, T.D., Bunde, C.J.W. and Fillmore, B.J. (2000) Mechanism of action in thalidomide teratogenesis. *Biochem. Pharmacol.* 59: 1489–1499.

Stephens, T.D. and Fillmore, B.J. (2000) Hypothesis: thalidomide embryopathy – proposed mechanism of action. *Teratology* 61: 189–195.

Chapter 2

Organ-selective toxicity

Contents

When the organism is exposed to a potentially toxic compound at critical concentrations, a toxic response is often evoked locally, at the site where the xenobiotic first gets into contact with the body, such as skin, airways, lungs, gastrointestinal tract, etc. This makes sense, in particular if the chemical is highly reactive. However, in most cases, xenobiotics are absorbed and distributed throughout the body, where they cause either general systemic effects or effects that occur predominantly in certain specific target organs. Such a target organ-selective toxicity, often independent of the route of uptake, is called organotropic toxicity.

2.1. Biological basis of organ-selective toxicity

The biological causes by which such organotropic effects can often be explained comprise mechanisms which are based on both toxicokinetic and toxicodynamic factors (Table 2.1).

For many xenobiotics, the underlying mechanisms which govern their organotropy or make a particular tissue prone to succumb to the resulting toxic effects are not known. However, for other compounds, the mechanisms explaining organ-selective toxicity have been unraveled in the past years and have greatly helped our understanding of the tissue-specific effects. One such mechanism is molecular homology.

Table 2.1 Biological basis of organ-selective toxicity

Target tissue-specific toxicokinetic factors	■ Organ-selective uptake, distribution, accumulation of xenobiotics through multi-specific transporters and/or molecular homology ■ Organ-selective metabolism and bioactivation
Target tissue-specific toxicodynamic factors	■ Tissue-specific expression of receptors ■ Tissue-specific binding of xenobiotics to macromolecules ■ Tissue-specific expression of transcription factors ■ Increased susceptibility of cell populations ■ Tissue-specific adaptive response ■ Tissue-selective deficiencies in pathways of detoxication and repair

2.2.1. Molecular homology

Molecular homology (also called molecular mimicry) is a term that describes how a xenobiotic mimics, by its chemico-physical properties, the characteristics and behavior of an endogenous compound. Due to this molecular resemblance, a foreign compound can make use of physiological pathways normally designed for essential cell function. For example, a xenobiotic, by mimicking endogenous chemicals which play an essential role in selective tissues, can become a substrate of physiological entrance mechanisms, resulting in tissue-selective cellular uptake and possible accumulation. This is illustrated by the toxic metal, mercury.

Mercury in all its chemical forms causes toxic effects, and there is a distinct tissue selectivity. For example, inorganic mercury (Hg^{2+}) preferentially causes nephrotoxicity, in particular to the proximal tubular epithelia. On the other hand, organic mercury (e.g. methyl-Hg) typically is neurotoxic.

Methylmercury intoxication was first observed in Japan in the 1950s and 1960s and has been attributed to the consumption of heavily contaminated fish. The cause was found to be the release of mercury-containing compounds from a chemical plant, and the disease was named after the bay where the contaminated fish were caught (Minamata). Intoxication with methyl mercury starts with paresthesia (abnormal sensibility); later, ataxia (disturbed coordination), dysarthria (difficulty in articulation), and loss of vision may occur. These neurotoxic symptoms result from the destruction of neurons in certain areas of the brain. The reason for this brain-selective toxicity has remained a mystery for a long time.

In contrast, acute intoxication with mercuric salts (e.g. $HgCl_2$) from ingestion will acutely damage the gastrointestinal tract (primary exposure) but later affect the epithelial cells of the pars recta of the proximal tubules. This results in tubular necrosis, changes in kidney function, and can even culminate in acute renal failure.

What are the reasons for this tissue-selective toxicity? The fact that mercury is not equally distributed in the body but rather accumulates in these critical tissues, i.e. the proximal tubules (inorganic Hg salts) and the CNS (methyl-Hg), has provided some mechanistic clues to this question.

Mechanisms of the nephrotropic toxicity of mercury and CNS-selective toxicity of methyl mercury: At the molecular level, cellular injury is most probably due to the strong binding of mercury to thiol groups of amino acid residues of critical proteins (see section 5.3.3). In the periphery, this high affinity of Hg for sulfhydryl groups is also responsible for the avid binding of the metal to albumin. In organs where small, non-protein thiol-containing compounds are abundant, mercury is bound to and 'inactivated' by these scavengers. For example, glutathione (GSH; see section 5.3.1) binds Hg^{2+} to form diglutathionyl mercury (GS–Hg–SG). Accordingly, in the liver, which contains high concentrations of GSH, there is extensive GS–Hg–SG formation, followed by release of the complex into bile or the bloodstream. By a similar mechanism, methyl-Hg is complexed to GSH and forms methyl-Hg–SG.

These glutathionyl complexes reach the kidney and easily pass through the glomerular filtration barrier. In the lumen of the proximal tubule, the glutathione tripeptide is enzymatically cleaved, first by γ-glutamyltranspeptidase (which cleaves off the glutamyl moiety), and then by cysteinyl-glycinase (which removes the glycine moiety).

The remaining dicysteinyl–Hg complex (Cys–Hg–Cys) is the critical molecular species because it mimics an endogenous compound, cystine (Cys–Cys). Uptake of cystine into the proximal tubular epithelia is mediated by both an Na^+-dependent and an Na^+-independent transporter. It is this selective transport system that cannot distinguish between the normal amino acid dimer substrate and the foreign substrate (Cys–Hg–Cys), which, once inside the cell, unfolds its toxic effects like the warriors hidden in the Trojan horse (see Figure 2.1).

A similar mechanism accounts for methyl mercury toxicity in the CNS. The methyl-Hg–Cys complex, at the molecular level, mimics methionine and gains access to the brain across the blood–brain barrier (see section 3.3.3). This is in part because the xenobiotic is lipophilic, but more importantly because it makes use of a specific amino acid transporter. Specifically, the metal complex easily crosses the endothelial cell barrier and enters astrocytes. Once in the brain, methyl-Hg can fully elicit its thiol-reactive effects.

2.1.2. Tissue-selective transcription factors

An increasingly recognized factor contributing to cell- or tissue-specific responses to toxicants is the tissue-selective expression of transcription factors. These transcription factors regulate in a tissue-restricted, but also in a temporal-restricted, manner

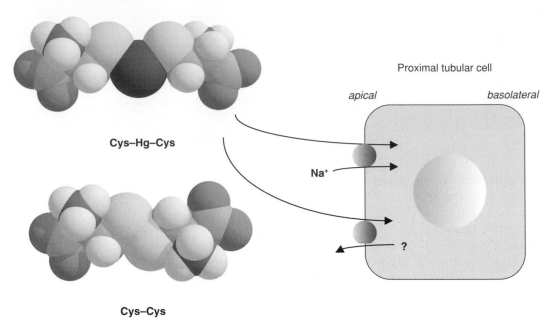

Figure 2.1. Molecular homology of cysteine–Hg–cysteine with cystine. The Cys–Hg–Cys complex is selectively transported into renal proximal tubular cells by the same transporters that normally carry cystine (Cys–Cys). This leads to selective uptake of Hg into the kidneys.
Source: Adapted from Zalups, R.K. (2000) Molecular interactions with mercury in the kidney, *Pharmacol. Rev.* 52: 113–143, with permission of the publisher.

the expression of tissue-specific functions. For example, a vast array of xenobiotic-metabolizing enzymes, which are distributed in a time- and organ-selective way (see Chapter 4), can largely determine the bioactivation and/or bioinactivation of drugs and other chemicals. Although the expression of such transcription factors is not wholly restricted to one tissue, the organ-selective distribution nevertheless is responsible for many of the effects of toxicants in liver, kidney, lung, heart, or the central nervous system.

An example of liver-selective transcription factors is the hepatocyte nuclear factor (HNF) family. HNF1, HNF3, and HNF4, each with a number of subtypes, are structurally different proteins. Some of them are critical for normal development, but also are implicated in the expression of liver-specific genes including β-fibrinogen, albumin (HNF1), or transthyretin (HNF3) (see section 12.2). Importantly, they regulate the expression of a number of enzymes involved in drug metabolism.

Hepatocyte nuclear factor-1 (HNF1), for example, is a transcription factor that is abundantly expressed in liver (HNF1α), but also in kidney (HNF1β) and, at lower expression levels, in other organs. Its expression in liver parallels the development of adult, differentiated hepatocytes. The protein features a DNA-binding domain and a transactivation domain. HNF1 binds either as a homodimer

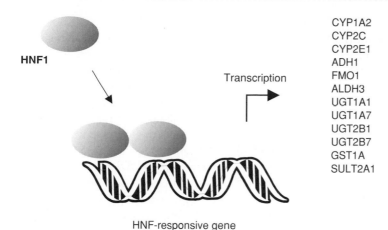

CYP1A2
CYP2C
CYP2E1
ADH1
FMO1
ALDH3
UGT1A1
UGT1A7
UGT2B1
UGT2B7
GST1A
SULT2A1

HNF1

Transcription

HNF-responsive gene

Figure 2.2. Hepatocyte nuclear factor-1 (HNF1) regulates the transcription of a vast array of xenobiotic-metabolizing enzymes which are involved in tissue-selective responses to toxicants. CYP, cytochrome P450; ADH, alcohol dehydrogenase; FMO, flavin monooxygenase; ALDH, aldehyde dehydrogenase; UGT, UDP-glucuronosyltransferase; GST, glutathione-*S*-transferase; SULT, sulfotransferase.

or as a heterodimer (with co-factors). Genes responsive to HNF1 include a number of cytochrome P450s, as well as several phase II enzymes involved in conjugation reactions, e.g. glucuronosyltransferase, glutathione-*S*-transferase, and sulfotransferase forms (see Figure 2.2). Taken together, because all these enzymes play a pivotal role in the metabolism and toxicity of many xenobiotics (see Chapter 4), the tissue-selective distribution of such transcription factors that tightly regulate the expression of drug-metabolizing enzymes is one of the crucial factors contributing to tissue-specific toxicity (see Figure 2.2).

2.1.3. Tissue-restricted expression of molecular targets

Among the driving forces of organ-selective toxicity, selective expression of molecular targets which are involved in mediating the toxicity plays an important role. For example, the tissue-selective distribution of receptors with which certain xenobiotics interact, and the degree of expression of these receptors at the protein level, can largely determine the extent of toxicity and gate the xenobiotic-induced adverse effects to certain organs while others are not affected.

The first example focuses on the molecular forces that govern the tissue-selective toxicity of synthetic estrogens and which are dependent on the tissue-specific distribution of molecular targets. This issue has become extremely important in view of the general discussion about a possible impact of environmental contaminants with estrogen-like activity (see section 13.2). The estrogenic potency of most of these environmental contaminants is low, but a rationally synthesized compound, diethylstilbestrol, featuring much higher estrogenic potency, has taught us an important lesson.

Diethylstilbestrol (DES) is a potent synthetic estrogen which was used extensively up to the 1970s. The main purpose of this estrogen was to increase weight gain in cattle or to caponize chickens, and it was therefore included in livestock feed. DES was also therapeutically used in humans to treat prostate cancer in men and prevent miscarriage in women. At that time it was simply not known that estrogenic substances (being 'natural' chemicals) could have deleterious effects like those seen a number of years or decades later in the children of mothers who were treated with DES during pregnancy.

Some of these daughters, many years after exposure to DES *in utero*, developed rare forms of cervical and vaginal cancers (the most common form was clear cell adenocarcinoma, which occurred in approximately 0.1% of exposed women). In the DES-exposed sons, there was a higher incidence of testicular changes than in non-exposed men. These included undescended testes, cysts in the epididymis, and sperm abnormalities, but also prostatic inflammation.

Similar forms of toxicity in the reproductive tract could be reproduced in experimental animals, and many studies have been performed with mice exposed to DES either *in utero* or in the postnatal phase. Today we know that at least some of these effects of DES are due to an estrogenization mediated by the estrogen receptor.

Mechanisms of DES-induced developmental changes of the reproductive tract: Diethylstilbestrol is distributed in the maternal organism, but is also able to cross the placenta and reach the fetal circulation, where it causes developmental changes in some of the primordial reproductive organs. The long-term changes in both males and females are due to estrogenic effects mediated by interaction of DES with the estrogen receptor (ER) (see section 13.2.1). This seems plausible since DES is an estrogen-type hormone with high affinity for both ERα and ERβ. The two ER subtypes exhibit a differential developmental expression profile and distinct tissue distribution. For example, in the reproductive tract ERα is expressed in rat epididymis and testis, while ERβ predominates in prostate, and both types are present in rat ovary and uterus.

Importantly, the ER is already expressed in the mouse fetus before sexual differentiation is terminated, and the receptor's tissue distribution is similar in males and females. Compelling evidence indicating that the ER is mechanistically involved in the delayed DES-induced toxicity and carcinogenesis stems from experiments with mice genetically deficient in ERα. Newborn pups from normal, wild-type mice exposed to DES will develop, many months later, uterine changes (atrophy, smooth muscle disorganization, epithelial squamous cell metaplasia) and proliferative lesions of the oviduct, as well as vaginal changes, and also exhibit differential expression of estrogen-responsive genes. In contrast, ERα-null mice are completely resistant against DES and do not exhibit any of these changes in the reproductive tract. The widely used newborn mouse model mimics the human situation, because until postnatal day 5 the maturity level of the newborn mice resembles that of a human embryo in the second trimester.

How the synthetic estrogen causes the feminization of genes at the molecular level is still incompletely known. One can surmise that, like in many other cases of gene imprinting during critical periods of development, DNA is methylated, which leads to a differential regulation of these genes later in life. DES could thus sensitize target cells (e.g. cells of the primordial female reproductive tract, the Müllerian duct) to subsequent postnatal exposure to endogenous estrogens.

At this point the intriguing question may arise as to why it is the synthetic estrogen, but not the maternal estrogens normally present at high concentrations during pregnancy, that induces these changes in fetuses. There are a number of facts that can mechanistically explain this paradox.

1 Endogenous estrogen-binding proteins normally shield the embryo from the endogenous estrogens. In contrast to estradiol, DES has a poor affinity to these estrogen-binding proteins and therefore exhibits higher circulating concentrations of the 'free' (active) compound.
2 DES is an extremely potent ligand of the ER; its binding affinity is several-fold higher than that of estradiol.
3 The differential effects of estrogens and estrogen-like xenobiotics are dependent on many factors other than binding and include receptor conformational changes upon binding, differential binding to response elements on DNA, recruitment of co-regulatory proteins, and cross-talk with other signaling systems.
4 Some of the effects of DES are caused by non-ER mechanisms.

Collectively, however, it has become clear that it is the tissue-selective ER expression which is responsible for the organ-selective toxicity induced by estrogenic xenobiotics (see Figure 2.3).

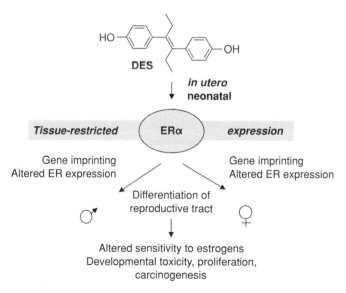

Figure 2.3. Binding of diethylstilbestrol to the estrogen receptor, which is already expressed in the primordial reproductive tract, triggers a series of downstream effects that are receptor-mediated and can culminate in severe developmental toxicity and cancer of the female reproductive system.

The second example is the tissue-selective toxicity attributed to a group of plasticizers including di-(2-ethylhexyl) phthalate and other phthalates. These compounds have been reported to cause hepatic changes and even liver tumors in rodents; they belong to the class of 'peroxisome proliferators' (see section 13.3.1). Because humans are also potentially exposed to these chemicals, elucidation of the mechanisms is important in assessing the risk for human health.

Di-(2-ethylhexyl) phthalate (DEHP) is a widely used plasticizer which has found broad application in the manufacturing of polymers and plastics and in dispersions. Due to its heavy use, DEHP is found ubiquitously in the environment. Because the compound may leak out from containers, tubing, and wastes, or because it may be released by burning of these plastics, it is important to analyse the potential risk to humans.

Mice treated with high doses of DEHP typically develop toxic lesions in the liver, including hepatomegaly and liver tumors (toxicity is also seen in the kidney and other target organs including the testes, but this will not be discussed here because different mechanisms are involved). The typical liver-restricted lesions were never observed in guinea pigs or non-human primates treated with high doses of DEHP. Thanks to the deeper insights into the underlying mechanisms that we have gained over the years, it was concluded that humans, too, are unlikely to develop such liver toxicity, even at high exposure. In fact, in 2000, DEHP was re-classified as a 'non-carcinogen in humans'. What is the rationale for this bold prediction and what is the mechanistic basis for the organ-selective toxicity in rodents?

Mechanisms of DEHP-induced liver toxicity: In search of the molecular basis that would explain the organotropic effects of these plasticizers in rodents, it was found that these compounds are ligands and activators of the nuclear receptor, peroxisome proliferator-activated receptor-α (PPARα) (see section 13.3.1). This receptor subtype is particularly abundant in liver. Activation of the receptor is associated with a pleiotropic response that includes decreases in the rates of apoptosis, increases in cell proliferation, proliferation of peroxisomes in hepatocytes with concomitant induction of enzymes involved in peroxisomal fatty acid β-oxidation, increased production of oxidative stress, and eventually the development of hepatic tumors.

The proof of concept for a crucial role of tissue-selective, and perhaps species-selective, distribution of PPARα again has been derived from models with a genetic deficiency in the receptor. While wild-type mice develop the typical signs of liver toxicity, PPARα-null mice exposed to DEHP do not develop any of these changes (while the effects in the other organs are still there). This points to a critical role of PPARα in the hepatotropic toxicity. The fact that DEHP does not induce any of these liver changes in non-human primates, guinea pigs and humans has a two-fold reason. First, it is known that humans (and guinea pigs) express hepatic PPARα at an approximately ten-fold lower level than rodents (quantitative factor). Second, most humans express truncated or mutant variants of PPARα, which are functionally inactive (qualitative factor). Even if there is transcriptional activity, the actual transcription rate in humans is very low, due to differences in promoter sequence and activity and due to the absence of PP response elements in the promoter region of many relevant genes. Hence, the transactivation of PPARα-responsive genes may be limited to those therapeutic and desired effects that mediate the hypolipidemic response (induced by PPARα agonists), but the down-stream effects are not sufficient to induce the undesired hepatic changes. Taken together, there is ample evidence that the toxic response in the liver secondary to DEHP and other plasticizers is determined by the organ-specific distribution and abundance of functional PPARα receptor expression, which can explain the liver-restricted toxicity in rodents.

2.2. Selective hepatotoxicity and nephrotoxicity

Liver and kidneys are particularly frequent target organs of toxicity that are often injured (and selectively injured) by xenobiotics, both experimentally and clinically. There are several reasons for these organotropic effects, which are based on a number of biological factors shared by liver and kidneys.

1 Both organs receive large amounts of blood (delivering the xenobiotics) per time unit and are therefore extensively exposed to the compounds.
2 Both organs harbor a large variety of xenobiotic-metabolizing enzymes, including cytochrome P450s, and many of them abundantly. If a compound is bioactivated to a reactive metabolite by these enzymes, then it often interacts with and damages the tissue in which it has been generated.
3 Both hepatocytes and proximal tubular epithelia are polarized cells, featuring a basolateral membrane and an apical membrane domain. Both cell types have excretory function. Xenobiotics are selectively taken up by these cells via spe-cific carriers and subsequently exported by other transmembrane transporters. Such primary or secondary active transport systems (see section 3.1) can highly up-concentrate xenobiotics or their metabolites in certain compartments.

For the liver in particular, a number of organ-specific features have been implicated in mediating organ-selective toxicity (see Table 2.2). Two of these characteristics, the bioactivating enzymes and vectorial transport of xenobiotics, are particularly important in driving organ-selective toxicity and are highlighted below.

2.2.1. Xenobiotic-bioactivating enzymes

The liver is the major site of xenobiotic biotransformation (see Chapter 4). In particular, the cytochrome P450 (CYP) enzyme superfamily is crucial for the metabolism of a diverse group of xenobiotics (see section 4.2.1). One possible con-sequence of this metabolism is that reaction products that are generated can be more toxic than the parent compound. If the chemical reactivity of these meta-bolites is high, then these reactive metabolites can potentially elicit toxicity in the liver itself, before they are translocated to another site or inactivated.

Table 2.2 Biological basis of the hepatotropic toxicity of xenobiotics

- The liver receives a large volume of blood (approximately 1.5 L/min).
- The portal system accounts for ~$^2/_3$ of the total hepatic blood supply (the rest is provided by the hepatic artery). Therefore, the liver is the first organ that is exposed to orally absorbed xenobiotics after passage across the intestinal mucosa. In fact, portal concentrations of a xenobiotic taken by the oral route can be several-fold (≤50×) higher than those in peripheral blood.
- Active transport systems can transport and excrete xenobiotics against a concentration gradient. For example, certain drug metabolites (e.g. acyl glucuronides; see section 4.2.2.) are first up-concentrated in hepatocytes by approximately 50-fold, and then further up-concentrated in the biliary tree by another factor of ~100, resulting in a ~5,000-fold higher biliary concentration of these xenobiotics as compared to that in peripheral blood!
- The liver is the major site (both quantitatively and qualitatively) of xenobiotic biotransformation.
- The endothelia outlining the liver sinusoids, which supply the hepatic parenchyma with blood, do not possess a basal membrane, and the cells are fenestrated, so that compounds and certain cells in the bloodstream come into direct contact with the hepatocytes.
- The liver harbors a large percentage of resident macrophages (Kupffer cells) and specific resident T cells (γδ T cells) which have been implicated in certain forms of immune cell-mediated toxicity induced by xenobiotics (see section 10.1).

The pivotal role of metabolic bioactivation of xenobiotics in the liver is exemplified by the hepatic toxicity of acetaminophen (APAP) (see section 9.2.1). Liver damage induced by APAP is primarily mediated by CYP2E1, an important CYP form in the liver.

Among the many CYP isoforms, **CYP2E1** has received much attention because of its toxicological relevance in the biotransformation and activation of small and lipophilic compounds to toxic or carcinogenic intermediates. For example, acetaldehyde, acrylamide, aniline, benzene, butanol, carbon tetrachloride, ethyl carbamate, ethylene chloride, halothane, ethylene glycol, N-nitrosodimethylamine, and vinyl chloride and all substrates for CYP2E1. This CYP form is abundantly expressed in liver (but occurs also in lungs or brain).

Role of hepatic CYP2E1-dependent bioactivation of APAP: The crucial role of this enzyme in triggering the initial steps of APAP hepatotoxicity can be demonstrated if the expression and/or activity of this enzyme is modulated. For example, if the metabolism of APAP is blocked by chemical inhibitors of CYP2E1, then no hepatic toxicity will occur.

The most compelling evidence for a crucial role of CYP in the toxicity of APAP stems from recombinant deletion experiments of the gene coding for CYP2E1. Mice in which the *cyp2e1* gene was knocked out and which phenotypically did not express

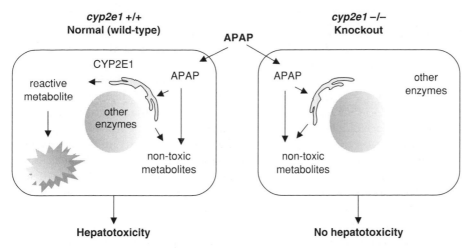

Figure 2.4. Acetaminophen (APAP) at high dose is toxic to mouse hepatocytes featuring normal expression of CYP2E1, but is non-toxic to hepatocytes of *cyp2e1*-null mice.

CYP2E1 in the liver were refractory to the hepatotoxic effects of APAP. Doses of APAP that were highly toxic to wild-type mice did not alter the parameters indicative of liver injury in *cyp2e1*-null mice. Even otherwise lethal doses of 600 mg/kg were well tolerated (however, at higher doses other, non-CYP2E1 isoforms, featuring a higher K_m for the substrate, accept APAP as a substrate and will activate the compound, see Figure 2.4).

Because bioactivation of many xenobiotics to a reactive metabolite is the first step which entails a vast and complex network of secondary reactions ultimately converging in lethal cell injury (if not compensated by rescue mechanisms), the role of hepatic and renal xenobiotic-metabolizing enzymes is of paramount importance in mechanistic toxicology.

2.2.2. Vectorial transport of xenobiotics

The kidney is a major site of excretion for xenobiotics and/or their metabolites. Small compounds (<50 kD) can pass the glomerular filtration barrier and are excreted in the urine. However, if their size exceeds the molecular mass threshold, then they are excreted via other pathways, including active secretion by the tubular epithelia. In fact, specific carriers located on the basolateral membrane of proximal tubular cells can transport compounds from the blood into the epithelial cells against a concentration gradient. Other transporters at the opposite (apical) membrane domain then excrete the compounds into the tubular lumen (urine).

In some cases, however, especially if the uptake rate into cells greatly exceeds the transport capacity for the subsequent excretory steps, a compound can accumulate in the proximal tubular cells and attain dangerous levels. A typical example is the nephrotoxicity of cephalosporin antibiotics.

One important clue to the mechanism of toxicity came from early observations indicating that the toxic cephalosporins, but not their non-toxic congeners, accumulate in the renal cortex (see Table 2.3).

Cephalosporins belong to a group of β-lactam antibiotics that are structurally related to penicillins. They are derived from cephalosporin C, a naturally occurring product of the fungus *Cephalosporium*, and are produced semi-synthetically. A well-recognized potential adverse effect of the first generation cephalosporins was their clinical nephrotoxicity. One of the first compounds was cephaloridine, the use of which was associated with damage to the proximal tubular epithelia. Since then, more than four generations of cephalosporins have been developed, and nephrotoxicity has become less frequent. Nevertheless, kidney liability is still an important challenge related to this class of antibiotics.

Structurally, the cephalosporins are carboxylic acids which are ionized at physiological pH. Some cephalosporins, e.g. the toxic cephaloridine, feature in addition a cationic group at the nitrogen, making it a zwitterion. These structural differences can explain, mechanistically, why cephaloridine is toxic in experimental animals (and in humans), while cephalothin is not nephrotoxic, even when given at a ten-fold higher dose (see Figure 2.5).

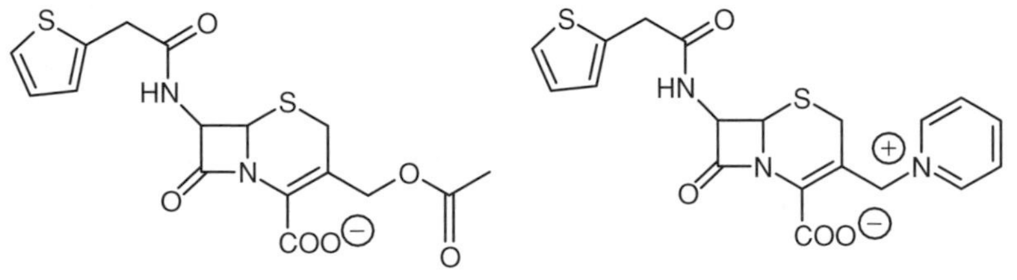

Cephalothin
(not nephrotoxic)

Cephaloridine
(nephrotoxic)

Figure 2.5. Chemical structures of typical cephalosporins.

***Table 2.3* Accumulation of cephaloridine in the renal cortex**

Drug	Concentration in cortex (µg/g)	Concentration in serum (µg/ml)	Cortex/Serum	Nephrotoxic dose (mg/kg)
Cephaloridine	$2{,}576 \pm 267$	$167 + 12$	15.1 ± 0.8	90
Cephalothin	431 ± 122	$127 + 16$	3.2 ± 0.4	>1,000

Note: The numbers are steady state concentrations after infusion of 100 mg/kg body weight of the cephalosporin to female rabbits. Mean ± SE.
Source: data are from Tune, B.M. (1998) The renal toxicity of beta-lactam antibiotics: Mechanisms and clinical implications, Clinical Nephtotoxins. Renal Injury from Drugs and Chemicals, DeBroe, M.E. *et al.* (eds), Kluwer Academic, Dordrecht, The Netherlands, pp. 121–134.

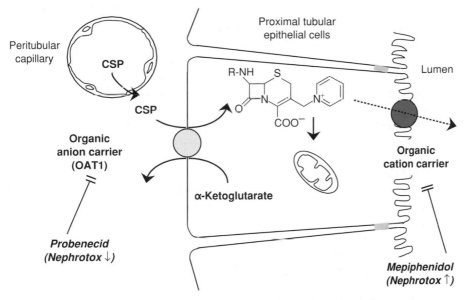

Figure 2.6. Transmembrane carriers involved in both uptake of cephalosporins (CSP) from blood into the proximal tubulular cells and subsequent excretion into the tubular lumen. The involvement of the specific carriers has been indirectly demonstrated by chemical inhibitors of these transporters; probenecid, a specific inhibitor of the organic anion carrier system, decreases the toxicity of cephaloridine, while mepiphenidol, a specific inhibitor of the organic cation carrier system, increases the extent of cephaloridine nephrotoxicity.

Mechanisms underlying cephalosporine nephrotoxicity: At the cellular level, the mechanism of cephalosporine toxicity is based on concentrative uptake of the drug into proximal tubular epithelia in the kidney cortex. Specifically, cephaloridine is rapidly transported across the basolateral membrane via the organic anion transporter, OAT1. The transport at the apical side is less well characterized, but it is clear that the movement of cephaloridine across the cell-to-tubular lumen membrane is greatly restricted, probably due to the cationic group within the same molecule, leading to a considerable intracellular accumulation of the drug. In contrast, the anionic cephalothin molecule rapidly moves across the epithelia from the blood into urine (see Figure 2.6).

> The human **organic anion transporter 1 (OAT1)** belongs to a family of transport proteins which have a key role in the renal secretory pathways of xenobiotics. One of the most widely studied substrates for OAT1 is the marker compound, p-aminohippuric acid (PAH). Substrate uptake is in exchange with intracellular α-ketoglutarate; uphill xenobiotic uptake is driven by the down-hill flux of α-ketoglutarate. OAT1 is expressed at high level specifically in the kidney; it is localized at the basolateral membrane.

OAT1 exhibits broad substrate specificity and transports a number of chemically unrelated compounds. The common structural requirements for a substrate include a hydrophobic moiety, the ability to form hydrogen bonds, and the presence of ionic or partial electrical charges. Compounds with one or two negatively charged sites interact preferentially with OAT1, but zwitterionic xenobiotics can also be transported, provided they are hydrophobic enough. Cephalosporins clearly fall into this category.

Further downstream, at the molecular level, the toxicity of cephalosporins has multiple causes. These include redox cycling of the pyridine ring (see section 5.1.1), acylation and inactivation of tubular cell proteins through the spontaneous reactivity of the β-lactam ring (see section 10.3), and inhibition of mitochondrial fatty acyl carnitine transport (see section 15.1).

The same mechanisms of renal accumulation, due to rapid uptake at the basolateral membrane coupled with inefficient export at the apical membrane of tubular cells, have been implicated in the toxicity of other xenobiotics. For example, cidofovir or adefovir, nucleoside analogs (acyclic nucleoside phosphonates) and anti-retroviral drugs used against HIV share the same vectorial transport characteristics with cephalosporins. The drugs are avidly taken up via OAT1, but poorly excreted into the urine and therefore accumulate in proximal tubular cells. Indeed, the potential for clinical nephrotoxicity of cidofovir and adefovir has become evident in patients.

Learning points

- It is striking that toxic effects of xenobiotics are often manifested in a tissue- or organ-selective manner (organotropic toxicity). The mechanisms underlying this differential targeting include toxicokinetic factors (tissue-selective uptake or accumulation) and toxicodynamic factors (tissue-restricted expression of receptors or other macromolecular targets).
- Xenobiotics can mimic (in size, charge, etc.) endogenous compounds and thus become transported like a physiological substrate. Mercury is taken up into tubular epithelial cells in the kidney using the cystine transport system (molecular homology).
- Xenobiotics which act as specific ligands for nuclear receptors can mediate toxicity through the activation of these receptors. The tissue-restricted distribution and expression of the estrogen receptor is responsible for the disruption of the reproductive system by synthetic estrogens like diethylstilbestrol. Similarly, the liver-selective and species-specific expression of PPARα determines the hepatotropic injury induced by phthalate plasticizers.
- Liver and kidney are frequently targeted. The biological basis of this susceptibility includes high exposure, abundance of drug-bioactivating enzymes, and expression of many xenobiotic-transporting proteins that can up-concentrate compounds in certain compartments.
- The nephrotropic toxicity of cephalosporins can be explained mechanistically by avid uptake of these drugs via the organic anion transporter, coupled with poor efflux rates at the apical side, resulting in high intracellular drug exposure.

Further reading

Tissue-selective transcription factors

Cereghini, S. (1996) Liver-enriched transcription factors and hepatocyte differentiation, *FASEB J.* 10: 267–282.

Hines, R.N. and McCarver, D.G. (2002) The ontogeny of human drug metabolizing enzymes: Phase I oxidative enzymes, *J. Pharmacol. Exp. Ther.* 300: 355–360.

Tissue-restricted expression of molecular targets

Couse, J.F., Dixon, D., Yates, M., Moore, A.B., Ma, L., Maas, R. and Korach, K.S. (2001) Estrogen receptor-α knockout mice exhibit resistance to the developmental effects of neonatal diethylstilbestrol exposure on the female reproductive tract, *Develop. Biol.* 238: 224–238.

McLachlan, J.A., Newbold, R.R., Burow, M.E. and Li, S.F. (2001) From malformations to molecular mechanisms in the male: Three decades of research on endocrine disrupters, *APMIS* 109 (Suppl. 103): S1–S11.

Roberts, R. (1999) Peroxisome proliferators: Mechanisms of adverse effects in rodents and molecular basis for species differences, *Arch. Toxicol.* 73: 413–418.

Ward, J.M., Peters, J.M., Perella, C.M. and Gonzalez, F.J. (1998) Receptor and nonreceptor-mediated organ-specific toxicity of di(2-ethylhexyl)phthalate (DEHP) in peroxisome proliferator-activated receptor-alpha-null mice, *Toxicol. Pathol.* 26: 240–246.

Vectorial transport of xenobiotics

Burckhardt, G. and Wolff, N.A. (2000) Structure of renal organic anion and cation transporters, *Am. J. Physiol. (Renal Physiol.)* 278: F853–F866.

Cihlar, T., Ho, E.S., Lin, D.C. and Mulato, A.S. (2001) Human renal organic anion transporter 1 (hOAT1) and its role in the nephrotoxicity of antiviral nucleotide analogs, *Nucleosides Nucleotides Nucl. Acids* 20: 641–648.

Dresser, M.J., Leabman, M.K. and Giacomini, K.M. (2001) Transporters involved in the elimination of drugs in the kidney: Organic anion transporters and organic cation transporters, *J. Pharm. Sci.* 90: 397 421.

Sweet, D.H., Bush, K.T. and Nigam, S.K. (2001) The organic anion transporter family: From physiology to ontogeny and the clinic, *Am. J. Physiol. (Renal Physiol.)* 281: F197–F205.

Tune, B.M. (1998) The renal toxicity of beta-lactam antibiotics: Mechanisms and clinical implications, *Clinical Nephrotoxins. Renal Injury From Drugs and Chemicals*, DeBroe, M.E. *et al.* (eds), Kluwer Academic, Dordrecht, The Netherlands, pp. 121–134.

Xenobiotic-bioactivating enzymes

Guengerich, F.P., Kim, D.H. and Iwasaki, M. (1991) Role of human cytochrome P-450 IIE1 in the oxidation of many low molecular weight cancer suspects, *Chem. Res. Toxicol.* 4: 168–179.

Lee, S.S.T., Buters, J.T.M., Pineau, T., Fernandezsalguero, P. and Gonzalez, F.J. (1996) Role of CYP2E1 in the hepatotoxicity of acetaminophen, *J. Biol. Chem.* 271: 12063–12067.

Chapter 3

Cellular transport and selective accumulation of potentially toxic xenobiotics

Contents

3.1. Transmembrane transport of xenobiotics

Xenobiotics often exert their toxic effects inside a cell, implying that the uptake of such compounds involves transport across the plasma membrane. Likewise, for a xenobiotic to be excreted from a cell into a specific compartment, it has to cross the cell membrane, sometimes even against a concentration gradient. However, cell membrane lipid bilayers are physico-chemical barriers and do not favor a facile exchange between two compartments, in particular for bulky molecules and polar, hydrophilic structures. Therefore, specific transmembrane transport systems have evolved that allow for a much more rapid and efficient, and sometimes more select-ive, way of transporting endogenous and exogenous compounds.

There is increasing awareness that such transport systems may be important regu-lators of toxicity and play a crucial role in explaining the underlying mechanisms. For example, organ-selective toxicity (see Chapter 2) can often be explained by a tissue- or cell-specific expression of a particular transport system which accepts certain xenobiotics as a substrate and which delivers the compound to potential intracellular targets. In particular, organs with a high capacity of metabolizing foreign compounds are endowed with such transporters. While many transport systems feature a relatively broad substrate specificity and recognize and transport a large variety of xenobiotics, others are more narrow and restricted in their substrate selectivity.

Four basic mechanisms have been implicated in **transmembrane transport** of xenobiotics.

1 Diffusion is an important mechanism for small and lipophilic compounds. It is a passive process, and the driving force for the transport across the membrane is the concentration gradient between the two compartments. This gradient is either a chemical potential (for non-ionic diffusion) or an electrochemical potential (for ionic diffusion).

2 Facilitated diffusion is a much more efficient means of transmembrane transport. Specific mediators that are associated with the cell membrane greatly facilitate the transport rate for selective compounds. These mediators are large membrane proteins which deliver xenobiotics from one side of the membrane to the other by specific binding of the substrate, followed by a change of molecular conformation, and subsequent release of the compound. They are termed carriers, or channels (for ions). Importantly, similarly to diffusion, facilitated diffusion is a passive process. The driving force is a chemical or electrochemical potential difference. However, major differences to free diffusion are the following characteristics: (i) high selectivity for molecules that are transported; this even includes enantiomer selectivity, e.g. differential transport of D- and L-sugars; (ii) saturability of transport; (iii) the transport rate can be inhibited or activated by other compounds; and (iv) temperature dependence of transport. Often the transport of two distinct substrates is coupled (co-transport), e.g. transport of a large molecule is often accompanied and even driven by the co-transport of Na^+. Alternatively, the transport of one compound can be driven by the counter-transport of another substrate in the opposite direction.

3 Active transport is involved in transporting xenobiotics across cell membranes against a concentration gradient. This is only achieved under energy expenditure (ATP hydrolysis). Primary active transporters are directly ATP-dependent. In a further step, secondary active transporters indirectly use this energy; for example, concentration gradients of Na^+, which had been previously generated and maintained by a primary active transporter (the Na^+, K^+-ATPase). Such primary active transporters are often termed 'pumps' to indicate their activity in the vectorial transport of substrates against a concentration gradient. Of increasing toxicological relevance are a number of transporters genetically related to the ABC transporters (ABC for ATP-binding cassette). These proteins are multifunctional transporters and serve as 'export pumps'. They are located at the excretory domain of the plasma

membrane in organs with excretory function, e.g. at the apical side of hepatocytes or renal tubular epithelial cells (see section 3.3).

4 Endocytosis is a mechanism of transmembrane transport for large molecules or particles. This process is ATP- (and Ca^{2+}-) dependent and involves invagination of the plasma membrane. Such formed vesicles containing the enclosed xenobiotics are then shed off inside the cell. Endocytosis is induced either after binding of a xenobiotic to a membrane receptor (e.g. in the case of cholera toxin) or independently of a receptor (fluid-phase endocytosis).

3.2. Cell-specific delivery of xenobiotics to intracellular targets by physiological uptake systems

There are many examples where xenobiotics are substrates for multispecific transmembrane transporters. In most cases, the foreign compounds are then metabolically converted and excreted. The metabolism of certain compounds can, however, intracellularly produce potentially toxic intermediates. Tissue- or cell type-specific metabolic activation is therefore an important mechanism of organ-selective toxicity and will be discussed in detail below (see Chapter 4).

In this context, the focus is on the cell-selective transmembrane transport mechanisms, rather than cell-selective metabolism, which can determine the ensuing organ toxicity. Evidence indicates that in specific tissues toxic responses can be induced by the delivery of certain xenobiotics to intracellular targets, often based on molecular homology with a physiological substrate (see section 2.1.1). In other cases, it is the vectorial transport of xenobiotics to extracellular compartments that is an important toxicokinetic factor governing the compound's toxicity.

3.2.1. Multispecific hepatic bile salt uptake systems

A classical example of specific transport-mediated organ toxicity is the *Amanita* toxins.

Intoxications with the mushroom *Amanita phalloides* (toadstool) are due to a number of naturally occurring oligopeptide toxins, including the amanitins. The most important species of this group is **α-amanitin**. Amanitins are bicyclic octapeptides and are the sole cause of lethal human poisoning after ingestion of this mushroom (if not antagonized by antidotes). This toxin exerts its most dramatic effects in the liver, which is exposed to high concentrations of the compound, while most other organs are spared. Another group of toxins produced by *Amanita* mushrooms are the phalloidins, which are bicyclic heptapeptides. In contrast to amanitins, phalloidins are not toxic when ingested (but they are toxic when given parenterally). The reason for this differential effect is poor enteral absorption of phalloidins, while amanitins have a much higher oral bioavailability.

Typical for intoxications with amanitins is the relatively late onset of symptoms (8–24 h) resulting in death after several days, due to hepatic failure. The molecular mechanism of hepatic toxicity, at the toxicodynamic level, is a specific inhibition of RNA polymerase II by α-amanitin, which results in a block of mRNA synthesis and, hence, overall protein synthesis. At the toxicokinetic level, the liver-selective toxicity can be explained by specific uptake of α-amanitin into hepatocytes.

Mechanisms of hepatocyte-selective uptake of α-amanitin: Octapeptides can certainly not just diffuse across cell membranes. Instead, α-amanitin binds to and is transported by a polyspecific transporter located at the hepatocellular basolateral membrane. The normal function of this transporter is to extract bile salts from the circulation and to mediate their uptake into hepatocytes. Indeed, in cultured hepatocytes or in isolated membrane vesicles, the transport of α-amanitin is temperature-sensitive and saturable, indicating that facilitated diffusion is involved. Furthermore, the transport can be stimulated by an out-to-in Na^+ gradient and is inhibited by taurocholate. Although only indirectly demonstrated, it is therefore highly likely that it is the Na^+-dependent taurocholate co-transporting peptide (NCTP) that mediates amanitin uptake into hepatocytes (see Figure 3.1).

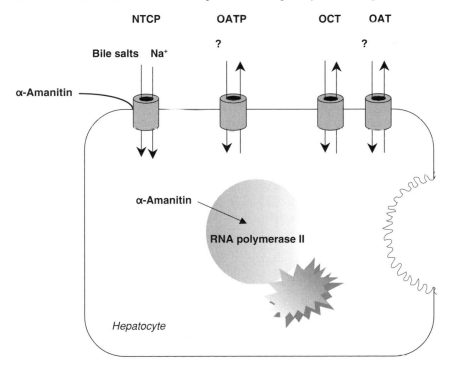

Figure 3.1. Putative hepatocellular uptake systems for α-amanitin responsible for the hepatotropic toxicity of the mushroom toxin. These include the bile salt carrier system (NTCP, possibly others).

In the liver, four families of transport proteins have been identified and cloned, all of which are involved in the **hepatocellular uptake of organic anions** (including bile salts) and cations. They are expressed at the basolateral (sinusoidal) membrane domain of hepatocytes. These proteins are (i) the Na$^+$-taurocholate cotransporting peptide (NCTP), (ii) the organic anion transporting peptides (OATP), (iii) the organic cation transporters (OCT), and (iv) the organic anion transporters (OAT). While the NCTP functions unidirectionally, the other proteins are bidirectional transporters.

3.2.2. *Pulmonary epithelial cell polyamine carrier*

Another example of specific carrier-driven toxicity is the lung-selective injury associated with paraquat exposure. The pulmonary effects can be readily explained by the participation of a transport system abundantly expressed in certain cell types in the lung.

Paraquat is a non-selective contact herbicide of the dipyridinyl class. After its introduction in the 1960s, the use of paraquat rapidly expanded worldwide. However, it was soon recognized that paraquat, following accidental or suicidal ingestion, but also after incorrect use, caused selective (but not exclusive) pulmonary injury in humans. Following exposure, lung damage develops over a period of many days or weeks. At first, the pulmonary alveolar cells are injured, followed by the development of edema, inflammation, and hemorrhage. Interestingly, it is only the alveolar cells type I and II that are affected; the capillary endothelial cells remain intact. In a second phase, lung fibrosis can develop, which is probably a compensatory repair mechanism for the damaged alveolar epithelial cells.

Because of these well defined pulmonary adverse effects, the use of paraquat has been restricted in many countries, and rigorous tolerance limits on foods have been established. Instead, a congener of paraquat, diquat, which is much less toxic, has been widely used. Elucidation of the molecular mechanisms of paraquat toxicity has led to a concept that plausibly explains the differential pulmonary liability of these two compounds (see Figure 3.2).

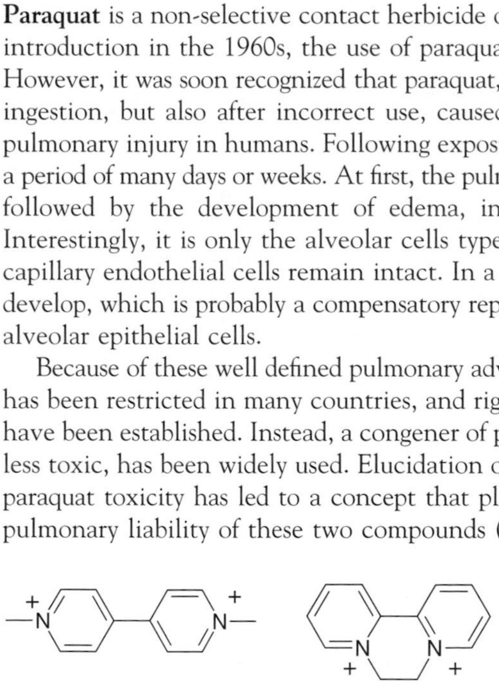

Figure 3.2. Chemical structures of paraquat (left) and diquat. Paraquat is used as the dichloride, diquat as the dibromide.

Mechanisms of paraquat injury to alveolar cells: After oral ingestion of paraquat, only a small fraction is absorbed. Interestingly, however, the blood levels remain constant over many hours as paraquat is not metabolized in the liver. Paraquat typically accumulates in the lung (pulmonary concentrations can be six to seven times higher than those in the plasma), and the compound is retained in the lung even when blood levels are starting to decrease.

In search of the underlying mechanism, it was found that the lungs accumulate paraquat in an energy-dependent manner. In addition, its accumulation features saturability, which is compatible with the concept of carrier-mediated transmembrane transport. But how is paraquat selectively up-concentrated in the lung?

A number of physiological substrates were found to inhibit paraquat uptake into lung tissue. Among these, polyamines are powerful inhibitors. This has led to the hypothesis that the polyamine transport system might be the gate for paraquat uptake.

Polyamines are diamines (putrescine and cadaverine) or oligoamines (spermidine and spermine) that occur in all eukaryotic and prokaryotic cells. Polyamines are positively charged at physiological pH and therefore have a high affinity for negatively charged cellular targets. In particular, they exert strong electrostatic interactions with DNA and RNA. Polyamines have multiple physiological functions and have been implicated in cell growth, proliferation, and differentiation. They also play a role in antioxidant defense and in immune reactions.

In the lung, polyamines are taken up by active transport leading to high cellular concentrations. Specifically, alveolar cells I and II have a much more efficient polyamine uptake system than any other major organ. However, to date, neither the nature of the carrier protein nor the reason for its high expression in alveolar cells is known. A possible gene coding for a polyamine transporter (TPO1) was isolated from eukaryotic cells and introduced into yeast cells. Yeast cells heterologously expressing TPO1 indeed become sensitive to polyamines. For mammals, though, it is not known whether the transporter(s) is (are) located at the apical or basal side of the cells, and how the expression of the gene is regulated.

When one compares the chemical structures of these diamines with that of paraquat, it is striking that the two compounds share some similarities. In particular, both have two quaternary nitrogen atoms, separated by an alkyl chain or by aromatic rings with a similar spacer size. Therefore, many pieces of evidence have led to the current concept that paraquat is indeed a substrate for the polyamine carrier located in the membrane of alveolar cells type I and II.

The substrate specificity is quite rigorous. In order to act as a substrate for the pulmonary polyamine transport system, a xenobiotic must exhibit a number of characteristics. First, it must possess two (or more) charged nitrogen atoms; the maximal positive charge must surround these nitrogens. In addition, a nonpolar group must separate these charges, and there must be minimal steric hindrance. Furthermore, the optimal distance between the two nitrogens is four carbons (methylene groups), as it occurs in putrescine, which features an N–N distance of 6.6 Å (but up to seven carbons are tolerated). Matching these prerequisites, the distance between

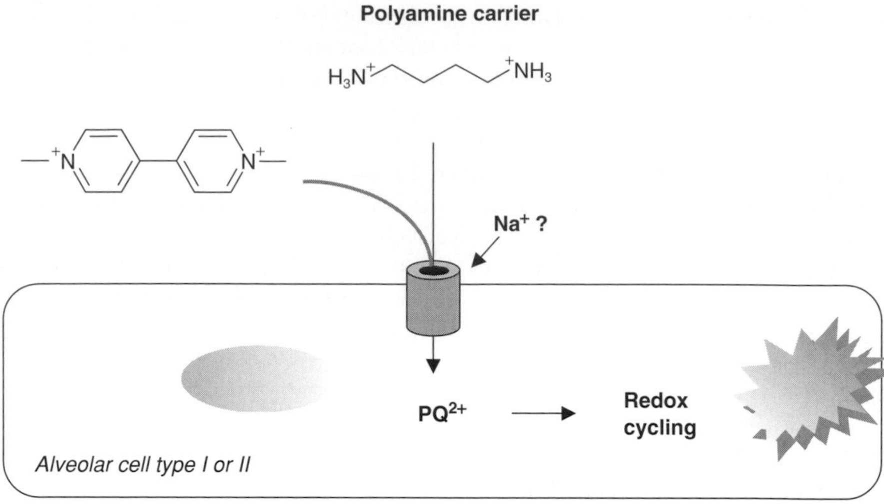

Figure 3.3. Uptake of paraquat (PQ^{2+}) via the polyamine transport system in alveolar type I and type II cells. The physiological substrate depicted here is putrescine. The molecular characteristics of the transporter have not been identified in mammals. However, substrate selectivity includes two charged nitrogens, an ideal distance between these nitrogens, and a nonpolar spacer.

the two charged nitrogen atoms of paraquat is 7.0 Å, which explains its affinity for the carrier. The two pyridine rings, however, somewhat pose a steric hindrance, making paraquat a less ideal substrate for the carrier and featuring a somewhat lower affinity (higher K_m) than polyamines. Nevertheless, substantial amounts of paraquat are taken up into the lung through this uptake system. In contrast, diquat, which is not pneumotoxic and which does not accumulate in alveolar cells, exhibits a much smaller intramolecular distance between the two charged nitrogen atoms, which makes this compound a poor substrate for the transporter, and which explains its much greater safety margin (see Figure 3.3).

Further downstream at the toxicodynamic level, the molecular mechanism of paraquat cytotoxicity to alveolar cells I and II is based on redox cycling and intracellular oxidative stress (see section 5.1.1).

Alveolar (A) cell types I and II are the epithelia that line the airways of the lung alveoli. The main function of the A I cells, which are flat and actually form the alveolar vesicle, is gas exchange between the air space and the vessels. The A II cells are more round and located at the distal border of the alveolar vesicles. Their main functions are surfactant secretion, active transport of water and ions, and epithelial regeneration. The role of the surfactant (phospholipids, mainly phosphatidylcholine) is to form a thin film on top of a thin aqueous layer that covers the epithelial cells. This decreases the surface tension and also acts as a defense against noxious agents.

Alveolar cells are exposed to xenobiotics from two sides. First, all inhaled xenobiotics have to pass the pulmonary epithelia before they gain access to the blood. Second, not only inhaled compounds but also xenobiotics in the circulating blood (such as paraquat) come into close contact with the pulmonary epithelia, which can have toxic implications for the lung.

3.2.3. The neuronal dopamine transporter and xenobiotic-induced Parkinsonism

A paradigm of cell-type selective accumulation of a toxic compound in the brain, which sets the stage for the subsequent development of toxic neuronal injury, is MPTP.

In the early 1980s, designer drug users in California who synthesized a type of 'new heroin' (meperin) were unexpectedly found to develop neurotoxic properties that resembled the symptoms otherwise typical for Parkinson's disease. These symptoms included slowed movements, 'frozen' features, gait problems, and other disorders. Therefore, the drug addicts who had administered themselves meperin and who exhibited Parkinson-like symptoms were given the usual treatment for Parkinson's disease, i.e. a combination treatment of L-DOPA (a precursor of dopamine which passes the blood–brain barrier) and a decarboxylase inhibitor. This promptly resulted in improvement of the condition. There were relapses, though, some of them with fatal outcome. Puzzling at first and only later understood, the autopsy of the brain of people who died from the abuse of this drug revealed that, like in Parkinson's disease, dopaminergic neurons located in the substantia nigra pars compacta (an area in the mesencephalon) had undergone site-specific cell death.

Later it turned out that it was not meperin itself that had caused the neurotoxicity, but that a contaminant, **1-methyl-4-phenyl-1,2,3,6-tetrahydropyridine (MPTP)** was involved. MPTP had been unexpectedly generated as a side-product during the synthesis of the new heroin. The ultimate toxic species, however, is **1-methyl-4-phenylpyridine (MPP$^+$)**, which is a metabolite generated from MPTP in the brain (see Figure 3.4).

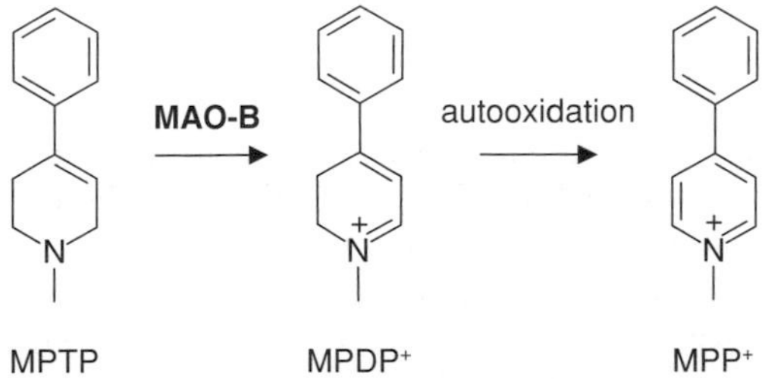

Figure 3.4. Metabolic conversion of MPTP to MPP$^+$.

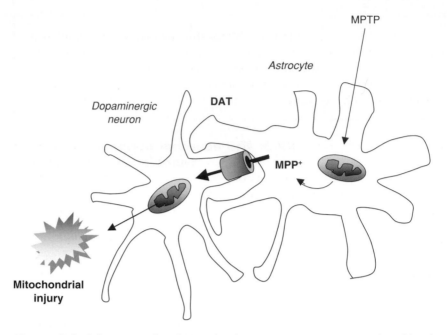

Figure 3.5. Selective uptake of MPP$^+$ by dopaminergic neurons is mediated by the dopamine transporter.

Mechanisms of MPTP injury to dopaminergic neurons: MPTP, which is a lipophilic compound, can cross the blood–brain barrier and reach the CNS, where it is taken up by glial cells. In astrocytes, MPTP is converted by monoamine oxidase (MAO)-B, a mitochondrial enzyme, to MPDP, which then autooxidizes to MPP$^+$. That MAO-B is indeed critically involved in bioactivating MPTP was shown in experiments in which chemical inhibitors of MAO-B prevented the toxicity of MPTP. With this knowledge, it can also be readily explained mechanistically why the rat is a species that is not sensitive to MPTP neurotoxicity; in rats the expression of MAO-B in astrocytes is poor.

But how can the selective toxicity of MPP$^+$ to dopaminergic neurons be explained? Again, selective transport phenomena provide the clue to the puzzle. It turned out that MPP$^+$ is a good substrate for a transporter that is located on the plasma membrane of dopaminergic neurons and which normally transports dopamine into these neurons. The accumulation of MPP$^+$ inside the neurons explains the cell-selective cell death (see Figure 3.5).

The carrier that transports dopamine into dopaminergic neurons is known as the **dopamine transporter (DAT)**. The DAT is situated at the plasma membrane and fulfills a crucial function; it terminates the action of dopamine by rapidly removing dopamine from the synaptic cleft. It is a member of the Na$^+$ and Cl$^-$-coupled neurotransmitter transporter family. The transporter is differentially expressed in dopaminergic neurons; it has a distinctly greater expression in cells of the substantia nigra than in other areas. Furthermore, the density of the DAT on these cells strongly correlates with the extent of dopaminergic cell loss. Although the DAT exhibits high selectivity for this neurotransmitter, it can also transport synthetic or natural analogs of dopamine, MPTP, and structurally related compounds including pyridine, isoquinoline, and β-carboline derivatives.

More downstream, at the molecular and toxicodynamic level, the ultimate mechanism of MPP$^+$ toxicity is based on the compound's ability to bind to and inhibit complex I activity in mitochondria. This results in the generation of reactive oxygen species (see section 5.1), which poses an oxidative stress and causes damage to mitochondria. In addition, the neuron will face an acute energy crisis (see section 15.1).

Intensified research on MPP$^+$ has triggered a host of unresolved questions. For example, is it possible that environmental compounds could be involved, at least in part, in the pathogenesis of Parkinson's disease through similar mechanisms?

While the etiology of Parkinson's disease is still idiopathic (i.e. having an unknown cause), and as some of the underlying causative factors are only slowly emerging, it has been suggested that perhaps xenobiotics in the environment could be a major cause of this disease. Indeed, MPP$^+$ structurally resembles dipyridyl pesticides, such as paraquat (see section 3.2.2), and environmental contamination with pesticides has been considered a possible cause. However, a number of arguments speak against this assumption. For example, the incidence of morbus Parkinson has not been increasing since its discovery in the middle of the nineteenth century, although the use of pesticides worldwide had been greatly expanded. In addition, paraquat and structurally related pesticides are not neurotoxic.

Nevertheless, there is evidence that specific exposure to compounds in the environment can be related to the occurrence of Parkinson's disease. For example, it is known that the Chamorro population in Guam in the Western Pacific had an approximately 50-fold higher incidence of Parkinson's disease prior to the Second World War. After adaptation to the American lifestyle, the incidence nearly dropped to the average. A likely explanation is the involvement of a neurotoxin that is contained in the palm nuts of the *Cycas* tree and the consumption of which has drastically decreased in the past decades. Indeed, an amino acid, β-N-methylamino-L-alanine, has been identified in these nuts as a potent neurotoxin.

Furthermore, rotenone, a mitochondrial toxin (see section 15.4) is a compound which has been traditionally extracted from plants and used to catch fish by native populations in South and Central America. It turned out that rotenone causes a similar loss of dopaminergic neurons and induces the development of Parkinson's disease when injected into rats. Although rotenone is rapidly degraded and has been regarded as harmless in the environment, its potential toxicity should be revisited.

3.3. Xenobiotic export pumps

'Xenobiotic export pumps' is a term that describes a number of primary active transporters which mediate the vectorial export of endogenous and exogenous compounds from the cell to the extracellular space. Because this process is not driven by a chemical gradient but rather by ATP consumption, this uphill transport can indeed occur very efficiently against a steep concentration gradient.

Xenobiotic export pumps logically play a central role in liver and kidney, and it is in these organs that they have also been implicated in being mechanistically related to toxicity.

In the liver, a number of export pump systems have been identified which are involved in bile formation and in the excretion of xenobiotics. The transport proteins are located on the apical membrane domain of hepatocytes. All these proteins belong to the **ATP-binding cassette (ABC) transporter superfamily** and share common structural and functional characteristics.

1 The **multidrug resistance P-glycoprotein** (encoded by the gene **MDR1**) transports a wide range of xenobiotics (see section 3.3.2). No endogenous substrates have been identified yet for this carrier. It is relatively weakly expressed in liver but abundant in other organs.
2 The **phospholipid export pump (MDR3)** is a transporter that functions as a flippase to translocate phospholipids from the inner to the outer leaflet of the membrane. Biliary phospholipids are used in forming vesicles and mixed micelles.
3 The **conjugate export pump (MRP2**; the canalicular isoform of the multidrug resistance-associated protein) transports a large number of organic anions into bile. Among these are a number of endogenous compounds, including bilirubin conjugates, glutathione, and glutathione conjugates. Importantly, MRP2 is the transporter that exports xenobiotic glucuronide or sulfate conjugates and therefore plays a critical role in drug metabolism.
4 The canalicular **bile salt export pump (BSEP)** mediates the transport of bile acids from hepatocytes into the bilary tree.

Other isoforms of some of these carriers (e.g. MRP1 and MRP3 to 6) are located on the basolateral membrane rather than the apical domain. Their function is not yet clearly determined, but they could take over rescue transport function under conditions of severe impairment of canalicular secretion, in order to avoid accumulation of potentially toxic compounds within the cell.

3.3.1. Hepatobiliary conjugate export pump and cholestasis

A number of examples have illustrated in the past how hepatobiliary export pumps can form the molecular basis, and are the actual driving force, for a xenobiotic to become toxic in the biliary tree. A recent and clinically relevant case is the hepatic toxicity induced by the drug benoxaprofen.

Benoxaprofen is a nonsteroidal anti-inflammatory drug (NSAID) that was used efficiently to treat rheumatoid disorders. However, soon after its introduction in the 1980s, the drug had to be withdrawn from the market due to rare but unpredictable cases of severe hepatic toxicity. Liver toxicity presented as cholestatic jaundice, with minimal damage to the hepatic parenchyma. Unusually for this phenotypic pattern, the development of benoxaprofen-associated intrahepatic cholestasis was fatal in some cases. The mechanism underlying the hepatic injury had remained unknown for a long time. Because the latency period from start of treatment until onset of the disease was long (several months), an immunoallergic mechanism directed against the drug was unlikely (for drug allergies in the liver, the latency period usually is one to five weeks).

Several pieces of evidence soon raised the possibility that a pharmacokinetic factor might be involved. Indeed, the fatal disease occurred mainly in elderly people who often exhibit a compromised excretory rate for drugs or their metabolites. In addition, benoxaprofen exhibits an unusually long elimination half-life ($t_{1/2} > 100$ h). The possibility of the formation of a reactive metabolite was considered; however, it turned out that bioactivation by cytochrome P450 was unlikely to be involved in this case.

Because benoxaprofen, like many other acidic NSAIDs, features a carboxylic acid group, it is metabolized in the liver by an alternative pathway. In fact, carboxylic acids are readily conjugated to glucuronic acid, mediated by UDP-glucuronosyltransferase (UGT), which is abundant in the liver. This process of coupling a sugar to a xenobiotic's phenolic or carboxylic acid group is a major way of detoxication, allowing for a more rapid elimination of many xenobiotics due to their increased water solubility (see section 4.2.2). Acyl glucuronides are usually excreted either across the basolateral membrane of hepatocytes into the blood, or else across the canalicular membrane into the bile canaliculus. This efficient elimination by a xenobiotic export pump is a likely explanation for the lack of damage to the parenchymal cell itself. In contrast, the conjugate export pump-mediated up-concentration of the metabolite in the biliary compartment has yielded a clue to a possible mechanism underlying the induction of cholestasis.

The powerful up-concentration capacity of xenobiotics, driven by some of these export pumps, can be appreciated if one looks at the relative concentrations of acyl glucuronides in the different compartments. Compared to the circulation, the concentrations of acyl glucuronides in the liver can be ~50-fold higher, and in bile even ~5,000-fold increased. Therefore, intracellular macromolecules, but even more so membrane components facing the lumen of the bile canaliculus, and also biliary ductular epithelia, are exposed to very high concentrations of these xenobiotics. This might lead to damage and intrahepatic cholestasis.

Cholestasis is defined differentially by pathologists, physiologists, or toxicologists. While the pathological picture is defined as the presence of bile plugs in canaliculi, and of accumulated bile pigment in hepatocytes (in humans, but not detectable in rats), the physiological viewpoint defines cholestasis as a reduction or even cessation of bile flow. From the toxicological angle, the term mainly relates to the retention in the liver of cholephilic compounds (that is, compounds that are normally excreted into bile). Inefficient excretion can lead to toxic concentrations in the hepatocyte, and impaired bile flow can cause high intracanalicular levels of cholephilic excretory products. These compounds are not only xenobiotics but also include physiological substrates, such as bile salts. Bile salts and other endogenous compounds are continually secreted and fulfill a vital physiological function: they provide the driving force for the generation of bile flow (unlike in the kidney, there is no hydrostatic pressure for bile production).

A large number of xenobiotics can induce intrahepatic cholestasis, and this occurs through different mechanisms. However, recently it has become clear that in many cases it is the transmembrane transporters that are involved. Often these transporters become functionally impaired, or their expression is down-regulated, and thus they exhibit markedly decreased functional capacity and impaired overall transport rates.

Mechanisms of benoxaprofen-induced cholestasis: Most likely, the cause of the specific injury of the hepatobiliary system is selective accumulation of benoxaprofen glucuronide in the biliary tree, which results in very high local drug concentrations. At least three factors contribute to the toxicity.

1 Benoxaprofen acyl glucuronide is poorly water-soluble and might precipitate in the biliary tree as a function of its increasing concentration.
2 Due to the slightly more alkaline pH of bile (as opposed to the intracellular milieu in hepatocytes), the alkali-labile acyl glucuronide is more readily hydrolyzed. In fact, this hydrolytic degradation of acyl glucuronides is tightly coupled with their chemical reactivity towards nucleophilic residues on protein targets (see section 9.2.2.3). Benoxaprofen acyl glucuronide is indeed protein-reactive; administration of benoxaprofen to mice forms covalent adducts to canalicular proteins at the apical membrane lining the bile canaliculi.
3 Most importantly in this context, it is the vectorial transport of the acyl glucuronide metabolite of benoxaprofen which causes dramatic increases in the biliary concentrations of the drug. This is mediated by the canalicular isoform of the conjugate export pump, Mrp2 (see Figure 3.6).

The reason why cholestasis developed in only a very small percentage of patients receiving benoxaprofen, while the vast majority of recipients tolerated the drug well, is still enigmatic. One can only speculate that genetic and/or environmental

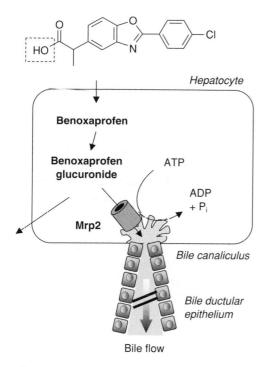

Figure 3.6. Up-concentration of benoxaprofen acyl glucuronide in the bile canaliculus is mediated by Mrp2.

factors might have altered the expression of canalicular Mrp2. For example, experimental induction of Mrp2 in rats readily entails higher biliary concentrations of acyl glucuronides exported from hepatocytes. Alternatively, it is well known that other conditions, e.g. the release of bacterial lipopolysaccharide (LPS) from the gut, can greatly down-regulate the expression of canalicular Mrp2. This might lead to a retention of the xenobiotic in hepatocytes and to a recruitment of alternative, basolateral carriers to get rid of the accumulating drug.

3.3.2. Multidrug resistance in cancer cells

In contrast to the previous examples, where transmembrane uptake or export systems were involved in the development of *undesired* cellular effects, this example describes the opposite. Sometimes therapeutic approaches are aimed at actively killing cells, and targeted cellular toxicity is a *desired* effect, as it occurs with chemotherapeutic compounds used to treat certain forms of cancer.

Unfortunately, failure of such chemotherapeutic agents to damage cancer cells is a common problem and poses a big challenge in the clinic. Many of these drugs simply do not reach the critical cellular target. Among the possible explanations at the pharmacokinetic level, transmembrane transport plays a pivotal role. This is a key mechanism in the phenomenon of 'multidrug resistance'.

Multidrug resistance is a phenomenon that describes the resistance of tumor cells to a wide range of anticancer agents. This phenomenon not only is observed in cultured transformed cell lines but also occurs *in vivo*. Multidrug resistance can be induced by one specific anticancer agent, and it may even be associated with cross-resistance against other therapeutics. These agents include many compounds which are structurally unrelated to each other; common molecular features are high lipophilicity and often an amphipathic character.

It was soon discovered that it is a highly increased cellular efflux rate of these agents that is responsible for the cells' resistance to the toxic drugs. The first export protein involved in this mechanism was identified as the **P-glycoprotein (pgp)** (see also section 3.3). Initially it was suspected that P-glycoprotein may somehow alter the cell membrane's overall permeability to drugs (hence the 'P'). Today we know that P-glycoprotein functions as a transmembrane pore-forming protein, leading to an energy-dependent drug efflux. This efflux is so efficient that the carrier has been compared with a 'hydrophobic vacuum cleaner', implying that it can remove drugs from the plasma membrane before they can even reach the cytoplasm (or the DNA, a major target of antineoplastic agents) (see Figure 3.7).

P-glycoprotein is not only up-regulated in cancer cells, where it is responsible in part for multidrug resistance, but it is also expressed in many normal tissues. The transport protein is typically present in organs that are involved in xenobiotic absorption (intestine), elimination (kidney and liver), but also in tissue-selective exclusion of entrance (brain, testes). The transporter is typically localized at the apical pole of cells. For example, it is expressed on the brush border of renal tubular epithelial cells, at the canalicular membrane of

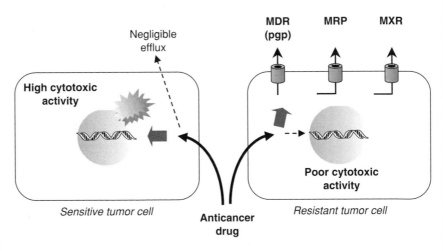

Figure 3.7. Transmembrane transporters involved in multidrug resistance. A number of export pumps with partly overlapping substrate selectivity expel the chemotherapeutic agents before these can reach their cellular targets (e.g. DNA). MDR, multidrug resistance; pgp, P-glycoprotein; MRP, multidrug resistance-associated protein; MXR, mitoxantrone resistance protein.

hepatocytes, and at the luminal side of the small and large intestine. In addition, P-glycoprotein is found at the capillary endothelial cells of the brain and testes, where it forms the blood–brain barrier and the blood–testes barrier, respectively.

The second protein that has been implicated in cancer cell resistance is the **multidrug resistance-associated protein (MRP)** subfamily (MRP1 to 7). These proteins exhibit partly overlapping activity towards the substrates for P-glycoprotein, but they feature additional functions. While P-glycoprotein exhibits greatest affinity for large hydrophobic cations, MRP is very effective in exporting large organic anions. In normal liver, MRP2 is expressed at the canalicular membrane of hepatocytes and is identical with the conjugate export pump (see section 3.3.1).

Recently, a third member of multidrug resistance proteins has been identified, the **mitoxantrone resistance protein (MXR)**. The resistance phenotype greatly overlaps with P-glycoprotein. It is a half-transporter member as it is has only half the size of the full-length ABC transporters and probably requires dimerization to become fully functional. This protein is expressed in many cancer cells but is also abundant in placenta, liver (canalicular membrane of hepatocytes), small intestine, colon, lung, kidney, and the endothelia of veins and capillaries.

Attempts to reverse the multidrug resistance phenotype in patients by chemical inhibitors of these transporters have been disappointing. For example, several drugs including calcium channel blockers and cyclosporin A can efficiently inhibit P-glycoprotein activity and thus reverse multidrug resistance *in vitro*, but many of these agents are simply too toxic at doses that would be needed to reverse the multidrug resistance phenomenon.

3.3.3. Permeability of the blood–brain barrier

Xenobiotic export pumps, and in particular P-glycoprotein, play a pivotal role in the maintenance of the blood–brain barrier, the blood–testes barrier, and other barriers, shielding sensitive organs from the potential toxicity of xenobiotics (see Figure 3.8).

The **blood–brain barrier (BBB)** is an efficient system in the brain of all vertebrates that protects the CNS from many xenobiotics. The BBB is based on a number of anatomical and physiological characteristics that make this barrier impermeable for a large number of compounds, except for small and lipophilic ones. For example, the vascular endothelial cell lining in the brain is tight and non-fenestered, and endocytosis is rare. Only receptor-mediated uptake occurs to provide the brain with essential physiological substrates. In addition, and importantly, abundant expression of the P-glycoprotein export pump is a major component of this barrier. This transporter, encoded by the MDR1 gene, is located at the vascular endothelial cell membrane. Its main function is to keep out xenobiotics that will cross the endothelial cell membrane in the vascular space and to prevent them from entering the brain.

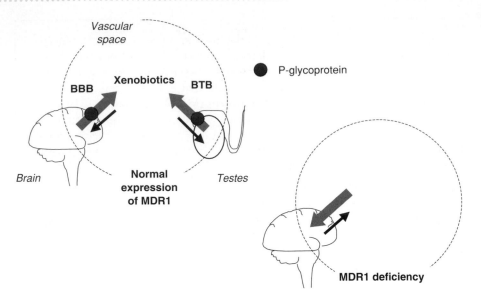

Figure 3.8. P-glycoprotein is a key factor in the integrity of the blood–brain barrier (BBB) and the blood–testes barrier (BTB) and protects these organs against influx and accumulation of xenobiotics.

The difference in the potency of many pharmaceutical drugs acting on the CNS often parallels their relative affinity to and transport rates by the P-glycoprotein in the brain. Similar compounds, or even enantiomers of the same compound, can be differentially transported into or expelled from the brain by this transport system. Clinical examples where a xenobiotic exerts clear neurotoxic effects because of an insufficient function of the P-glycoprotein are rare, but will become increasingly important as the significance of P-glycoprotein and other export pumps will become more appreciated.

The importance of P-glycoprotein can be illustrated in experimental models in which the gene for MDR1 has been knocked out and which are thus deficient in P-glycoprotein. The brain/plasma ratio of normally impermeable xenobiotics (e.g. digoxin, cyclosporin A) can be increased up to 50-fold or more in these *mdr1*-null mice as compared to that in normal mice. An example which actually links increased drug concentrations in the brain with downstream adverse effects resulting from these increased drug levels is the neurotoxicity of ivermectin. Ivermectin is an antiparasitic drug widely used as an acaricide and anthelmintic in animals and also in humans. In the P-glycoprotein-deficient murine model, the *mdr1a*-null mice displayed an increased sensitivity to the centrally neurotoxic action of ivermectin. In fact, the symptoms of ivermectin toxicity (immobilization, inability to right themselves, recumbency, tremors, decreased breathing frequency, and in extreme cases coma and death) became manifest in the P-glycoprotein-deficient mice at a 100-fold lower dose as compared to the dose which induced similar symptoms in wild-type mice. This greatly increased toxicity was reflected by a 87-fold higher brain level of the drug as compared to wild-type control mice which had received the same dose. Interestingly, the dose which is lethal in *mdr1a*-null mice is dangerously close to the human therapeutic dose used to

Table 3.1 Increased concentrations of ivermectin in the brain of P-glycoprotein-null mice as compared to wild-type mice

Tissue	Ivermectin concentrations (ng/g tissue)	
	mdr1a −/− mice	mdr1a +/+ mice
Brain	131 ± 16	1.5 ± 1.2
Liver	497 ± 74	130 ± 45
Kidney	141 ± 27	47 ± 14
Plasma	52 ± 8	16 ± 6

Note: Tissue levels were measured 24 h after oral administration of 0.2 mg/kg ivermectin. Data are mean ± SD ($n = 3$).
Source: data are from Schinkel, A.H., Wagenaar, E., Vandeemter, L., Mol, C.A.A.M. and Borst, P. (1995) Absence of the mdr1a P-glycoprotein in mice affects tissue distribution and pharmacokinetics of dexamethasone, digoxin, and cyclosporin A, *J. Clin. Invest.* 96: 1698–1705.

treat river blindness (onchocerciasis); there are, however, no reports of a similar sensitivity in patient subsets. Thus, not only the disposition of centrally acting drugs, but also the downstream toxicological consequences, i.e. the potential neurotoxicity of xenobiotics, can be greatly influenced by the lack of activity of this efflux pump.

Learning points

- Tissue or cell-selective accumulation of xenobiotics is often the underlying toxicokinetic force explaining cell-specific toxicity. This is mediated by transport proteins that have a high affinity for a xenobiotic and which facilitate compound-selective uptake and up-concentration to toxic levels.
- Examples include the liver toxicity induced by the mushroom poison α-amanitin, which is transported via the hepatocellular bile salt carrier OAT1; pulmonary toxicity associated with the pesticide paraquat, which is transported into alveolar cells I and II by the polyamine carrier; and induction of Parkinson-like disease by MPP⁺, a metabolite of a contaminating product in a designer drug, which is taken up into dopaminergic neurons by the dopamine transporter.
- Xenobiotic export pumps are ATP-dependent transporters involved in the excretion of many endogenous and exogenous compounds and their metabolites. They can highly up-concentrate these compounds in extracellular compartments, e.g. the biliary canaliculi, causing toxicity. Alternatively, if transporter function is compromised, xenobiotics may accumulate intracellularly.
- Multidrug resistance in cancer cells can be explained in part by overexpression of MDR and/or MRP and related proteins, causing increased efflux of cytotoxic drugs from targeted cancer cells.
- Transmembrane transporters (e.g. P-glycoprotein) are important components of the blood–brain barrier or blood–testes barrier; loss of function of these carriers can cause xenobiotics to cross this barrier and induce undesired toxic effects in these otherwise well-shielded organs.

Further reading

Multispecific hepatic bile salt uptake systems

Kröncke, K.D., Fricker, G., Meier, P.J., Gerok, W., Wieland, T. and Kurz, G. (1986) α-Amanitin uptake into hepatocytes. Identification of hepatic membrane transport systems used by amatoxins, *J. Biol. Chem.* 261: 12562–12567.

Kullak-Ublik, G.A. (1999) Regulation of organic anion and drug transporters of the sinusoidal membrane, *J. Hepatol.* 31: 563–573.

Pulmonary epithelial cell polyamine carrier

Foth, H. (1995) Role of the lung in accumulation and metabolism of xenobiotic compounds – implications for chemically induced toxicity, *Crit. Rev. Toxicol.* 25: 165–205.

Hoet, P.H.M. and Nemery, B. (2000) Polyamines in the lung: Polyamine uptake and polyamine-linked pathological or toxicological conditions, *Am. J. Physiol. (Lung Cell. Mol. Physiol.)* 278: L417–L433.

Smith, L.L. (1997) Paraquat, *Comprehensive Toxicology. Toxicology of the Respiratory System* 8: 581–589.

Tomitori, H., Kashiwagi, K., Sakata, K., Kakinuma, Y. and Igarashi, K. (1999) Identification of a gene for a polyamine transport protein in yeast, *J. Biol. Chem.* 274: 3265–3267.

Neuronal dopamine transporter and Parkinsonism

Aschner, M. and Kimelberg, H.K. (1991) The use of astrocytes in culture as model systems for evaluating neurotoxic-induced injury, *Neurotoxicol.* 12: 505–518.

Chen, N. and Reith, M.E.A. (2000) Structure and function of the dopamine transporter, *Eur. J. Pharmacol.* 405: 329–339.

Cleeter, M.W., Cooper, J.M. and Schapira, A.H. (1992) Irreversible inhibition of mitochondrial complex I by 1-methyl-4-phenylpyridinium: Evidence of free radical involvement, *J. Neurochem.* 58: 786–789.

Jenner, P. and Marsden, C.D. (1987) Parkinsonian syndrome caused by 1-methyl-4-phenyl-1,2,3,6-tetrahydropyridine (MPTP) in man and animals, *Selectivity and Molecular Mechanisms of Toxicity*, DeMatteis, F. and Lock, E.A. (eds), Macmillan Press, Basingstoke, pp. 213–248.

Miller, G.W., Gainetdinov, R.R., Levey, A.I. and Caron, M.G. (1999) Dopamine transporters and neuronal injury, *Trends Pharmacol. Sci.* 20: 424–429.

Storch, A. and Schwarz, J. (2000) The dopamine transporter: Involvement in selective dopaminergic neurodegeneration, *Neurotoxic Factors in Parkinson's Disease and Related Disorders*, Storch, A. and Collins, M.A. (eds), Kluwer Academic Press, New York, NY, 17–40.

Xenobiotic export pumps

Dong, J.Q., Etheridge, A.S. and Smith, P.C. (1999) Effect of selective phase II inducers on glucuronidation of benoxaprofen in rats, *Drug Metab. Dispos.* 27: 1423–1428.

Keppler, D. and König, J. (2000) Hepatic secretion of conjugated drugs and endogenous substances, *Sem. Liver Dis.* 20: 265–272.

Oude Elferink, R.P.J., Meijer, D.K.F., Kuipers, F., Jansen, P.L.M., Groen, A.K. and Groothuis, G.M.M. (1995) Hepatobiliary secretion of organic compounds; molecular mechanisms of membrane transport, *Biochim. Biophys. Acta (Rev. Biomembranes)* 1241: 215–268.

Sallustio, B.C., Sabordo, L., Evans, A.M. and Nation, R.L. (2000) Hepatic disposition of electrophilic acyl glucuronide conjugates, *Current Drug Metab.* 1: 163–180.

Seitz, S., Kretz-Rommel, A., Oude Elferink, R.P.J. and Boelsterli, U.A. (1998) Select-ive protein adduct formation of diclofenac glucuronide is critically dependent on the rat canalicular conjugate export pump (Mrp2), *Chem. Res. Toxicol.* 11: 513–519.

Stieger, B., Fattinger, K., Madon, J., Kullak-Ublik, G.A. and Meier, P.J. (2000) Drug- and estrogen-induced cholestasis through inhibition of the hepatocellular bile salt export pump (Bsep) of rat liver, *Gastroenterology* 118: 422–430.

Trauner, M., Meier, P.J. and Boyer, J.L. (1998) Molecular pathogenesis of cholestasis, *New Engl. J. Med.* 339: 1217–1227.

Trauner, M., Meier, P.J. and Boyer, J.L. (1999) Molecular regulation of hepatocellular transport systems in cholestasis, *J. Hepatol.* 31: 165–178.

Multidrug resistance in cancer cells

Ambudkar, S.V., Dey, S., Hrycyna, C.A., Ramachandra, M., Pastan, I. and Gottesman, M.M. (1999) Biochemical, cellular, and pharmacological aspects of the multidrug transporter, *Annu. Rev. Pharmacol. Toxicol.* 39: 361–398.

Bellamy, W.T. (1996) P-glycoproteins and multidrug resistance, *Annu. Rev. Pharmacol. Toxicol.* 36: 161–183.

Kavallaris, M. (1997) The role of multidrug resistance-associated protein (MRP) expres-sion in multidrug resistance, *Anti-Cancer Drug* 8: 17–25.

Litman, T., Druley, T.E., Stein, W.E. and Bates, S.E. (2001) From MDR to MXR: New understanding of multidrug resistance systems, their properties and clinical signific-ance, *Cell. Mol. Life Sci.* 58: 931–959.

Permeability of the blood–brain barrier

Ayrton, A. and Morgan, P. (2001) Role of transport proteins in drug absorption, dis-tribution and excretion, *Xenobiotica* 31: 469–497.

Matheny, C.J., Lamb, M.W., Brouwer, K.L.R. and Pollack, G.M. (2001) Pharmacokinetic and pharmacodynamic implications of p-glycoprotein modulation, *Pharmacother.* 21: 778–796.

Schinkel, A.H., Smit, J.J., van Tellingen, O., Beijnen, J.H., Wagenaar, E., van Deemter, L., Mol, C.A.A.M., van der Valk, M.A., Robanus-Maandag, E.C. and te Riele, H.P. (1994) Disruption of the mouse mdr1a P-glycoprotein gene leads to a deficiency in the blood–brain barrier and to increased sensitivity to drugs, *Cell* 77: 491–502.

Schinkel, A.H., Wagenaar, E., Vandeemter, L., Mol, C.A.A.M. and Borst, P. (1995) Absence of the mdr1a P-glycoprotein in mice affects tissue distribution and phar-macokinetics of dexamethasone, digoxin, and cyclosporin A, *J. Clin. Invest.* 96: 1698–1705.

Smith, B.J., Doran, A.C., McLean, S., Tingly, F.D., O'Neill, B.T. and Kajiji, S.M. (2001) P-glycoprotein efflux at the blood–brain barrier mediates differences in brain disposi-tion and pharmacodynamics between two structurally related neurokinin-1 receptor antagonists, *J. Pharmacol. Exp. Ther.* 298: 1252–1259.

Chapter 4

Bioactivation of xenobiotics to reactive metabolites

Contents

In many cases it is not the parent compound itself that confers toxicity on a cell, but rather one or several of its metabolites. This chapter deals with the mechanisms of formation of such reactive metabolites from pro-toxicants and the consequences of reactive metabolite formation. A large number of enzymes are involved in catalyzing reactive metabolite generation; only a few of them will be highlighted here.

4.1. Biotransformation and bioactivation/-inactivation

After a xenobiotic has entered the body, higher organisms have the capacity to get rid of the compound (unless it is used for the organism's intermediate metabolism), thus avoiding accumulation. If the xenobiotic is hydrophilic, it can be readily excreted in the urine. However, the more hydrophobic a xenobiotic is, the more difficult it becomes to excrete it via the kidneys.

The body has basically two ways of handling such lipophilic compounds. The first option is to store it in the body's lipophilic compartments. This happens with many extremely lipophilic compounds, e.g. polychlorinated xenobiotics, which are difficult to metabolize. Normally, such a sequestered compound poses no harm and can remain in these lipophilic compartments for many months or years. It is only upon rapid release of the body's fat stores that the compound may suddenly reach high systemic concentrations.

The second option is to enzymatically convert the lipophilic compound to a more hydrophilic species. This process is called biotransformation (xenobiotic metabolism) and can proceed by two major pathways:

1 by the addition, or cleavage, of a functional group (called functionalization, or 'phase I' metabolism)
2 by coupling the xenobiotic (or its primary metabolite) with an endogenous substrate (termed conjugation, or 'phase II' metabolism – although phase II reactions can also occur without a preceding phase I reaction).

Often, a pharmaceutical drug loses its pharmacologic activity after being metabolized, and toxic compounds may be readily inactivated by this process. Nevertheless, metabolism is not always a detoxication or bioinactivation process. Instead, it has been well known for a long time that many xenobiotics are metabolically converted to a potentially more reactive and more toxic species. In this case, the metabolic step is called bioactivation. This can be brought about by phase I and/or phase II reactions. The resulting bioactivated species are reactive metabolites (also called biological reactive intermediates).

Because reactive metabolites have been implicated in many cases, often plausibly explaining an underlying mechanism of toxicity, xenobiotic metabolism and the disposition of the metabolites are crucial toxicokinetic determinants of a compound's toxicity (see section 1.2).

In this chapter, only the basic concepts and principles of reactive metabolite formation, from a mechanistic point of view, and their downstream biological effects will be discussed. Comprehensive overviews on the chemistry of a variety of possible reactions, as well as the systematic biotransformation profiles of many chemical groups, are found in many excellent books and reviews.

4.2. Phase I (functionalization) and phase II (conjugation) reactions

The major types of phase I or II reactions that are toxicologically relevant (and examples of which are discussed in the following sections) are summarized in Table 4.1. It is important to note that most of these enzymes are enzyme families, having branched out during evolution. Due to the advent of novel techniques in genomic analysis, we are increasingly aware of an increasing number of subfamilies and individual enzyme forms. Some of these are true isoenzymes, i.e. the individual members are encoded and regulated differently while catalyzing the same reactions. For others, in particular for cytochrome P450, some members of an enzyme family do not necessarily catalyze the same reactions and are therefore termed isoforms.

Table 4.1 Overview of the major functionalization and conjugation reactions involved in xenobiotic biotransformation

Enzyme (families)	Function
Phase I	**Substrate functionalization**
■ Cytochrome P450 (CYP)	■ Oxidation or reduction, including aliphatic or aromatic hydroxylation, epoxidation, N-, O-, or S-dealkylation, N-hydroxylation, sulfoxidation, desulfuration, oxidative dehalogenation
■ Flavin-dependent monooxygenase (FMO)	■ N- and S-oxidation (not C)
■ Peroxidase (Px)	■ Reduction of hydroperoxides to alcohol
■ Carboxylesterase, amidase	■ Hydrolysis of ester or peptide bonds
■ Alcohol dehydrogenase (ADH)	■ Oxidation of alcohols to aldehyde
■ Epoxide hydrolase (EH)	■ Hydrolysis of epoxides to dihydrodiols
Phase II	**Substrate conjugation**
■ UDP–glucuronosyltransferase (UGT)	■ Transfer of glucuronic acid (from UDP–glucuronic acid) to xenobiotic
■ Sulfotransferase (SULT)	■ Transfer of sulfate (from phosphoadenosine phosphosulfate) to xenobiotic
■ N-Acetyltransferase (NAT)	■ Transfer of acetate (from acetyl-CoA) to xenobiotic
■ Glutathione-S-transferase (GST)	■ Transfer of glutathione to xenobiotic

4.2.1. Cytochrome P450 (CYP)

Cytochrome P450 is undoubtedly the most important enzyme family in mechanistic toxicology. Therefore, its role, regulation, and genetic variability will be highlighted with selected examples.

Cytochrome P450 (CYP, P450) is a superfamily of enzymes found in some prokaryotes and in all eukaryotes. They are important in oxidative, reductive, and peroxidative biotransformation of many endogenous (e.g. steroids, bile acids, fatty acids, prostaglandins) and exogenous (natural products contained in plants, drugs, environmental pollutants) compounds. CYP evolved and greatly diversified during the evolutionary transition from aqueous life to terrestrial life. Although CYP phylogenetically was first involved in endogenous metabolism, these enzymes later in the evolution have been playing a paramount role in metabolizing xenobiotics that are contained in plants and that could be potentially harmful when ingested.

More than 400 genes for CYP have been identified (approximately 90 different CYP genes in *Drosophila*!), and many isoforms with different but partly overlapping substrate specificity are present in mammals and insects. This diversification during the evolution also created ecological niches allowing access to foodstuffs and plants that would otherwise be toxic for other competing organisms.

CYPs are not classified and named after their catalytic function (the actual outcome of the catalytic reaction depends mostly on the nature of the substrate; all that CYP does is to bind and bring together the substrate and activated oxygen). Instead, CYPs are classified according to their genetic relationship. For example, the term 'CYP2E1' means gene family 2 (>40 percent homology among members), gene subfamily E (>55 percent homology, and all genes of a subfamily are located in the same chromosome and in the same gene cluster), and finally, 2E1 is the individual gene. Some of these CYP families, in particular CYP1, 2, and 3, play a particularly important mechanistic role in mediating bioinactivation, bioactivation, and toxicity of xenobiotics.

CYPs are hemoproteins (red color!) which have an Fe^{2+} moiety that can bind molecular oxygen, but also carbon monoxide. The original name ('P450') stems from the early observation that this hemoprotein features maximal absorption at 450 nm (the number has nothing to do with a protein or a molecular mass).

The enzyme is found predominantly in the liver, but also in intestine, nose epithelia, lung, and skin. This organ-selective distribution suggests that CYP is abundantly expressed in those organs through which xenobiotics enter the body first, providing a checkpoint before they reach the circulation. However, CYPs are also expressed in kidney, sertoli cells of the testis, ovary, placenta, and other organs.

In the cell, CYPs are associated primarily with the membrane of the smooth endoplasmic reticulum (forming microsomes after homogenization), but are also expressed at the plasma membrane and mitochondrial inner membrane.

The overall function of CYP is that of a monooxygenase, implying that the enzyme inserts one atom of oxygen into a substrate (oxygenation). This oxygen atom stems from molecular oxygen, which first binds to the heme moiety and is subsequently cleaved. The remaining atom of oxygen is reduced to yield water. For this reduction, two electrons are required, which stem from NADPH, one of the biologically most important reductants. However, as the ferrous iron can only accept one electron at a time, the two electrons are not transferred simultaneously but sequentially via an associated protein adjacent to CYP, the NADPH–P450 reductase. This reductase thus takes the role of a 'transformer' (see Figure 4.1).

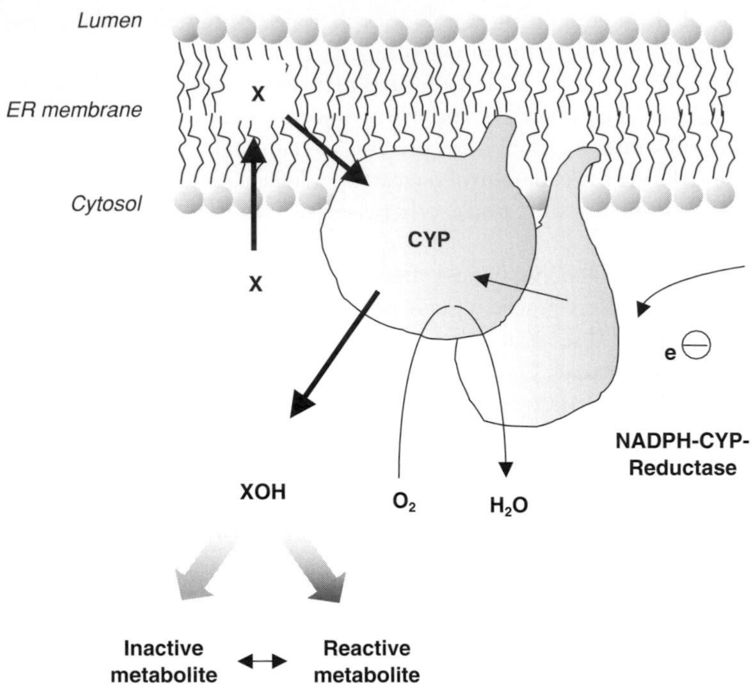

Figure 4.1. Topology and general function of cytochrome P450 (X = xenobiotic).

Two features associated with CYPs are toxicologically important: their regulation and induction potential, and genetic variability including polymorphisms.

First, CYPs are tightly regulated and can be induced upon need by many substrates and xenobiotics. For most CYPs, the regulation is transcriptional, but for some others pretranslational, translational and posttranslational regulation also occurs. The result is that enhanced expression of P450 activity can greatly augment the bioinactivation/-activation rates of potentially toxic compounds.

An impressive example, used to illustrate the profound consequences of CYP induction on the extent of toxicity of a xenobiotic, is cocaine toxicity to hepatocytes and its potentiation by the multiple CYP form inducer, phenobarbital.

Cocaine is an alkaloid which is converted in hepatocytes to a sequence of reactive metabolites that have been implicated in the hepatotoxic effects of cocaine in experimental animals (and possibly in humans) (see section 5.1.6). In rat liver, it is CYP2B that bioactivates cocaine (in mice or humans, other isoforms including CYP3A and CYP2A are involved). Although the exact mechanism underlying cocaine hepatotoxicity is still enigmatic and possibly involves multiple mechanisms, the manifestation of toxicity clearly requires

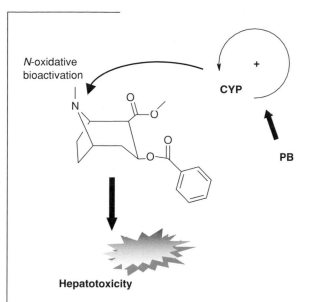

Figure 4.2. Induction of rat CYP2B by phenobarbital (PB) results in an increased rate of cocaine bioactivation and potentiation of cocaine-induced hepatotoxicity.

initial *N*-oxidative metabolic activation (*N*-demethylation and subsequent steps) catalyzed by CYP (see Figure 4.2).

Cultured hepatocytes from normal rats are largely resistant to cocaine exposure, and cell injury can only be achieved by very high concentrations. In contrast, hepatocytes isolated from rats which had been pretreated with phenobarbital (PB) for a few days (in order to induce CYP) were greatly sensitized to cocaine. In fact, induction of P450 by PB can amplify the toxicity by a factor of 100–1,000! In naive female ICR mice, administration of cocaine (45 mg/kg) is without any apparent effects on the liver, while the same dose given to PB-pretreated mice causes extensive liver necrosis. The marker enzyme activity for the integrity of hepatic parenchymal tissue, alanine aminotransferase (ALT) in the plasma, was increased >100-fold over vehicle control values (from approx. 20 U/L to 2,500 U/L, which is indicative of severe hepatotoxicity). Thus, induction of CYPs can have profound effects on the expressivity of a toxic effect that otherwise is not manifest at identical exposure.

Molecular mechanisms of CYP induction: Transcriptional activation of different CYPs is regulated by distinct mechanisms. For example, CYP1A1, CYP1A2, and CYP1B1 are regulated via the aryl hydrocarbon receptor (AHR) (see section 12.1). In contrast, CYP3A is regulated by the pregnane X receptor (PXR) (see section 4.2.1.1). Finally, CYP2B6, CYP3A, and CYP2C induction is mediated by the constitutively active receptor (CAR). Elucidation of the last of these mechanisms has finally shed some light on the mechanism underlying phenobarbital induction.

Phenobarbital (PB), a barbiturate derivative and anticonvulsant drug, has gained broad application as an experimental compound because it is one of the most powerful inducers of CYPs (and other enzymes as well). PB can co-induce a variety of CYPs; the most responsive ones are members of the CYP2B subfamily (human 2B6). The mechanism of induction has been elusive for many years, and no receptor had been identified to which PB might bind. Although much has been learned since, the exact mechanism of induction is still unclear.

Today we know that the induction is mediated by a nuclear receptor, **CAR (constitutively active receptor)**. This receptor can transactivate CYPs without prior binding of a ligand. Therefore, unlike most other nuclear receptors involved in CYP induction, PB is an inducer but not a ligand for CAR. PB may mediate two regulatory steps: (1) dephosphorylation of CAR to its active form, so that CAR can migrate into the nucleus, and (2) phosphorylation of CAR, once it is in the nucleus, to its active form so that it can bind to DNA response elements. This is done by forming a heterodimer with RXR, the retinoid receptor X. The heterodimer binds to PBREM (phenobarbital-responsive enhancer module), after which the transcription of CYP2B6 is increased. So-called inverse agonists can deactivate the receptor and suppress transcription (such inverse agonists include steroids related to androstanol). Compelling evidence for the role of CAR stems from gene knockout experiments; in fact, CAR-null mice are unable to respond to PB and do not up-regulate CYP.

CAR is down-regulated by proinflammatory cytokines, which could explain the negative acute phase response evoked by these cytokines (see Figure 4.3).

The second toxicologically relevant feature associated with CYPs is the genetic variability in humans. There are several known polymorphisms (defined as occurring in >1 percent of a population) and other, less frequent allele variations for individual CYP genes. Again, these individual differences in the potency to metabolize xenobiotics could readily explain many of the observed differential reactions to xenobiotics among individuals and different populations. The first CYP polymorphism was detected by serendipity, and its elucidation was triggered by initially unexplained pharmacological responses with the drug debrisoquine.

In the 1970s it was incidentally found that a human volunteer exhibited an exaggerated pharmacologic effect after taking **debrisoquine**, an antihypertensive drug. This effect was manifested by a marked and sustained fall in blood pressure. It turned out that this effect was due to a low rate of debrisoquine hydroxylation in this individual, due to low activity of the involved CYP isoform. Later, debrisoquine was taken off the market, but this same phenomenon of differential response to a large number of drugs was soon the basis for intensive research on individual expression of CYP forms.

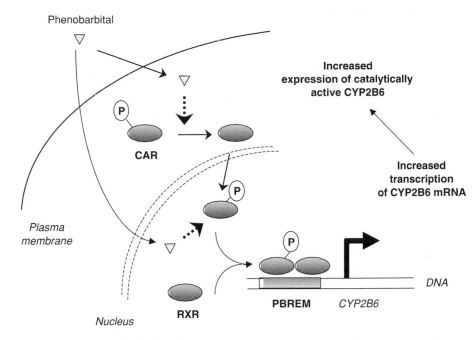

Figure 4.3. Phenobarbital induces CYP2B by activating, but not by binding to, the nuclear receptor CAR.

Today it is known that it is the human CYP2D6 that exhibits a distinct genetic polymorphism due to the presence of various mutations of the *CYP2D6* gene. The molecular basis of these mutations has been elucidated. Loss of function of some alleles leads to the phenotype of 'poor metabolizer'. Heterozygotes often are 'intermediate metabolizers'. On the other hand, duplication or amplification of an active gene may lead to the 'ultrarapid metabolizer' phenotype.

Similar polymorphisms have been found for other CYPs and for phase II enzymes. In fact, many altered genotypes result in the poor metabolizer phenotype. Because the metabolism by these enzymes has been implicated in the activation, toxicity, and carcinogenicity of certain xenobiotics, a correlation between the genotype and the development of individual expression of toxicity caused by a xenobiotic is likely.

4.2.1.1. Mechanisms and toxicological consequences of isoform-selective CYP induction

Among the many implications of CYP activity in mechanistic toxicology, one consequence of xenobiotic metabolism by highly expressed levels of CYP is the undesired increased rate of clearance of a xenobiotic. If this is a therapeutic drug, rapid loss of therapeutic function can ensue, possibly entailing pathophysiological effects. This may occur when one drug induces a CYP form for which a second drug is a substrate, too, leading to drug–drug interactions. An example is St John's wort.

St John's wort (*Hypericum*) extracts are therapeutically used as a herbal anti-depressant. In some cases, treatment with St John's wort has been associated with greatly decreased plasma levels of other drugs taken at the same time. This decrease in plasma level has caused a loss of the desired therapeutic efficacy of these other drugs and, in some cases, entailed medical complications. For example, concomitant use of St John's wort extracts and cyclosporin A has caused organ rejection, and co-medication with ethinyl estradiol has resulted in irregular bleeding in women.

The basis for the obviously increased clearance of these drugs, caused by *Hypericum* extracts, has been suspected to be an increased expression and activity of the CYP isoform(s) that metabolize these drugs. Both cyclosporin A and ethinyl estradiol are substrates for the human CYP3A4, and increased expression of CYP3A4 would cause these drugs to be metabolically eliminated too rapidly. Indeed, hyper-forin, the active component of St John's wort, is a strong inducer of CYP3A4 in the liver.

The logical consequences of such an unrecognized CYP induction could be far-reaching: for example, if enzyme induction were to alter the disposition of an oral contraceptive, then the failure of contraception might lead to a fetus being exposed inadvertently to a new drug. Therefore, there is an urgent need to estab-lish the enzyme-inducing properties of all new chemical entities.

But how can the liver cell 'sense' the presence of a possible inducing agent, and how can the transcription and increased expression of the CYP be regulated? This is achieved by the PXR.

Pregnane X receptor (PXR) (also called steroid- and xenobiotic-sensing recep-tor, SXR) is a nuclear receptor. Its recent detection provided the missing link between the long-known inducing capacity of many chemicals and drugs and the increased *de novo* synthesis of specific CYP forms, in particular CYP3A4 (see Figure 4.4). This receptor is primarily expressed in liver, the small intestine, and the colon. The name of the receptor is derived from its avidity to bind steroid hormones and their metabolites, including progesterone, estrogen, and corticosterone. In addition, other ligands include xenobiotics such as rifampicin, phenobarbital, nifedipine, clotrimazole, and metyrapone, all well-known inducers of CYP3A4 in humans. The most potent PXR lig-and known to date, however, is hyperforin, a component of St John's wort. Hyperforin binds with an EC50 of $\sim 2 \times 10^{-9}$ M!

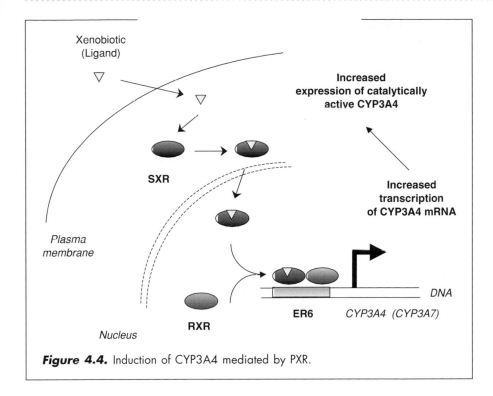

Figure 4.4. Induction of CYP3A4 mediated by PXR.

Similarly to other nuclear receptors, PXR forms a heterodimer with the retinoid X receptor-α (RXRα). It binds to ER6 (everted repeat with a 6 bp spacer) elements, and transactivates CYP genes. Co-activators can also participate in the induction of transcription.

Both PXR and RXR can be induced by activation of another receptor, the glucocorticoid receptor (GR). This explains why glucocorticoids (indirectly) induce the transcription of CYP3A4. On the other hand, PXR is down-regulated by pro-inflammatory cytokines (e.g. IL-6), which is the basis for the well-known observation that these cytokines exert a negative acute phase response and cause a decrease in some P450s. PXR-null mice were unable to respond to inducing agents by up-regulating CYP3A, but the basal expression was not changed.

4.2.1.2. Mechanisms and consequences of isoform-selective CYP inhibition

Another mechanistically relevant aspect is inhibition of a particular CYP isoform by a xenobiotic. In contrast to the phenomenon of CYP induction by a compound, which requires several doses and several days to reach maximal effects, inhibition is an immediate effect. Enzyme inhibition might result in the accumulation of other substrates for this CYP form, due to impaired metabolic clearance, and, in rare cases, in toxicity. As underlying mechanisms of CYP inhibition, an irreversible destruction of CYP by a compound (e.g. carbon tetrachloride, see section 5.2.3) or competitive interactions of two substrates for the same CYP form (e.g. CYP3A4 and drug–drug interactions; see section 1.2.1) are possible.

While in many cases a competitive inhibitor of CYP is a second therapeutic drug, there are also compounds in our daily diet that can modulate CYP activities, such as grapefruit juice.

Grapefruit juice has long been known to contain certain components that can interact with the metabolism of xenobiotics. For example, a single glass of grapefruit juice in patients taking the calcium antagonist nifedipine has caused an approximately five-fold increase in the AUC of nifedipine. This could become toxicologically relevant; studies with other calcium channel blockers have revealed that grapefruit juice not only caused an increase in the AUC of the drug but also greatly influenced the pharmacodynamics (lowering blood pressure and increasing the heart rate).

Interactions of one or several components in the grapefruit with the hepatic metabolic clearance of nifedipine were first suspected. However, as the juice has little effect on the availability of intravenously adminstered drug and does not change its elimination half-life, it appears now that grapefruit juice effects are at the level of the intestine and not the liver.

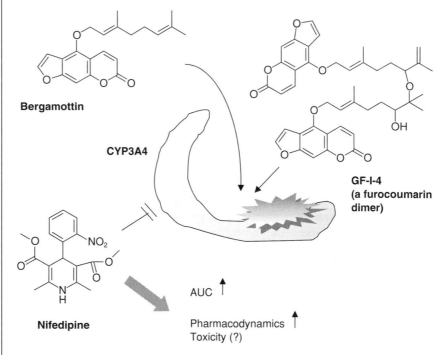

Figure 4.5. Mechanism-based inactivation of CYP3A4 by furanocoumarin constituents (monomers and dimers) contained in grapefruit juice leads to inhibition of nifedipine metabolism and increases in nifedipine AUC.

Initially naringine and other flavonoids, major constituents of grapefruit juice, were considered to be the crucial compounds. However, it has become clear that there are a number of other compounds that are responsible for this interaction. In particular, furanocoumarin monomers (e.g. bergamottin) and dimers (e.g. GF-I-4), although present in graperfruit juice at much lower concentrations than flavonoids, were found to be more than 100-fold more potent inhibitors of CYP than flavonoids. The furanocoumarins also exhibit isoform specificity; the dimers in particular inhibit CYP3A4 (the CYP isoform involved in nifedipine metabolism), with half-maximal rates of inactivation value (K_i) of as low as 100–300 nM. Bergamottin, in contrast, also inhibits selectively CYP1A2, CYP2C9, CYP2C19, and CYP2D6, other important human CYPs involved in the metabolism of xenobiotics (see Figure 4.5).

Mechanisms of furanocoumarin-induced CYP3A4 inactivation: Because the inhibition of CYP3A4 is both concentration- and time-dependent and also an irreversible effect, the type of inhibition by grapefruit juice constitutents is termed 'mechanism-based' inhibition (also called 'suicide inactivation'). This term implies that a compound is bioactivated by CYP to a reactive metabolite which in turn destroys the enzyme that has been involved in the biactivation process. Obviously, the reactive metabolite in this case must be extremely reactive.

Indeed, the reactivity of a metabolite generated by CYP can greatly determine the site and extent of the downstream consequences of these reactive metabolites. If the stability (half-life) of the metabolite is extremely short, it may interact with the molecule right at the site of generation, i.e. the enzyme itself. The logical consequence of such a mechanism-based inactivation is a self-limitation of the reaction, because the CYP involved is irreversibly damaged and needs to be resynthesized.

Mechanism-based CYP inactivation also occurs with other reactive furanocoumarins (psoralens), including those involved in photoactivated toxic reactions (see section 4.3). For example, the most widely studied furanocoumarin, 8-methoxypsoralen (8-MOP), is a potent inhibitor of human CYP2A6. The mechanism of inhibition has been elucidated; it proceeds through bioactivation of 8-MOP to a reactive epoxide, which in turn covalently modifies an amino acid residue of the CYP apoprotein (see Figure 4.6).

4.2.1.3. Bioactivation of xenobiotics by CYP

In many cases cytochrome P450 has been implicated in bioactivating xenobiotics that are initially harmless and non-reactive into reactive and potentially harmful metabolites. Because of the involvement of specific CYP isoforms, this bioactivation, and hence toxicity, can be organ-selective and also species-selective.

Among the host of examples that are known today, 4-ipomeanol is selected, because this example not only illustrates the role of cell-specific bioactivation but also delineates some of the difficulties and caveats in extrapolating from one species to another (humans).

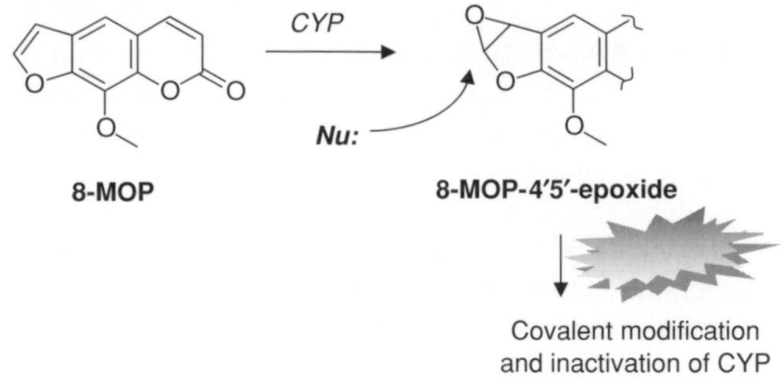

Figure 4.6. Suicide inactivation of CYP apoprotein by the epoxide of the activated 8-methoxypsoralen.

4-Ipomeanol (IPO) is a furane derivative naturally occurring in common sweet potatoes (*Ipomea batatas*) infected with the fungus *Fusarium solani*. The compound was first isolated from mold-infected potatoes as it was the puzzling cause for a severe pulmonary disease in cattle. This toxin is extremely organotropic; following ingestion of 5–10 mg/kg IPO, cattle exhibited lung edema and hemorrhages. Rats and mice are equally sensitive to IPO and develop pulmonary toxicity. For humans the risk is minimal, as exposure through food obviously is small. Nevertheless, the compound has been investigated for its potential to be therapeutically used as an anticancer agent against some forms of pulmonary cancer.

Mechanisms of 4-ipomeanol-induced lung injury: Ipomeanol is biotransformed by CYP to an α,β-unsaturated dialdehyde. This is a reactive species which can interact with and form covalent adducts to tissue protein (see Chapter 9). The major CYP form that biotransforms IPO in rodents is CYP4B1, found predominantly in the Clara cells and type II epithelial cells that line the terminal airways. Because the degree of covalent binding of this reactive intermediate to lung tissue has been proportional to the lung-selective toxicity *in vivo*, and because antibodies directed against the specific CYP form have precluded binding and toxicity, it was inferred that the reactive metabolite generated from P450 was directly responsible for the induction of toxicity. The highly reactive metabolite binds to and damages the tissue exactly at the site where it is generated (however, the exact toxicodynamic mechanisms underlying the killing of Clara cells and the sequelae in the lung have not been elucidated).

Clara cells are the non-ciliated cells of the bronchiolar epithelium. Their numerical density varies from species to species and can reach high numbers; in the terminal bronchiole Clara cells can account for >50 percent in rodents. They express a number of CYPs at high levels and have been implicated in being the primary site of xenobiotic biotransformation in bronchioli. Furthermore, this cell type is the stem cell for the distal bronchiolar epithelium and has been implicated in some forms of bronchogenic carcinomas (and therefore used as a target for IPO chemotherapy).

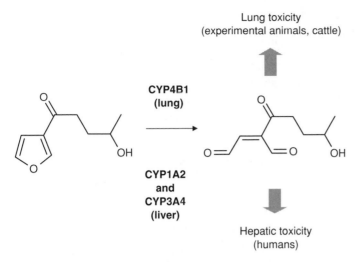

Lung toxicity
(experimental animals, cattle)

CYP4B1
(lung)

CYP1A2
and
CYP3A4
(liver)

Hepatic toxicity
(humans)

Figure 4.7. CYP-mediated bioactivation of 4-ipomeanol to a reactive metabolite produces toxicity. Clara cell-selective CYP4B1 activity in rodents and many animal species produces lung injury, while in humans, other CYP forms present in liver bioactivate the xenobiotic to a reactive metabolite that produces liver injury.

In many species including rabbits, rats, mice, guinea pigs, and dogs, IPO was indeed bioactivated in the lung by Clara cells, and to a lesser extent and only at higher doses also by type II epithelial cells, because both cell types abundantly express CYP4B1. This bioactivation sets the stage for bronchiolar cell necrosis. Therefore, IPO was initially considered for therapeutic use against lung cancer. Surprisingly, IPO had little activity towards these lung cancer cells. Furthermore, in a number of clinical trials, hepatotoxicity developed in most patients, characterized by transient elevations of aminotransferases (ALT) (see Figure 4.7). In view of these adverse effects, and also because there was no obvious clinical benefit in treating lung cancer, the drug was abandoned for this indication.

The reason underlying this species difference has been elucidated: the preponderance of hepatotoxicity, instead of pulmonary toxicity, indicates that IPO in humans is preferentially bioactivated in the liver. Indeed, human CYP1A2 and CYP3A4 (in liver) share overlapping substrate specificity with the rodent CYP4B1 (in Clara cells). In addition, although mRNA for CYP4B1 is expressed in human lung tissue (not in liver), heterologously expressed human CYP4B1 did not catalyze the oxidation of IPO! This illustrates that one has to be very careful with species extrapolation. As a logical step, IPO has been used in therapeutic trials to treat hepatocellular carcinoma (with moderate success so far).

4.2.2. UDP-glucuronosyltransferase (UGT)

Besides CYP-mediated bioactivation, there are many examples in which phase II enzymes have been mechanistically implicated in the toxicity of xenobiotics. Among these, UGT-mediated glucuronoconjugation reactions play an important role.

Uridine-diphosphate glucuronosyltransferase (UGT) is an enzyme super-family that catalyzes the transfer of a glucuronic acid moiety from 'activated' glucuronic acid (uridine-diphosphate glucuronic acid, UDPGA) to the accep-tor xenobiotic. The endogenous glucuronic acid can be conjugated to a phenolic group or a carboxylic acid group (O-glucuronides) or to an amino group (N-glucuronides) of a substrate. Because in rare cases sugars other than glucuronic acid are also conjugated with a substrate, the enzyme superfamily has also been termed 'glycosyltransferases', but this new name has not found widespread acceptance in the literature.

The major consequence of glucuronidation is an increase in the aqueous solubility of the xenobiotic. For example, phenol, which is poorly water-soluble and which features a pK_a of ~10 is converted to phenyl-β-D-glucuronide, featuring a pK_a of ~3.4. This means that at physiological pH the glucuronide carboxylic group is dissociated. Thus, in most cases, glucuronidation will facilit-ate elimination of the xenobiotic. Examples include physiological substrates, such as bilirubin or steroid hormones, but also a host of xenobiotics.

Glucuronidation of xenobiotics is, however, not always a detoxication reaction. On the one hand, the conjugation reaction can result in the gen-eration of reactive glucuronide intermediates. For example, glucuronidation of carboxylic acids to acyl glucuronides (see section 4.2.2.2) and the N-glucuronidation of aromatic amines (see section 4.2.2.3) are such bioactivating

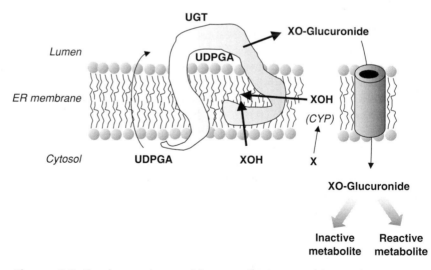

Figure 4.8. Topology and general function of UGT. Lipophilic xenobiotics (X) are hydroxylated by CYP, and the hydroxylated product binds to the catalytic site of UGT. After glucuronide conjugation (UDPGA binds to the sugar binding site at the UGT molecule), the glucuronide is released into the lumen of the ER. It is transported by a carrier back into the cytosol (and then exported from the cell by a carrier). UDPGA is synthesized in the cytosol and transported into the ER by a translocase.

processes. On the other hand, glucuronides can unmask or augment a potential toxicity of the parent compound by other mechanisms. Examples include steroid hormones, the glucuronides of which have been involved in cholestasis, and morphine glucuronide, which is more active than the aglycone, morphine. Thus, glucuronidation should not generally be considered a detoxication reaction.

UGTs are classified by sequence-based nomenclature. Isoforms belonging to one family (e.g. UGT1 or UGT2) share >60 percent sequence homology. The liver is the most important organ involved in xenobiotic glucuronidation, both in quantitative and qualitative terms, but UGTs are also expressed in extrahepatic organs. At the cellular level, UGT is a membrane-bound microsomal enzyme adjacent to CYP. It features a binding site for the aglycone (the substrate) and another binding site for the sugar (see Figure 4.8).

Similarly to CYP and other xenobiotic-metabolizing enzmyes, UGT is regulated and can be induced by a variety of substrates. Also, human polymorphisms in the genes coding for the UGT forms exist; for example, a genetic deficiency of UGT1 (the bilirubin-conjugating form) results in Crigler-Najar syndrome. These patients are not able to glucuronoconjugate sufficiently and thus excrete bilirubin; they are jaundiced and suffer from potential bilirubin neurotoxicity.

4.2.2.1. Mechanisms and toxicological consequences of UGT induction

UGT is regulated and can be induced by a variety of xenobiotics. Interestingly, this induction is often coordinated with the induction of CYP. For example, compounds that induce CYP1A often induce UGT forms that conjugate planar phenols. Alternatively, compounds that induce CYP2B forms (such as phenobarbital) often co-induce the UGT forms that glucuronoconjugate bulky substrates. Finally, other UGTs are coordinately regulated through the AHR (see section 12.1).

An example of how selective induction of UGT activity in the liver can modulate the toxicokinetics and toxicodynamics of a xenobiotic is the increased glucuronidation of carboxylic acid-containing nonsteroidal anti-inflammatory drugs. Increased glucuronoconjugation alters their disposition and, because these glucuronides are reactive metabolites, the potential toxicity of these metabolites at more distant sites.

Many **nonsteroidal anti-inflammatory drugs (NSAIDs)** are carboxylic acids which are conjugated to glucuronic acid in the liver. The resulting acyl glucuronides are delivered into bile and finally reach the intestine. Selective chemical induction of those hepatic UGT forms that conjugate these NSAIDs results in increased biliary output of the conjugates.

High exposure to NSAIDs has been associated with small intestinal irritation, bleeding, ulcers, and even perforation (see section 9.2.2.3). For example, a single dose of orally or parenterally administered diclofenac is able to induce

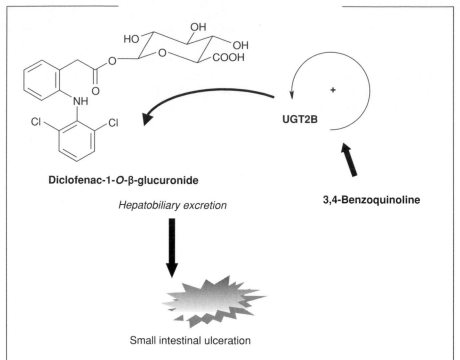

Diclofenac-1-*O*-β-glucuronide

Hepatobiliary excretion

3,4-Benzoquinoline

Small intestinal ulceration

Figure 4.9. Induction of hepatic diclofenac–UGT is associated with increased formation of the reactive acyl glucuronide, increased biliary excretion, and increased rates of small intestinal ulcers caused by diclofenac or its glucuronide.

small intestinal injury in rat models. Induction of UGT by 3,4-benzoquinoline was associated with an increased severity (>five-fold increase in total ulcer length) of intestinal ulcer formation as compared to that in non-induced rats given the same dose of diclofenac (whether this effect reflects the consequence of a direct toxicity of the reactive acyl glucuronide, or whether it is simply due to an increased rate of enterohepatic cycling and thus increased overall exposure to the drug, is not known but is irrelevant in this context) (see Figure 4.9).

4.2.2.2. Reactive acyl glucuronides and their positional isomers

One important group of xenobiotics that are biotransformed into reactive glucuronides is carboxylic acids. Many carboxylic acid-containing drugs, including nonsteroidal anti-inflammatory drugs (NSAIDs) or lipid lowering agents of the clofibrate type, form acyl glucuronides. This conjugation is catalyzed primarily by UGT2B7 (in humans) and by UGT2B1 in rats. These isoforms are most abundant in the liver.

Acyl glucuronides (ester glucuronides), in contrast to ether glucuronides (formed from, for example, phenols), are less stable and are prone to undergo hydrolysis, intramolecular rearrangements, and covalent interaction with cellular target molecules (proteins, nucleic acid) by covalent binding (see section 9.2.2.3).

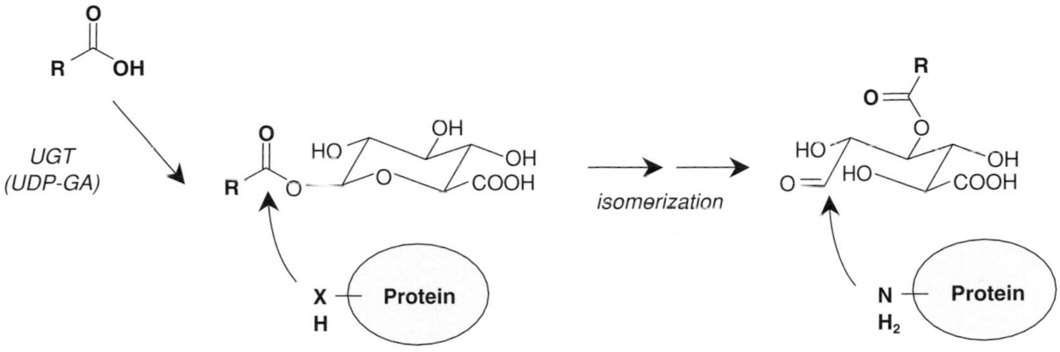

Figure 4.10. Acyl glucuronides are reactive metabolites (reactive site indicated by arrow). 1-O-β-Acyl glucuronides (left) can react with residues (X = NH, S, or O) on proteins. Alternatively, the aglycone can migrate from the 1-OH position of the sugar ring (here to the 3-OH position, right), followed by ring opening to expose another reactive carbon (arrow).

Interestingly, it is not only the primary glucuronide (1-O-β-glucuronide) that is protein-reactive. After formation of the conjugate, the xenobiotic moiety (the aglycone) can migrate along the sugar ring to the 2-hydroxy, 3-hydroxy, or 4-hydroxy position. Following this internal migration (rearrangement), by which positional isomers are formed, the sugar ring can transiently open and exist in the open chain form (unlike the ring in the original 1-O-position). This exposes another reactive site of the molecule, the aldehyde carbon. These positional isomers are also important because they are equally reactive, and their occurrence and significance have been demonstrated *in vivo* (see Figure 4.10).

4.2.2.3. N-Glucuronidation of aromatic amines

N-Glucuronidation of aromatic amines facilitates their renal excretion, because the conjugates are more water-soluble. However, this conjugation reaction results in the generation of reactive intermediates that play an established role in cancer formation. This mechanism was first recognized for 2-naphthylamine and related compounds.

2-Naphthylamine is an aromatic compound which is formed as an intermediate in the manufacturing process of aniline. Aniline itself is an important industrial chemical and was widely used in the dye industry. It was observed already in the nineteenth century that workers in dye factories exhibited a highly increased incidence of bladder cancer (this form of cancer was called 'aniline cancer') as compared to non-exposed workers. First, aniline was considered to be the culprit; however, decades later it was found experimentally that it was not aniline but 2-naphthylamine which was responsible for the carcinogenic activity.

Meanwhile, 2-naphthylamine and other aromatic amines are recognized human carcinogens acting through a similar mechanism that involves glucuronoconjugation.

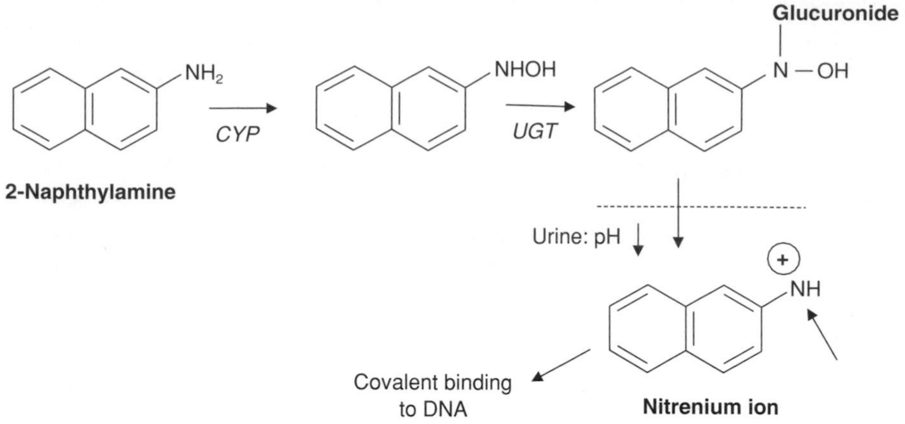

Figure 4.11. *N*-Glucuronidation of the *N*-hydroxy metabolite of 2-naphthylamine is the critical step in bioactivating the aromatic amine to a DNA-reactive (arrow) and carcinogenic intermediate.

Mechanisms of 2-naphthylamine bioactivation and carcinogenicity: The first and crucial metabolic step in the activation of aromatic amines is *N*-hydroxylation. There is clear evidence that aromatic amines that are readily *N*-hydroxylated (e.g. benzidine, 4-aminobiphenyl, and 2-naphthylamine) are also able to induce bladder cancer in humans (and dogs, which are a good animal model, in contrast to rodents, which are a poor animal model for this type of mechanism). Structural analogs that are not readily *N*-hydroxylated (e.g. 2-aminobiphenyl or 1-naphthylamine) do not cause bladder cancer. This first metabolic step is CYP-mediated and occurs in the liver.

Subsequently, UGT in the liver catalyzes the conversion of these *N*-hydroxylated aromatic amines to the corresponding *N*-glucuronide. These glucuronides are stable at physiological pH. They are excreted into the blood, transported to the kidneys, and excreted into the urine. As urine is slightly acidic, and as the *N*-glucuronides are acid-labile, they are hydrolyzed in the urine and degraded to the highly reactive nitrenium ion. Nitrenium ions are electrophilic species and DNA-reactive (see section 9.3.).

The reason why 2-naphthylamine does not induce bladder cancer in rodents is that rodents readily metabolize the *N*-hydroxylated compound via another competing pathway, *N*-acetylation (see section 4.2.3.). Dogs, in contrast, lack hepatic *N*-acetyltransferase activity (see Figure 4.11).

4.2.3. *Sulfotransferase (SULT)*

Sulfate conjugation has traditionally been considered a detoxication reaction, resulting in a more rapid elimination of a sulfated substrate. However, it has become clear that in many cases sulfation is a bioactivation step leading to the formation of reactive metabolites.

Xenobiotic-metabolizing sulfotransferases (SULT, or ST) belong to a super-family of cytosolic enzymes, featuring many isoforms with differential tissue distribution and substrate specificities. Polymorphisms and allelic variants in humans are known, as for other xenobiotic-metabolizing enzmyes.

One important feature that differentiates ST from other enzyme systems is the possibility of conjugation–deconjugation cycles. Once formed, the sulfuric acid esters can be readily hydrolyzed, followed by re-sulfation and continued cycling. This may increase the overall exposure to the potentially toxic intermediates.

Again, the formation of a reactive sulfoconjugate intermediate can be explained by the electron-withdrawing potential of the sulfate group, which, after heterolytical cleavage, can produce a strongly electrophilic cationic carbon center (see section 9.1). For example, safrol (a constituent of natural spices) is carcinogenic at high doses in rodents through this mechanism.

A clinically important example of a reactive sulfate intermediate, which also poses interesting considerations with regard to interspecies extrapolation, is tamoxifen.

Tamoxifen is an anti-estrogenic drug widely used in the treatment of breast cancer. The drug is also given prophylactically as a chemopreventive drug in healthy women at high risk of developing the disease. A first alert, however, is the fact that tamoxifen has turned out to be a liver carcinogen in rats. Importantly, it is a genotoxic carcinogen, i.e. it dose-dependently damages DNA by forming adducts (see section 9.3) both *in vitro* and *in vivo*. Tamoxifen also produces DNA adducts in mice, but at lower concentrations, and the drug is not hepatocarcinogenic in mice. This poses the pivotal question about the relative risk of such liver tumors developing in women.

Although there is a slightly increased risk of developing endometrial cancer after tamoxifen, there has been no indication that tamoxifen is hepatocarcinogenic in humans. What is the rationale for using the drug safely, and on what basis can this assumption be made? Again, elucidation of the molecular mechanisms that underlie the bioactivation of tamoxifen, and interspecies comparisons of these mechanisms, have yielded a plausible yet simple mechanistic explanation.

Mechanisms of tamoxifen bioactivation and carcinogenicity: Again, reactive metabolites are involved in the genotoxic activity of tamoxifen. Tamoxifen is α-hydroxylated and subsequently O-glucuronidated and eliminated. However, a second but more dangerous metabolic pathway represents the critical step: α-hydroxy-tamoxifen is a substrate for SULT and can readily undergo O-sulfation. Subsequently, the sulfate group of tamoxifen O-sulfate is readily cleaved off, and a carbocation is formed. In fact, the sulfate is a particularly good leaving group because the resulting cation is resonance-stabilized by its allyl group. The

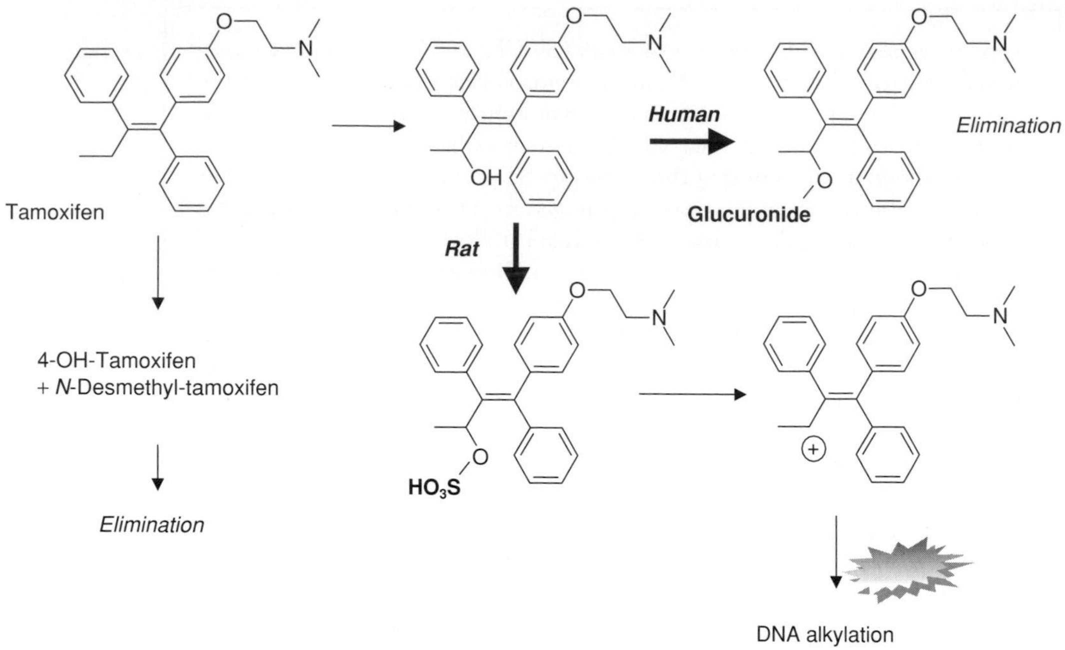

Figure 4.12. Pathways of tamoxifen bioactivation. O-Sulfation of α-hydroxy-tamoxifen leads to the formation of a reactive carbocation which can react with DNA bases and form covalent adducts. In contrast, in humans, O-glucuronidation prevails, leading to an inactive glucuronide.

carbocation is a strongly electrophilic intermediate which reacts with DNA bases and forms covalent adducts to DNA (see Figure 4.12).

The underlying reason for the species differences in tamoxifen metabolism can be found in the species-selective differential rates of activation and bioactivation. In the first place, rats can α-hydroxylate tamoxifen at a three-fold higher rate than humans. Next, and even more importantly, rats have no detectable glucuronosyl-transferase (UGT) activity towards α-hydroxy tamoxifen (which would be a clear detoxication pathway), while at the same time exhibiting a high SULT activity towards α-hydroxy tamoxifen (which is the critical bioactivation step). Fortunately, humans are at the other extreme; in fact, the rank orders for the relative activities (in microsomes) are, for the inactivating UGT, humans > mouse >> rat, and for the critical SULT, rat = mouse >> humans. Thus, the ~100-fold greater UGT activity in humans as compared to rats, in combination with the ~5-fold lower SULT activity towards tamoxifen, allows, on mechanistic grounds, a prediction of low levels of hepatic DNA adducts and, by implication, a low risk of liver tumors in patients. Indeed, no tamoxifen-specific adducts could be found in women treated with tamoxifen.

4.2.4. N-Acetyltransferase (NAT)

Acetylation of substrates is both an important detoxication and an important bio-activating reaction.

N-Acetyltransferase (NAT) is encoded by two genes (NAT1 and NAT2) in humans. NAT is a cytosolic enzyme (but also present in mitochondria and ER) that catalyzes the transfer of the acetyl group from acetyl-CoA to an aromatic amine or the terminal nitrogen of hydrazine. The two NAT forms have 87 percent sequence homology and only partly overlapping substrate selectivity, but also feature a certain degree of isoform-specific substrate selectivity. They are also independently regulated.

Many allelic variants are known. Also, there is well-known genetic polymorphism of both NAT1 and NAT2. Indeed, among individuals, NAT activity can vary more than 100-fold. This has been associated with the 'slow acetylator' and 'rapid acetylator' phenotypes. NAT2 is primarily expressed in liver but also present in the intestinal mucosa, while NAT1 is more ubiquitously expressed. Dogs do not express NAT.

NAT-mediated reactions can be mechanistically important in toxicology for two major reasons; first, the solubility of the acetylated xenobiotic may change dramatically, and second, the large differences in NAT expression in different human populations can modulate the metabolism and, hence, the toxicity of substrates that are subject to being acetylated.

In contrast to most other phase II reactions, acetylation is not associated with increased aqueous solubility of the conjugate. In fact, the N-acetylated substrates are much less water-soluble, as exemplified by sulfonamides. **Sulfonamides** which are N-acetylated by NAT and excreted in the urine (featuring a slightly acidic pH) are less water-soluble (>ten-fold) and often precipitate in the urinary tract. This leads to necrosis of the proximal tubular epithelial cells. To prevent this effect at high dosage, sulfonamides are increasingly used topically, or else given orally with alkalization of the urine to prevent precipitation.

4.2.4.1. Bioactivation of arylamines

N-acetylation can be a bioactivation step that has been related to carcinogenesis. This can be illustrated for aromatic amines (a structure that should always alert a toxicologist).

It has been known for a long time that aromatic amines can cause cancer. The multistep bioactivation pathways of these aromatic amines are, however, manifold, and a number of interdependent enzymes are involved. The tumorigenic potency of a given aromatic amine is dependent on, among other factors, the type of tissue and the species, each featuring specific patterns of enzyme expression.

> **Benzidine** is a compound formerly used for the production of azo dyes and is an example that nicely illustrates the mechanisms involved in the bioactivation process. Although benzidine is no longer produced or used, it is still present as a contaminant in wastewater as a result of bacterial conversion of other compounds. Benzidine is a recognized human carcinogen that has been associated with occupational bladder cancer and tumors in other organs.

Mechanisms of benzidine bioactivation: The first step in the activation of an aromatic amine is *N*-hydroxylation, followed by *N*-acetylation (the opposite sequence of events is also possible). The second step is a possible intramolecular acyl transfer to the acetoxyarylamine. This is a labile intermediate that can readily be degraded to the nitrenium ion. Alternatively, the acetylated *N*-hydroxylamine can be deacetylated back to the hydroxylamine. The latter readily decomposes under slightly acidic conditions, as may be present in urine, to the reactive nitrenium ion. Nitrenium cations are electrophilic species that can covalently bind to DNA (see sections 4.2.2.3 and 9.3 and Figure 4.13).

4.2.4.2. Toxicological consequences of individual NAT expression

N-Acetylation can be both a detoxication and a bioactivation process. Therefore, individual expression of NAT can greatly influence the fate of a xenobiotic. One of the best examples (and one of the first examples of a causative role of an enzyme polymorphism in explaining the individual variation in xenobiotic metabolism) is isoniazid.

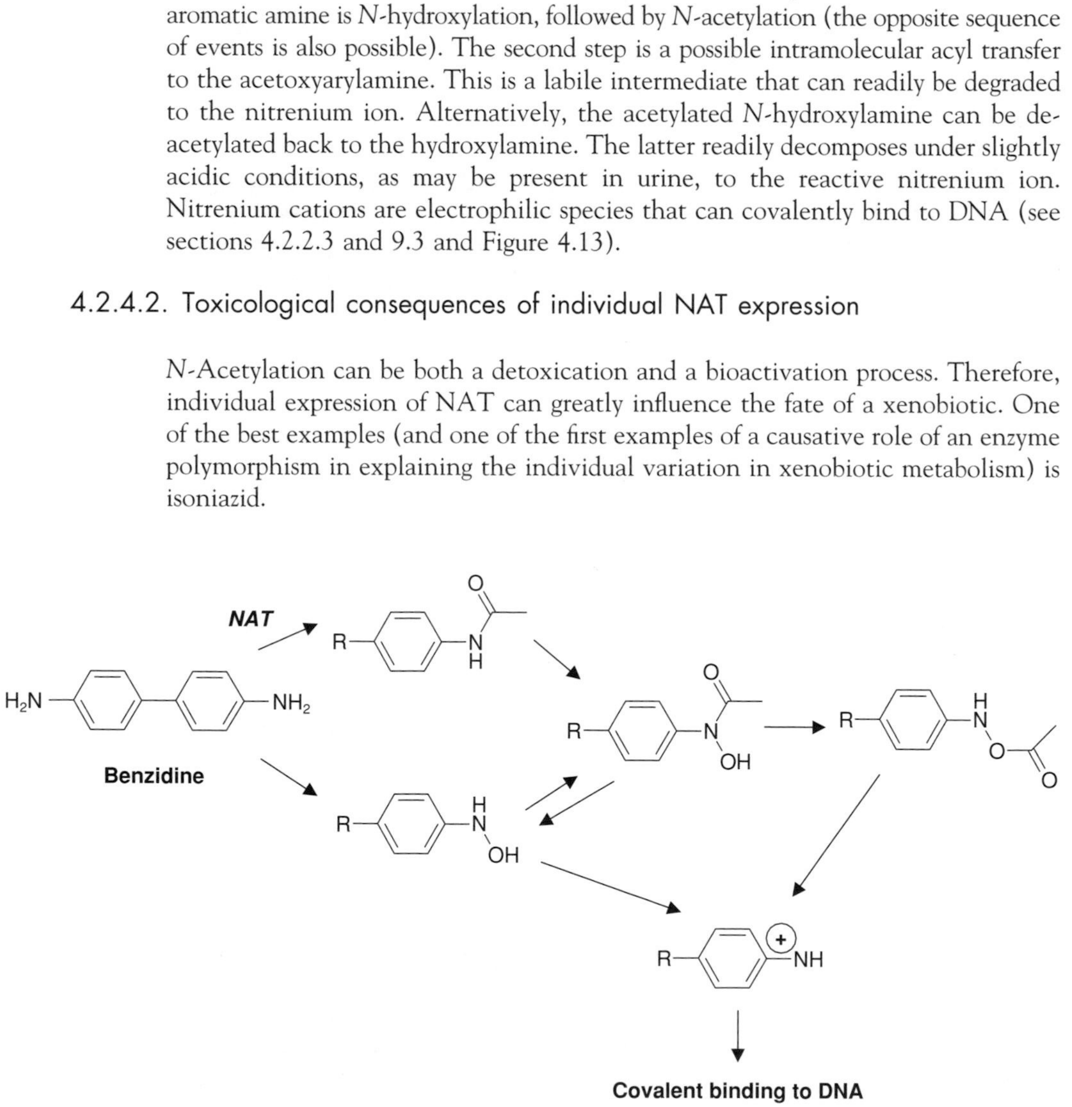

Figure 4.13 *N*-Acetylation of benzidine is a bioactivating step leading to a reactive nitrenium ion.

Isoniazid (INH) is a hydrazine derivative and anti-tuberculosis agent. It is an old drug but still the most widely used therapeutic in the treatment of tuberculosis. One of the rare but serious adverse effects of INH use is hepatotoxicity (significant toxicity in approximately 1–2 percent of recipients). In addition, INH is associated with a low incidence of peripheral neuropathy. These two adverse reactions are based on two distinct mechanisms and can be explained by INH metabolism.

The molecular mechanisms underlying INH-associated liver injury (at the toxicodynamic level) are incompletely known. The toxicity is not dependent on the dose, and its onset can be delayed by many weeks. What is known is that INH is N-acetylated in the liver to acetyl-INH, and that this NAT-mediated step is crucial for the development of liver injury. Acetyl-INH is then hydrolytically cleaved into isonicotinic acid and acetylhydrazine. The acetylhydrazine in turn is metabolically activated by CYP to a reactive electrophilic acylating and alkylating intermediate. Alternatively, a derivative of hydrazine has also been proposed to be involved in the generation of the ultimate reactive species that is responsible for precipitating liver injury.

Interestingly, NAT has recently been identified in the tuberculosis-causing microorganism, *Mycobacterium tuberculosis* itself. The expression of this INH-degrading enzyme is one important factor for the resistance of these bacteria to INH chemotherapy.

The peripheral neuropathy, on the other hand, is characterized by paresthesia (peripheral numbness) and ataxia (poor coordination of movements). This type of adverse reaction clearly is dependent on high plasma levels of INH, as it can occur after overdosage. Neurotoxicity can be explained by an interference of INH with vitamin B6 intermediary metabolism (see Figure 4.14).

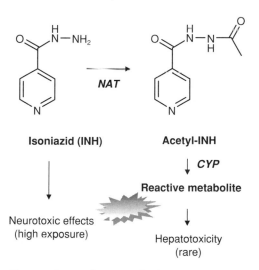

Figure 4.14. The type of adverse reaction associated with isoniazid is determined by the metabolic activation via N-acetylation.

> There are well known ethnic differences in the propensity to develop either hepatic adverse effects or peripheral neuropathies. Because toxicity is dependent on metabolism of INH, it is logical to assume that the risk of developing adverse reactions is coupled with a genetic predisposition for the expression of the xenobiotic-metabolizing enzymes involved. The major candidate gene is the NAT2 gene which underlies a genetic polymorphism.

Mechanisms of individual susceptibility to INH hepatotoxicity and peripheral neuropathy: As the rapid metabolic conversion (acetylation) of INH is associated with the generation of intermediates that can lead to hepatotoxicity, and as poor metabolic degradation of INH leads to sustained exposure, which may cause neuropathies, it is logical to assume that individuals featuring impaired NAT activity may be predisposed to develop neuropathies. Indeed, poor acetylators (featuring an elimination $t_{1/2}$ of INH of >3 h), which are frequently (90 percent) found among certain populations in Morocco, clearly exhibit this correlation. On the other hand, rapid acetylators (with an elimination $t_{1/2}$ of ~1 h) are frequently (95 percent) found among the North American natives and Japanese and Taiwanese populations. These latter also have an increased risk for developing INH-associated liver injury.

4.2.5. Glutathione-S-transferase (GST)

Conjugation to glutathione (GSH) is an extremely important mechanism in handling xenobiotics. In many cases, this conjugation step inactivates a reactive and therefore potentially dangerous metabolite and enables renal excretion of the xenobiotic. In other cases, however, GS-conjugation is a bioactivation step that leads to the formation of reactive intermediates which often exert their effect at sites distant from where they are generated.

> **Glutathione (GSH)** is an endogenous tripeptide (see section 5.3.1) which is abundant in most cells (i.e. present at mM concentrations!). Central to its biological properties is the cysteine residue with the reactive–SH group. Besides being an important antioxidant, reductant, and radical scavenger, GSH is also the co-substrate for glutathione-S-transferase.
> **Glutathione-S-transferase (GST)** is a superfamily of enzymes catalyzing the transfer of GSH to a broad variety of xenobiotics via the cysteine thiol. The enzyme is composed of homo- or heterodimer subunits and exists as four families (alpha, mu, pi, and theta). This classification reflects the composition of the subunits of GST and is based on the primary sequence. The enzyme is most abundant in the liver (≤5 percent of cytosolic protein is GST in human liver!). The greater part of GST is present in the cytosol, but other (structurally unrelated) isoforms have been found in the endoplasmic reticulum membrane and the inner mitochondrial membrane.

There are well-known polymorphisms for human GST. For example, approximately 45 percent of Caucasians do not have a functional gene for GST-M1. The lack of this gene is associated with an increased risk of bladder and lung cancer, indicating that GST exerts important protective functions.

Like other phase I or phase II enzymes, GST can also be induced by a number of xenobiotics. Often, it is a compound that produces a reactive metabolite and which is then detoxified by GST that can induce the enzyme.

4.2.5.1. Glutathione conjugation as a protective mechanism

GST is pivotal for detoxifying electrophilic metabolites. One toxicologically relevant example is the detoxication of aflatoxin.

Aflatoxins are naturally occurring products of the molds *Aspergillus flavus* and *Aspergillus parasiticus* which are abundant in the environment. Under warm and humid conditions, these molds may produce the toxins. Aflatoxins are difurocoumarins with a characteristic heterocyclic structure composed of five rings. The main aflatoxin is aflatoxin B_1, which is the most potent chemical carcinogen known so far. Aflatoxin B_1 has been causally associated with the occurrence of liver cancer in populations of China and Africa. High doses of aflatoxins can also be acutely toxic; a widely cited example is aflatoxin-related acute poisoning of poultry in England in 1960, where feeding of A. *flavus*-contaminated peanuts caused the death of approximately 100,000 turkeys.

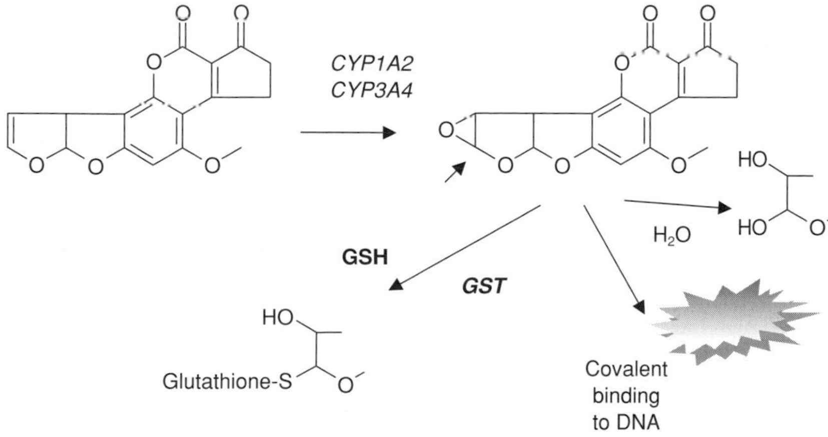

Figure 4.15. Metabolic activation of aflatoxin B_1 to the 8,9-epoxide produces a highly electrophilic species, which either is hydrolytically inactivated or else can react (arrow) with DNA bases and result in covalent binding. GST-mediated conjugation with GSH is therefore an important way of detoxication.

The mechanism behind the acutely toxic and carcinogenic potential is based on the bioactivation of aflatoxin. In the liver, aflatoxin B_1 is metabolized by CYP to the ultimate carcinogen intermediate, the 8,9-*exo*-epoxide. This metabolite is highly reactive and can covalently bind to proteins but, importantly, also to DNA, preferably to G:C-rich regions, forming adducts at the N^7-position of guanine (see section 9.3). If this happens to occur in the gene coding for p53 (a tumor suppressor gene), as is often the case, then this can result in a false base pairing upon DNA replication, a mutation, and, eventually, in cancer (see section 9.3 and Figure 4.15).

Mechanisms of aflatoxin inactivation by GST: GST can catalyze the rapid inactivation of aflatoxin B_1-8,9-epoxide by glutathione-S-conjugation (Figure 4.15). The thiol group of GSH thereby attacks the aflatoxin epoxide at the electrophilic carbon of the terminal furane ring.

Interestingly, mice (in contrast to rats) are largely resistant to aflatoxins and do not produce liver cancer even after high aflatoxin exposure. The most plausible reason for this species difference is the fact that mice have an approximately 100-fold higher activity of GST-A than rats, which results in an extremely efficient detoxication of the reactive intermediate. Unfortunately, humans exhibit, similarly to rats, a relatively low expression of GST-A, which makes humans highly susceptible to the toxic and carcinogenic effects of aflatoxin.

4.2.5.2. Bioactivation of xenobiotics by GST

Although generally GS-conjugation is considered a detoxication reaction, there are also examples where GST mediates a bioactivation pathway. Among these, there are several possibilities. For example, the GS-conjugate may be reactive by itself, as it occurs after conjugation of halo*alkanes*. If the newly formed conjugate is extremely reactive, it may directly target and damage the enzyme where it is generated. Alternatively, the GS-conjugate has to be activated by another enzyme system, the cysteine-conjugate β-lyase, as it is the case after conjugation of halo*alkenes*. For both cases, an example is given below.

Ethylene dibromide (dibromoethane) is a widely used industrial chemical involved in the synthesis of dyes and pharmaceuticals. It is also present in leaded gasoline, and has been used as a fumigant pesticide to protect foods. Ethylene dibromide is acutely toxic when inhaled, but after chronic use is also a carcinogen in experimental animals, and possibly in humans.

Besides the major CYP-mediated biotransformation pathway, ethylene dibromide is GS-conjugated through GST-A (abundant) and GST-T (high affinity).

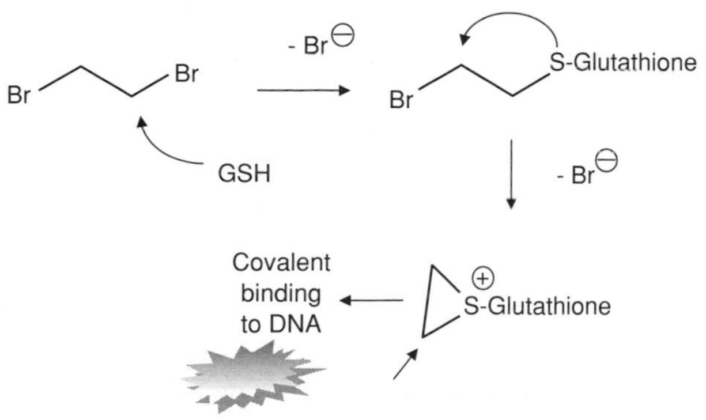

Figure 4.16. GS-conjugation of ethylene dibromide is a bioactivation step that results in the formation of a DNA-reactive episulfonium ion.

Mechanisms of ethylene dibromide-*S*-conjugate toxicity: The thiol group of GSH sequentially attacks the first and then the second carbon of ethylene dibromide, with the two bromide ions being released. The result is a ring-shaped episulfonium ion, which is a highly electrophilic species and can interact and covalently bind to DNA. In particular, N^7 of guanine is attacked, which can lead to mutations and, ultimately, tumor formation (see Figure 4.16).

When stable xenobiotic–GS-conjugates are formed hepatically, then one consequence of this reaction is their efficient export from the liver. Because specialized transport systems for GS-conjugates are present in hepatocytes (e.g. the canalicular conjugate export pump Mrp2, see section 3.3), the liver is not exposed to high concentrations of the conjugate and is therefore not necessarily a target organ of toxicity. However, because the conjugates are excreted via bile, reabsorbed in the gut, and finally transported to the kidneys, where the GS-conjugates are degraded and excreted, they may reach relatively high concentrations in these excretory organs. Importantly, because in many cases the GS-conjugated xenobiotics still retain the potential reactivity of the parent compound, or their reactivity even exceeds that of the non-conjugated compound, the kidney can become a frequent target organ of toxicity. An example of this transport of a reactive metabolite to the kidney, where the conjugate is accumulated and where it exerts its toxicity, is polyphenols, including hydroquinones.

Benzohydroquinone is an intermediate used in the chemical industry and a metabolite of benzene, and it also occurs naturally in cigarette smoke. Benzohydroquinone is nephrotoxic and also induces renal tubular adenomas. Current evidence suggests that the compound may induce tumors by a mechanism involving cytotoxicity, followed by sustained regenerative hyperplasia and ultimately tumor formation. Indeed, cell proliferation in the tubular epithelia is highly increased after benzohydroquinone.

> Benzohydroquinone is predominantly conjugated and excreted via glucuronidation and/or sulfation, which occurs in the liver. However, a small portion escapes conjugation and is oxidized to the benzoquinone. This benzoquinone can then be conjugated to glutathione. It is the GS-conjugate (and some of its secondary metabolites) that has been implicated as the ultimate toxicant in the kidney.

Mechanisms of benzohydroquinone–glutathione-S-conjugate nephrotoxicity: Following oxidation of the benzohydroquinone to the benzoquinone, this latter is conjugated to GSH. This can occur as a multistep process, leading from the mono-substituted conjugate to the di-, tri- and even tetra-GS conjugate. Generally, GS conjugation has been considered a cytoprotective step because GSH functions as a 'sacrificial' nucleophile sparing other, more critical cellular thiol groups from irreversible damage. However, the multisubstituted GS-conjugates exhibit differential toxicity; while the mono- and the tetra-GS-conjugates are essentially nontoxic, the di-GS-conjugate isomers show intermediate toxicity, and the 2,3,5-(triglutathionyl-S-yl) hydroquinone exhibits the highest toxicity in the kidney.

These multi-GSH substituted conjugates are actively transported from liver into bile. After reabsorption from the gut, the GS-conjugates reach the kidney, where they come into contact with the luminal side of the tubular epithelial cells. This pole of the cell is rich in two peptidases which sequentially cleave two amino acids off the GS moiety; first, γ-glutamyl transpeptidase (γGT), which cleaves off the glutamate residue, and then dipeptidase (DPP), which catalyzes the removal of glycine. As a result, the cysteine conjugate is left behind. This cysteine conjugate is readily taken up by the amino acid transporter into the proximal tubular epithelia. Inside the cell, the cysteine conjugate is oxidized to the substituted benzoquinone.

Quinones, including benzoquinone, are reactive species because they are electrophiles which can covalently bind to nucleophilic sites of target compounds, but also because they can undergo redox cycling during the reduction/oxidation cycle from the semiquinone to the quinone (see section 5.1.1). The (multi)-cysteine-S-conjugates of benzoquinone retain this molecular characteristic of the parent compound.

Thus, the key mechanism underlying the nephrotoxicity of benzohydroquinone and other polyphenols is the transport and delivery to the kidney as a result of GS-conjugation. Once in the kidney, the GS-conjugates are metabolically degraded and accumulate in the tubular cells (see Figure 4.17).

In some cases, renal metabolism can even further metabolize and bioactivate certain cysteine-S-conjugates, derived from GST-mediated conjugation of xenobiotics to glutathione. Typical examples of xenobiotics that exert a kidney-selective toxicity are haloalkenes such as hexachlorobutadiene.

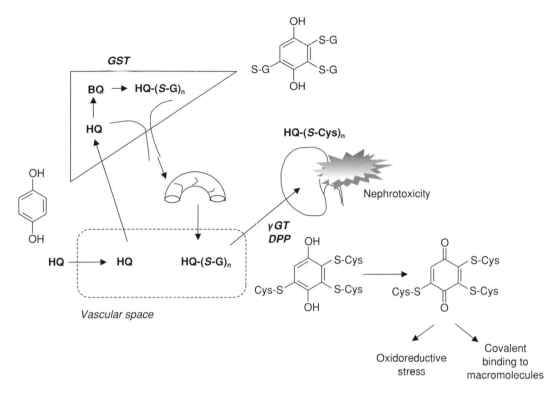

Figure 4.17. Multiple glutathione-S-conjugation of benzohydroquinone (HQ) in the liver leads to mono-, di-, tri-, or tetra-glutathionyl-benzoquinone (here, the 2,3,5,-tri-glutathionyl-HQ is shown). After active export from the liver into bile, the conjugate reaches the kidney, where the glutathionyl moieties are sequentially cleaved by γ-glutamyl transpeptidase (γGT) and dipeptidase (DPP). The cysteine conjugates are taken up in the kidney, where they cause injury to the proximal tubular epithelium due to covalent binding and redox stress.

Hexachlorobutadiene is an undesired but unavoidable industrial by-product that arises during the manufacturing of chlorinated hydrocarbons. The compound is also released into the environment and accumulates in freshwater and marine organisms, and it is a persistent pollutant.

Hexachlorobutadiene is minimally hepatotoxic, but it is a classical and dose-dependent nephrotoxicant in mice and rats, damaging the S_2-segment of the proximal tubule. Why is the kidney the target organ of toxicity, although the compound is metabolized in the liver?

The clue to anwering this question can again be found in glutathione-S-conjugation, followed by excretion, and transport to the lumen of the proximal tubular epithelia. At the apical membrane of the tubular cells, the pentachlorobutadiene–S-glutathione conjugate is degraded enzymatically to pentachlorobutadiene-S-cysteine. This latter compound is taken up into the

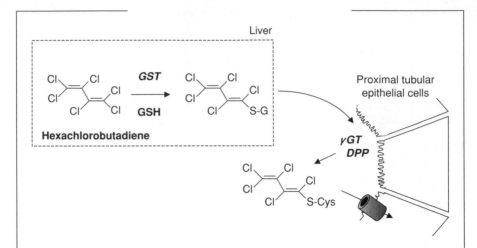

Figure 4.18. Glutathione-*S*-conjugation of hexachlorobutadiene leads to its elimination from the liver and delivery to the renal proximal tubular epithelia.

cells through the amino acid transporter system. In the cell, the cysteine conjugate can either be *N*-acetylated and excreted (detoxication step), or else bioactivated by β-lyase (see Figure 4.18).

Mechanisms of β-lyase-mediated hexachlorobutadiene nephrotoxicity: The cysteine-*S*-conjugate of pentachlorobutadiene (derived from its glutathione-*S*-conjugate) is a substrate for the enzyme β-lyase. The cleavage of the thioether bond results in the generation of a nephrotoxic metabolite which can cause covalent binding to macromolecules and toxicity. Again, organ selectivity is determined by the interorgan transport of the glutathione-conjugate and the rapid accumulation and bioactivation in the proximal tubular epithelia of the kidney (see Figure 4.19).

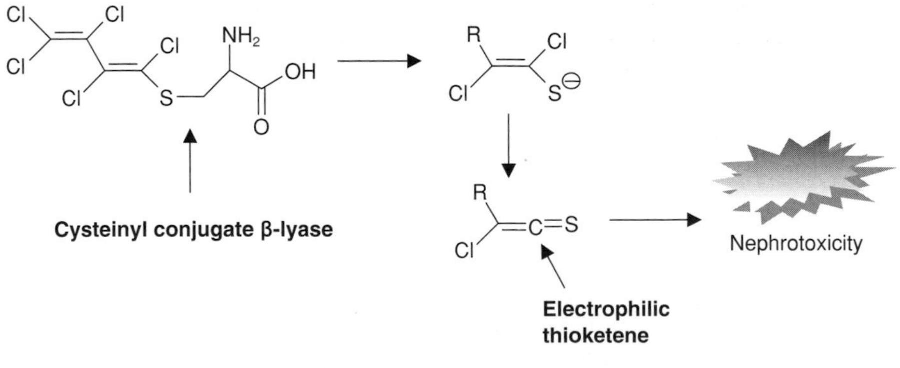

Cysteinyl conjugate β-lyase

Electrophilic thioketene

Nephrotoxicity

Figure 4.19. Cysteinyl conjugate β-lyase cleaves the sulfur–beta carbon bond, resulting in a reactive thioketene, which can form covalent binding with proteins.

Cysteine-S-conjugate-β-lyase is a mitochondrial, microsomal and cytosolic enzyme that catalyzes the metabolism of a wide variety of cysteine-S-conjugates. The name is derived from the fact that the enzyme cleaves carbon (C_3)-sulfur bonds of S-substituted cysteines ($R–S–CH_2–CH–(NH_2)–COOH$), leading to beta-elimination. Cleavage yields pyruvate, ammonia, and R-SH or a reactive intermediate.

The S_1, S_2, and S_3 segments of proximal tubuli all abundantly express β-lyase (but damage most often occurs at the S_3 segment, i.e. the pars recta of the proximal tubule). This site-specific expression of the enzyme can explain why the kidney is often a target of toxicity when β-lyase-mediated bioactivation of GS-conjugates is involved. Although human kidney exhibits only about 10 percent of the β-lyase activity of rat kidney, there is enough enzyme present, suggesting that humans are susceptible to long-term damage resulting from exposure to reactive cysteine conjugates.

4.3. Mechanisms of phototoxicity

Activation of xenobiotics to reactive metabolites can occur not only enzymatically but also by light energy. Phototoxicity (not to be confounded with photoallergy, which is an immune-mediated process) is a toxic effect that is triggered by photochemical activation of xenobiotics by UV and (less commonly) visible light. Such activated xenobiotics can exert their adverse effects at the site where they are generated, i.e. in the skin.

Photoactivation can occur by two distinct mechanisms.

1 UV absorption by a xenobiotic can lift the compound to a higher energy state. This high-energy intermediate can in turn activate molecular oxygen and convert it to a reactive oxygen species, e.g. singlet oxygen (see section 5.1). The resulting skin damage by reactive oxygen species derived from these reactions is mediated by keratinocytes and infiltrating leukocytes.
2 The second mechanism does not involve oxygen activation. Instead, UV can activate a xenobiotic which in turn undergoes a photochemical reaction with a target macromolecule. For example, it can interact and covalently bind to DNA bases and disturb DNA replication or repair (see Figure 4.20).

An example of a class of drugs where oxygen activation is involved in the phototoxicity is the fluoroquinolone antibiotics.

Fluoroquinolones, including ciprofloxacine, lomefloxacin, and moxifloxacin, are widely used antibacterial agents (they act by inhibiting gyrase, an enzyme involved in bacterial DNA replication). One adverse effect of these fluoroquinolones is phototoxicity. After exposure to sunlight, patients may present with a severe 'sunburn'.

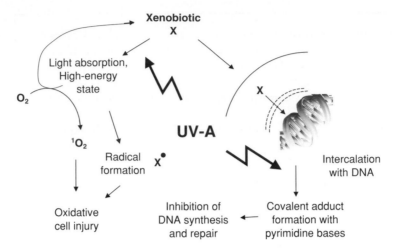

Figure 4.20. Oxygen-dependent and oxygen-independent phototoxic reactions.

Furthermore, *in vivo* experiments have revealed that UV radiation of cells in the presence of some of these fluoroquinolones causes oxidative DNA damage, as measured by the formation of 8-oxo-deoxyguanosine (see section 5.2.1). This DNA damage can cause mutations, and indeed some of these compounds have been found to be photomutagenic *in vitro* and photocarcinogenic in some murine models. How do fluoroquinolones turn into such reactive molecular species?

Mechanisms of fluoroquinolone phototoxicity: Several mechanisms are involved in oxidative DNA damage caused by fluoroquinolones. It is known that these compounds absorb UV energy and are promoted to an excited state. The activated molecules can become reactive through three different pathways (see Figure 4.21).

1 The activated fluoroquinolone can abstract an electron from the DNA base, deoxyguanosine (dG) to produce a radical cation. This species can react with water and form oxidized (8-oxo-) dG.
2 The activated fluoroquinolone can react with molecular oxygen to form singlet oxygen (see section 5.1), which is a reactive oxygen species and which can directly form 8-oxo-dG and induce strand breaks.
3 The activated fluoroquinolone can be homolytically degraded, forming a radical which can react with water to form hydroxyl radicals, an extremely reactive ROS that damages DNA.

Another toxicologically relevant group of notorious phototoxic compounds is the furanocoumarins (see section 4.2.1.2). These compounds exert their phototoxic effects by oxygen-independent DNA damage.

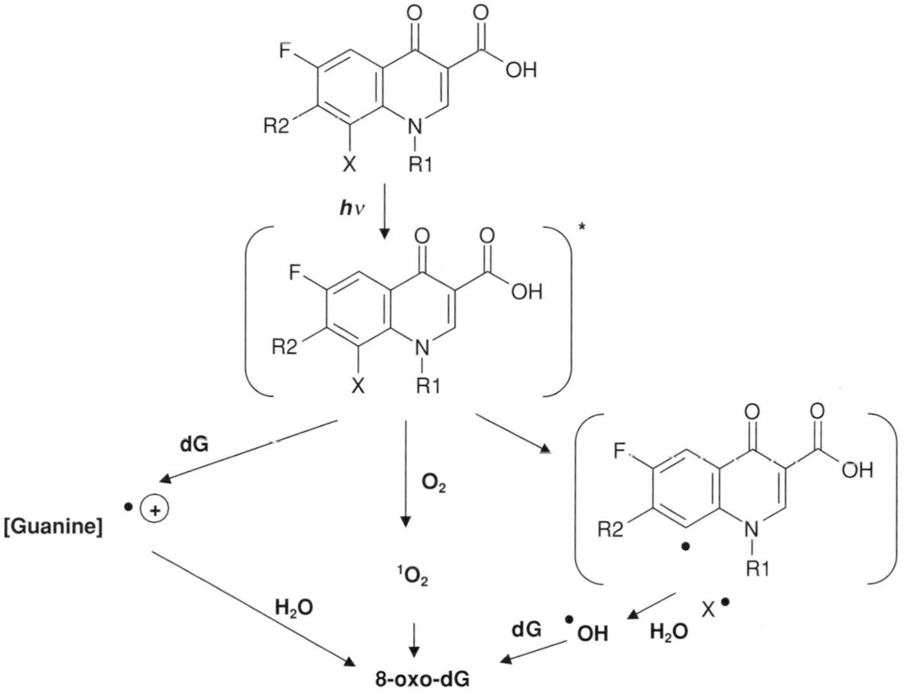

Figure 4.21. Mechanisms of phototoxicity of fluoroquinolones involving oxidative DNA damage.

Furanocoumarins (psoralens) are naturally occurring compounds found in a number of plants (e.g. umbelliferous plants, rutaceae). They have found use therapeutically for the treatment of cutaneous disorders and autoimmune disease. Their toxic potential, but also their therapeutic potential, resides in their ability to undergo photochemical activation.

Because phototoxic reactions are of a non-immunologic nature, they can occur in anybody given sufficient exposure to both the furanocoumarins and UV. Phototoxicity is characterized by erythema, edema, followed by hyperpigmentation. Typical reactions have been found with the furanocoumarins, 5-methoxypsoralen from the bergamot orange (*Citrus bergamia*) and 8-methoxypsoralen (xanthotoxin) from *Fagara* species.

Mechanisms of psoralen phototoxicity: Psoralens can intercalate into DNA. Because they absorb light with a maximum peak at 300 nm, they are activated by UV light and excited to a triplet state which renders them DNA-reactive. Specifically, the activated psoralens form covalent monoadducts to pyrimidine bases and can thus photoalkylate cytosine or thymidine in double-stranded DNA. The reaction

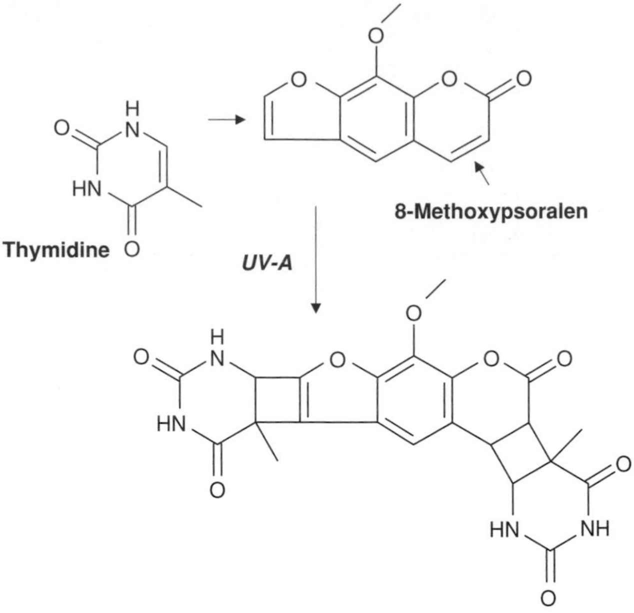

Figure 4.22. Cross-linking of DNA double strand by 8-methoxypsoralen.

takes place between the 3,4- (coumarin) or 4′,5′-(furane) double bonds of the psoralen and 5,6-double bond in thymidine. If the first reaction involves the furane double bond, then the reaction can continue to form bifunctional cross-links between pyrimidine bases. Possible consequences are mutations, inhibition of DNA replication and cell proliferation, and cell death (see Figure 4.22).

How can such phototoxic compounds become activated by UV? They are not always applied onto the skin, where they are exposed to light, but often administered orally.

The skin is composed of the epidermis, followed by the dermis (cutis), and the underlying subcutis. Blood vessels are not present in the epidermis but are found in the dermis. Hence, light that will activate a compound circulating in the bloodstream must be able to reach the dermis. While UV-B only reaches the corneal layer of the epidermis, UV-A can indeed penetrate into the dermis and thus activate compounds by photochemical reactions. In general, with increasing wavelength the light can penetrate more deeply into the skin layers. Therefore, xenobiotica can exert phototoxic effects not only when topically applied to the skin but also when ingested orally or after accumulation in the skin (see Figure 4.23).

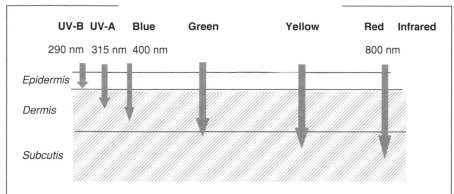

Figure 4.23. Increasing wavelength is associated with deeper penetration of light into the layers of the skin.

4.4. Protective mechanisms against reactive metabolites: the stress response

A complex array of cytoprotective mechanisms against the potentially deleterious actions of reactive metabolites has evolved. This is called the 'stress response' (stress being defined not only as reactive metabolites, but also including oxidative stress, radiation, increased temperature, etc.). Cells react by selective *de novo* synthesis of specific stress proteins. Importantly, these stress proteins are also expressed under physiological conditions, albeit at low level. They basically perform housekeeping functions, i.e. they fulfill essential roles in cell homeostasis. Under conditions of increased stress (e.g. by the production of reactive metabolites as discussed above), these stress proteins are up-regulated. Their central function under these conditions is now to help in cell survival.

4.4.1. Induction of heat shock proteins

The wide array of stress proteins are found not only in eukaryotes but also in prokaryotes, and they exhibit a remarkable homology. That their structure has been so highly conserved during evolution may be a sign that the function of these stress proteins is essential. Proteins that are up-regulated during the stress response include the glucose-regulated proteins (they are expressed if cells are deprived of glucose), immunophilins (involved in peptide rotation) and also binding proteins, metallothioneins (see sections 5.3.3 and 11.2), and acute phase proteins (produced in the liver). A very important group of stress proteins is the heat shock proteins.

Heat shock proteins (hsp), also called molecular chaperones, govern the folding, assembly, and transport of nascent polypeptides. They are classified according to their molecular mass. For example, hsp100 is a group of proteins whose molecular mass is approximately 100 kD. They are involved in heat tolerance and are induced for example by ethanol. The hsp90 proteins are associated with kinases or transcription factors and serve in proper protein folding. The hsp70 are a group of polypeptides that interact with other proteins. They bind to the unfolded proteins and present them to hsp60 for final folding. Importantly, this hsp group is also involved in facilitating proteolysis, in particular of abnormally folded proteins. Next, the hsp60 group (also called chaperonins) facilitate protein folding and are also involved in proteolysis of abnormally folded proteins. Finally, the hsp27/28 are involved in thermotolerance.

Besides this major function, heat shock proteins have more recently been recognized to play an important role in stress-induced immune responses. For example, hsp60 is immunogenic and can elicit protective cytotoxic T cell-mediated immunity even in the absence of helper T cells.

Because reactive metabolites often attack and inactivate proteins, such drug-altered proteins may be equivalent to proteins which are misfolded as a consequence of denaturing, oxidative stress, and other insults. Therefore, it is not surprising that many reactive metabolites induce the transcription of heat shock proteins. For example, mice treated with a single dose of cocaine respond with *de novo* synthesis of hsp70 and hsp25 in the liver (while the expression of other hsp remains unchanged). Because cocaine exerts cellular toxicity by several distinct pathways (see section 5.1.5) including the production of reactive oxygen species and oxidative stress, one might argue that the hsp response is an unspecific response, perhaps as a consequence of general cell injury. However, when mice were treated with antioxidants, cocaine toxicity could be totally prevented, while hsp79 was still induced. It can be inferred from this observation that it is the initial bioactivation and covalent binding of a cocaine metabolite, rather than a lethally damaged cell at a later stage, that triggers the induction of heat shock proteins.

4.4.2. Targeting of stress response proteins by reactive metabolites

Because reactive metabolites can attack many different cellular proteins, it has been speculated that such metabolites also might target and perhaps inactivate some of the protein components of the cytoprotective machinery. This intriguing possibility would have potentially fatal consequences, as an important rescue mission of the cell would be inactivated.

Indeed, one of the proteins that is covalently modified by cocaine administration to mice is hsp60 itself. Similarly, reactive metabolites of the anesthetic halothane (see section 10.2) or of the experimental nephrotoxin, tetrafluoroethyl–S-cysteine conjugate, both form covalent adducts to mitochondrial proteins that have been clearly identified as hsp60 and hsp70.

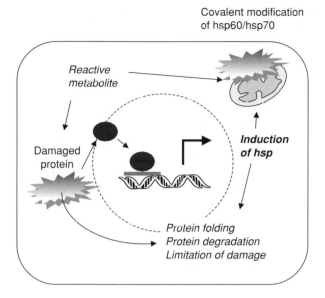

Figure 4.24. Stress proteins including heat shock proteins not only are induced by reactive metabolites but also are a target of covalent modification.

The underlying mechanism that would explain why the heat shock proteins are selective targets of these electrophilic metabolites is not entirely clear. Reasons may include the biochemical fact that hsps have a relatively high lysine content (approximately 10 percent of amino acid residues), to which the reactive metabolites preferentially bind. Alternatively, they could be targeted due to their function as recognizing damaged polypeptides. Finally, they could be targeted because many reactive metabolites arise in mitochondria (and >80 percent of hepatocellular hsp60 is located in mitochondria) (see Figure 4.24).

Collectively, an important means by which reactive metabolites damage cells is that they not only directly inactivate critical macromolecules but also can target and inactivate the cytoprotective machinery including heat shock proteins and other components of the stress response.

Learning points

- Many xenobiotics are bioactivated to reactive metabolites that can interact with cellular targets and are ultimately responsible for the toxicity. Such reactive intermediates can be generated not only by CYPs and other phase I enzymes, but also through conjugation reactions.
- Ultra-reactive metabolites can react right at the site where they are generated (inactivating the enzyme itself). More stable intermediates may diffuse away and react with more remote targets.
- Genetic polymorphisms and other variations in some of the drug-metabolizing enzymes may account for the differential susceptibility to potentially toxic xenobiotics in individuals and human populations.

- The expression of most CYP isoforms is tightly regulated and can be induced by xenobiotics. CAR, SXR and other transcription factors are involved in up-regulating gene expression. Induction of CYP can have profound consequences on the toxicity of xenobiotics (potentiation of toxicity by over-producing reactive metabolites; metabolic inactivation of a toxic compound).

- Acyl glucuronides (from carboxylic acids) and their positional isomers, or N-glucuronides (from aromatic amines), are important reactive glucuronide conjugates.

- Glutathione conjugation can effectively remove reactive intermediates (e.g. epoxides). Conversely, xenobiotic glutathionyl-S-conjugates can be further bio-activated in the kidney, the site of their excretion, and produce nephrotoxic effects.

- N-acetylation of hydroxylamines has been implicated as a bioactivating mechanism in carcinogenesis.

- UV light can activate xenobiotics in the skin and cause phototoxic effects by both oxygen-dependent and oxygen-independent mechanisms.

- An important protective mechanism against the toxicity of reactive metabolites is the stress response. Reactive metabolites can, however, inactivate components of the stress response (e.g. heat shock proteins) and thus enhance toxicity.

Further reading

Cytochrome P450

Aoki, K., Takimoto, M., Ota, H. and Yoshida, T. (2000) Participation of CYP2A in cocaine-induced hepatotoxicity in female mice, *Pharmacol. Toxicol.* 87: 26–32.

Boelsterli, U.A., Lanzotti, A., Göldlin, C. and Oertle, M. (1992) Identification of cytochrome P-450IIB1 as a cocaine-bioactivating isoform in rat hepatic microsomes and in cultured rat hepatocytes, *Drug Metab. Disp.* 20: 96–101.

Bornheim, L. (1998) Effect of cytochrome P450 inducers on cocaine-mediated hepatotoxicity, *Toxicol. Appl. Pharmacol.* 150: 158–165.

Guengerich, F.P. (2001) Common and uncommon cytochrome P450 reactions related to metabolism and chemical toxicity, *Chem. Res. Toxicol.* 14: 611–650.

Ingelman-Sundberg, M. (2001) Implications of polymorphic cytochrome P450-dependent drug metabolism for drug development, *Drug Metab. Dispos.* 29: 570–573.

Meyer, U.A. and Zanger, U.M. (1997) Molecular mechanisms of genetic polymorphisms of drug metabolism, *Annu. Rev. Pharmacol. Toxicol.* 37: 269–296.

Roberts, S.M., Pounds, J.G. and James, R.C. (1990) Cocaine toxicity in cultured rat hepatocytes, *Toxicol. Lett.* 50: 283–288.

Wormhoudt, L.W., Commandeur, J.N.M. and Vermeulen, N.P.E. (1999) Genetic polymorphisms of human N-acetyltransferase, cytochrome P450, glutathione-S-transferase, and epoxide hydrolase enzymes: Relevance to xenobiotic metabolism and toxicity, *Crit. Rev. Toxicol.* 29: 59–124.

Isoform-selective CYP induction

Park, K.B., Kitteringham, N.R., Pirmohamed, M. and Tucker, G.T. (1996) Relevance of induction of human drug-metabolizing enzymes: Pharmacological and toxicological implications, *Br. J. Clin. Pharmacol.* 41: 477–491.

Quattrochi, L.C. and Guzelian, P.S. (2001) CYP3A regulation: From pharmacology to nuclear receptors, *Drug Metab. Dispos.* 29: 615–622.

Watkins, R.E., Wisely, G.B., Moore, L.B., Collins, J.L., Lambert, M.H., Williams, S.P., Willson, T.M., Kliewer, S.A. and Redinbo, M.R. (2001) The human nuclear xenobiotic receptor PXR: Structural determinants of directed promiscuity, *Science* 292: 2329–2333.

Xie, W., Barwick, J.L., Downes, M., Blumberg, B., Simon, C.M., Nelson, M.C., Neuschwander-Tetri, B.A., Brunt, E.M., Guzelian, P.S. and Evans, R.M. (2000) Humanized xenobiotic response in mice expressing nuclear receptor SXT, *Nature*, 406: 435–439.

Furanocoumarin-induced CYP3A4 inactivation

Fuhr, U. (1998) Drug interactions with grapefruit juice. Extent, probable mechanism and clinical relevance, *Drug Safety* 18: 251–272.

Koenigs, L.L. and Trager, W.F. (1998) Mechanism-based inactivation of cytochrome P450 2B1 by 8-methoxypsoralen and several other furanocoumarins, *Biochemistry* 37: 13184–13193.

Schmiedlin-Ren, P., Edwards, D.J., Fitzsimmons, M.E., He, K., Lown, K.S., Woster, P.M., Rahman, A., Thummel, K.E., Fisher, J.M., Hollenberg, P.F. and Watkins, P.B. (1997) Mechanisms of enhanced oral availability of CYP3A4 substrates by grapefruit constituents. Decreased enterocyte CYP3A4 concentrations and mechanism-based inactivation by furanocoumarins, *Drug Metab. Dispos.* 25: 1228–1233.

Tassaneeyakul, W., Guo, L.Q., Fukuda, K., Ohta, T. and Yamazoe, Y. (2000) Inhibition selectivity of grapefruit juice components on human cytochrome P450, *Arch. Biochem. Biophys.* 378: 356–363.

4-Ipomeanol-induced lung injury

Gram, T.E. (1997) Chemically reactive intermediates and pulmonary xenobiotic toxicity, *Pharmacol. Rev.* 49: 297–341.

Lakhanpal, S., Donehower, R.C. and Rowinsky, E.K. (2001) Phase II study of 4-ipomeanol, a naturally occurring alkylating furan, in patients with advanced hepatocellular carcinoma, *Invest. New Drugs* 19: 69–76.

Verschoyle, R.D., Philpot, R.M., Wolf, C.R. and Dinsdale, D. (1993) CYP4B1 activates 4-ipomeanol in rat lung, *Toxicol. Appl. Pharmacol.* 123: 193–198.

UDP-glucuronosyltransferase (UGT)

Burchell, B., McGurk, K., Brierley, C.H. and Clarke, D.J. (1997) UDP-glucuronosyltransferases, *Compr. Toxicol.* 3: 401–435.

Ritter, J.K. (2000) Roles of glucuronidation and UDP-glucuronosyltransferases in xenobiotic bioactivation reactions, *Chem.-Biol. Interact.* 129: 171–193.

Tukey, R.H. and Strassburg, C.P. (2000) Human UDP-glucuronosyltransferases: Metabolism, expression, and disease, *Annu. Rev. Pharmacol. Toxicol.* 40: 581–616.

Mechanisms and toxicological consequences of UGT induction

Dong, J.Q., Etheridge, A.S. and Smith, P.C. (1999) Effect of selective phase II inducers on glucuronidation of benoxaprofen in rats, *Drug Metab. Dispos.* 27: 1423–1428.

Le, H.T. and Franklin, M.R. (1997) Selective induction of phase II drug metabolizing enzyme activities by quinolines and isoquinolines, *Chem. Biol. Interact.* 103: 167–178.

Le, H.T., Lamb, J.G. and Franklin, M.R. (1996) Drug metabolizing enzyme induction by benzoquinolines, acridine, and quinacrine; tricyclic aromatic molecules containing a single heterocyclic nitrogen, *J. Biochem. Toxicol.* 11: 297–303.

Seitz, S. and Boelsterli, U.A. (1998) Diclofenac acyl glucuronide, a major biliary metabolite, is directly involved in small intestinal injury in rats, *Gastroenterology* 115: 1476–1482.

Reactive acyl glucuronides

Bailey, M.J. and Dickinson, R.G. (1996) Chemical and immunochemical comparison of protein adduct formation of four carboxylate drugs in rat liver and plasma, *Chem. Res. Toxicol.* 9: 659–666.

Boelsterli, U.A. (2002) Xenobiotic acyl glucuronides and acyl CoA thioesters as protein-reactive metabolites with the potential to cause idiosyncratic drug reactions, *Current Drug Metab.* 3: 439–450.

Boelsterli, U.A. (2002) Acyl glucuronides in idiosyncratic toxicity, *Mechanisms, Models and Predictions of Idiosyncratic Drug Toxicity*, Subrahmanyam, V. (ed.), ISE Press, Brentwood, MO, in press.

Dickinson, R.G. (1993) Acyl glucuronide conjugates: reactive metabolites of non-steroidal anti-inflammatory drugs, *Proc. West. Pharmacol. Soc.* 36: 157–162.

Fenselau, C. (1994) Acyl glucuronides as chemically reactive intermediates, *Conjugation–Deconjugation Reactions in Drug Metabolism and Toxicity*, Kaufman, F.C. (ed.), Springer, Berlin, 367–389.

Ritter, J.K. (2000) Roles of glucuronidation and UDP-glucuronosyltransferases in xenobiotic bioactivation reactions, *Chem.-Biol. Interact.* 129: 171–193.

Sallustio, B.C., Harkin, L.A., Mann, M.C., Krivickas, S.J. and Burcham, P.C. (1997) Genotoxicity of acyl glucuronide metabolites formed from clofibric acid and gemfibrozil: a novel role for Phase-II-mediated bioactivation in the hepatocarcinogenicity of the parent aglycones?, *Toxicol. Appl. Pharmacol.* 147: 459–464.

Sallustio, B.C., Sabordo, L., Evans, A.M. and Nation, R.L. (2000) Hepatic disposition of electrophilic acyl glucuronide conjugates, *Current Drug Metab.* 1: 163–180.

Spahn-Langguth, H. and Benet, L.Z. (1992) Acyl glucuronides revisited – is the glucuronidation process a toxification as well as a detoxification mechanism?, *Drug Metab. Rev.* 24: 5–48.

Watt, J.A., King, A.R. and Dickinson, R.G. (1991) Contrasting systemic stabilities of the acyl and phenolic glucuronides of diflunisal in the rat, *Xenobiotica* 21: 403–415.

2-Naphthylamine bioactivation and carcinogenicity

Freudenthal, R.I., Stephens, E. and Anderson, D.P. (1999) Determining the potential of aromatic amines to induce cancer of the urinary bladder, *Int. J. Toxicol.* 18: 353–359.

Sulfotransferase (SULT)

Duffel, M.W. (1997) Sulfotransferases, *Biotransformation* 3: 365–383.

Glatt, H. (2000) Sulfotransferases in the bioactivation of xenobiotics, *Chem.- Biol. Interact.* 129: 141–170.

Tamoxifen bioactivation and carcinogenicity

Boocock, D.J., Maggs, J.L., Brown, K., White, I.N.H. and Park, B.K. (2000) Major inter-species differences in the rates of O-sulphonation and O-glucuronylation of α-hydroxytamoxifen *in vitro*: A metabolic disparity protecting human liver from the formation of tamoxifen-DNA adducts, *Carcinogenesis* 21: 1851–1858.

Boocock, D.J., Maggs, J.L., White, I.N.H. and Park, B.K. (1999) α-Hydroxytamoxifen, a genotoxic metabolite of tamoxifen in the rat: Identification and quantification *in vivo* and *in vitro*, *Carcinogenesis* 20: 153–160.

Individual susceptibility to INH hepatotoxicity

Grant, D.M., Hughes, N.C., Janezic, S.A., Goodfellow, G.H., Chen, H.J., Gaedigk, A., Yu, V.L. and Grewal, R. (1997) Human acetyltransferase polymorphisms, *Mut. Res. Fund. Mol. Mech. Mutagenesis* 376: 61–70.

Upton, A., Johnson, N., Sandy, J. and Sim, E. (2001) Arylamine N-acetyltransferases – of mice, men and microorganisms, *Trends Pharmacol. Sci.* 22: 140–146.

Vatsis, K.P. and Weber, W. (1997) Acetyltransferases, *Comprehensive Toxicology, Vol. 3, Biotransformation*, Guengerich, F.P. (ed.), Elsevier, New York, NY, pp. 385–399.

Aflatoxin inactivation by GST

Eaton, D.L. and Gallagher, E.P. (1994) Mechanism of aflatoxin carcinogenesis, *Annu. Rev. Pharmacol. Toxicol.* 34: 135–172.

Benzohydroquinone–glutathione-S-conjugate nephrotoxicity

Corley, R.A., English, J.C., Hill, T.S., Fiorica, L.A. and Morgott, D.A. (2000) Development of a physiologically based pharmacokinetic model for hydroquinone, *Toxicol. Appl. Pharmacol.* 165: 163–174.

Lau, S.S. (1995) Quinone-thioether-mediated nephrotoxicity, *Drug Metab. Rev.* 27: 125–141.

Monks, T.J. and Lau, S.S. (1998) The pharmacology and toxicology of polyphenolic-glutathione conjugates, *Annu. Rev. Pharmacol. Toxicol.* 38: 229–255.

Cysteine-S-conjugate-β-lyase

Armstrong, R.N. (1997) Glutathione transferases, *Biotransformation* 3: 307–327.

Cooper, A.J.L. (1994) Enzymology of cysteine S-conjugate β-lyases, *Conjugation-dependent Carcinogenicity and Toxicity of Foreign Compounds*, Anders, M.W. and Dekant, W. (eds), Academic Press, San Diego, CA, pp. 71–113.

Dekant, W. and Vamvakas, S. (1989) Bioactivation of nephrotoxic haloalkenes by glutathione conjugation: Formation of toxic and mutagenic intermediates by cysteine conjugate β-lyase, *Drug Metab. Rev.* 20: 43–83.

van Bladeren, P.J. (2000) Glutathione conjugation as a bioactivation reaction, *Chem.-Biol. Interact.* 129: 61–76.

Fluoroquinolone phototoxicity

Man, I., Traynor, N.J. and Ferguson, J. (1999) Recent developments in fluoroquinolone phototoxicity, *Photodermatol. Photoimmunol. Photomed.* 15: 32–33.

Spratt, T.E., Schultz, S.S., Levy, D.E., Chen, D., Schlüter, G. and Williams, G.M. (1999) Different mechanisms for the photoinduced production of oxidative DNA damage by fluoroquinolones differing in photostability, *Chem. Res. Toxicol.* 12: 809–815.

Psoralen phototoxicity

Epstein, J.H. (1999) Phototoxicity and photoallergy, *Sem. Cutan. Med. Surg.* 18: 274–284.

Induction of heat shock proteins

Hartl, F.U. (1996) Molecular chaperones in cellular protein folding, *Nature* 381: 571–580.

Moré, S.H., Breloer, M. and von Bonin, A. (2001) Eukaryotic heat shock proteins as molecular links in innate and adaptive immune responses: Hsp60-mediated activation of cytotoxic T cells, *Int. Immunol.* 13: 1121–1127.

Salminen, W.F., Roberts, S.M., Fenna, M. and Voellmy, R. (1997) Heat shock protein induction in murine liver after acute treatment with cocaine, *Hepatology* 25: 1147–1153.

Targeting of stress response proteins

Bruschi, S.A., West, K.A., Crabb, J.W., Gupta, R.S. and Stevens, J.L. (1993) Mitochondrial HSP60 (P1 protein) and HSP70-like protein (mortalin) are major targets for modification during S-(1,1,2,2,-tetrafluoroethyl)-L-cysteine-induced nephrotoxicity, *J. Biol. Chem.* 268: 23157–23161.

Butler, L.E., Thomassen, D., Martin, J.L., Martin, B.M., Kenna, J.G. and Pohl, L.R. (1992) The calcium-binding protein calreticulin is covalently modified in rat liver by a reactive metabolite of the inhalation anesthetic halothane, *Chem. Res. Toxicol.* 5: 406–410.

Chapter 5

Xenobiotic-induced oxidative stress: cell injury, signaling, and gene regulation

Contents

The importance of oxidative stress (oxidant stress) has been increasingly recognized as a pivotal mechanism contributing to the toxicity of many xenobiotics. Oxidative stress has also been implicated in the pathogenesis of many common diseases. One of the most widely used definitions of oxidative stress is an imbalance between the production of oxidizing molecular species (prooxidants) and the presence of cellular antioxidants, in favor of the prooxidants and leading to potential damage. Oxidative stress can be more correctly termed 'oxidoreductive stress' because some of the compounds involved can be both reductants and oxidants, depending on the molecular partner. Because thermodynamics requires that when something is oxidized, something else is reduced, reductive stress may also play a role.

Importantly, xenobiotic-induced oxidative stress not only can cause direct oxidative cell injury, due to the production of strong oxidants, but is also involved in signal transduction and the regulation of gene expression via redox-sensitive mechanisms (see Figure 5.1).

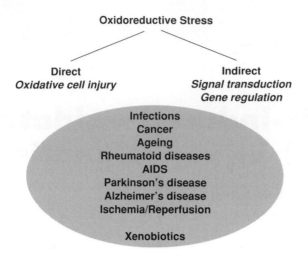

Figure 5.1. Role of oxidoreductive stress as a mechanism of xenobiotic-induced toxicity.

5.1. Reactive oxygen species (ROS) and oxidoreductive stress

One of the key players in the production of oxidoreductive stress is reactive oxygen species.

Although many xenobiotics can be oxidants or reductants, ultimately it is molecular oxygen (O_2) that is involved in the production of oxidoreductive stress. The reason for this is the fact that molecular oxygen (actually being a biradical) can be reduced with relative ease in biological sytems. This partial and stepwise reduction leads to the production of reactive intermediates that can pose an oxidoreductive stress. These oxygen intermediates (including the superoxide anion radical, hydrogen peroxide, and hydroxyl radical) are called reactive oxygen species (ROS) (see Figure 5.2).

Reactive oxygen species, also called reactive oxygen intermediates (ROI), are also often termed 'oxygen free radicals'. This latter term, although frequently used, is not correct for several reasons. First, not all ROS are radicals (e.g. hydrogen peroxide; radicals are atoms or groups of atoms with one or several unpaired electrons). Second, the suffix 'free' is no longer necessary (historically, radicals were functional groups).

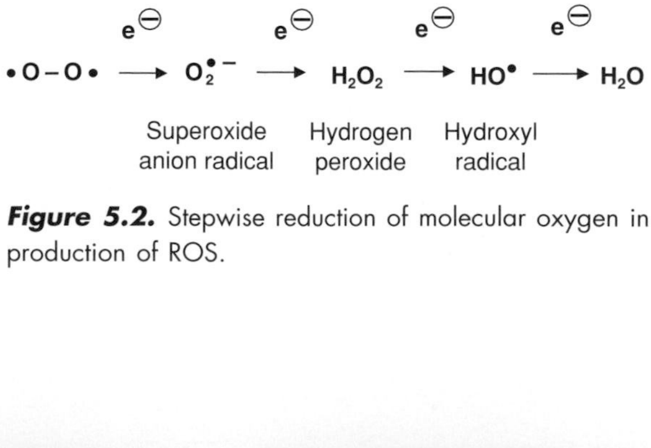

$$\cdot O{-}O\cdot \xrightarrow{\;e^{\ominus}\;} O_2^{\bullet\,-} \xrightarrow{\;e^{\ominus}\;} H_2O_2 \xrightarrow{\;e^{\ominus}\;} HO^{\bullet} \xrightarrow{\;e^{\ominus}\;} H_2O$$

Superoxide   Hydrogen   Hydroxyl
anion radical   peroxide   radical

Figure 5.2. Stepwise reduction of molecular oxygen in biological systems leads to the production of ROS.

The fact that many of these reduced oxygen species are chemically reactive seems paradoxical at first. Although during the evolution of aerobic life molecular oxygen has become an absolute prerequisite for life, the relative ease by which molecular oxygen is reduced and activated to ROS raises the question of why organisms can actually survive in this potentially dangerous environment. The obvious answer is, of course, that in parallel with the development of aerobic life a host of protective (antioxidant) mechanisms have evolved which can be regulated and tightly kept in balance with the prooxidants.

ROS can be generated either by UV radiation or enzymatically. The next questions are where in the cell, and how, are partially reduced oxygen species generated, and how do xenobiotics increase oxidative stress?

5.1.1. Mechanisms of xenobiotic-induced intracellular ROS production

Normally, small amounts of ROS are constantly generated inside cells by physiological processes. These include enzyme-catalyzed electron transfer, e.g. in mitochondria (electron transport chain) or during CYP-mediated oxidation processes. In addition, other enzyme systems (e.g. xanthine oxidase, cyclooxygenase) are also able to produce ROS.

In mitochondria, partially reduced oxygen species may escape the normal electron transfer process. For example, it is estimated that during normal cell respiration a small portion (probably <1 percent) of molecular oxygen, instead of being fully reduced to water, exits the electron transport chain as superoxide anion (earlier *in vitro* experiments using submitochondrial particles with succinate as the only reducing substrate had measured higher rates of 'physiological' ROS production, but *in vivo* the amount of ROS released is definitely lower). However, normally these small amounts of ROS are either readily scavenged or further metabolized and inactivated.

Xenobiotics can dramatically enhance ROS production if they are able to penetrate into mitochondria and interact with one or several of the electron transport chain complexes in the inner mitochondrial membrane, thus blocking the normal electron flow. As a consequence, and especially if the compounds are electron acceptors, they divert the normal electron flow and increase the production of ROS. Typical examples are doxorubicin (see section 15.4) and MPP$^+$ (see section 3.2.3).

The electrons needed to reduce molecular oxygen stem from the pyridine nucleotides, NADH and NADPH, the most important biological reductants (because they are pairs with a highly negative redox potential, facilitating the electron flow to an acceptor molecule). Importantly, xenobiotics can function as electron acceptors, taking up the electron from NAD(P)H via reductase-catalyzed reactions. Such cellular xenobiotic-reducing enzymes are abundantly present in the cytosol, the ER, and in mitochondria. If the reduced xenobiotic in turn reduces a second molecular species, it is ready to be reduced by these cellular reductases a second time, and so on. The resulting cyclic process is called *redox cycling*.

Repeated reduction and oxidation of a xenobiotic can have a number of toxicological consequences.

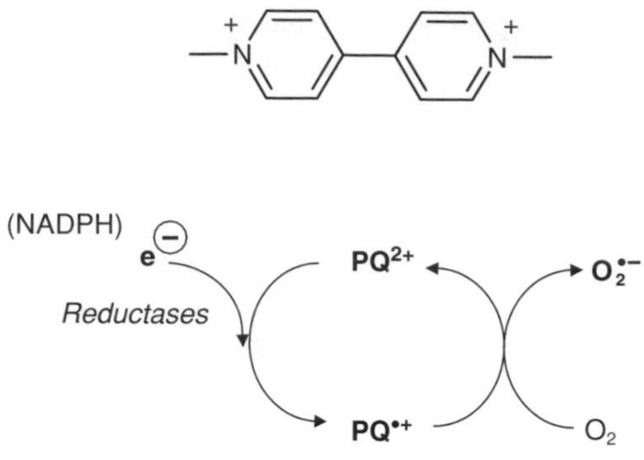

Figure 5.3. Redox cycling of paraquat.

1 If the redox potential allows it, the reduced xenobiotic can in turn reduce molecular oxygen to yield superoxide anion. This is an important pathway of ROS generation; in this case, the reduced xenobiotic poses a reductive stress in a cell.
2 Because this is a cycling process, a single molecule of a redox cycling xenobiotic may produce numerous molecules of superoxide. Thus, redox-cycling chemicals can greatly amplify the generation of ROS.
3 This process will continue until the supply of reducing equivalents (NADPH) is exhausted or can no longer be regenerated.

A typical example for a redox cycling xenobiotic is the herbicide paraquat (PQ) (see section 3.2.2). That paraquat is selectively accumulated in alveolar cells of the lung explains the organ- and cell-specific toxicity of this compound. The toxicodynamic mechanism of cell injury in these tissues, however, can be explained by the high redox-cycling activity of paraquat. The redox potential of paraquat ($PQ^{2+}/PQ^{\bullet+}$) is indeed very high ($E_0 = -0.45$ V), while that of molecular oxygen ($O_2/O_2^{\bullet-}$) is lower ($E_0 = -0.16$ V), thus facilitating electron flow from the reduced PQ to oxygen. In addition, oxygen is available in much higher concentrations in the lung than in any other organ (see Figure 5.3).

Another toxicologically important group of compounds that is involved in redox cycling and oxidative stress is quinones.

Quinones are a large group of ubiquitously occurring compounds found in bacteria, fungi, plants, and higher organisms. Many endogenous quinones exert biologically important functions (for example, in mitochondria, ubiquinone plays a central role as a redox-active component of the electron transport chain). Plants have developed toxic quinones probably to fight insect attacks. Many pharmaceutical drugs are *para-* or *ortho-*quinones (or contain a pivotal quinone moiety), for example doxorubicin (see section 15.4) or menadione, a vitamin K analog (see section 7.2.3). All this may reflect the fact that quinones are considered chemically reactive species; partly because they

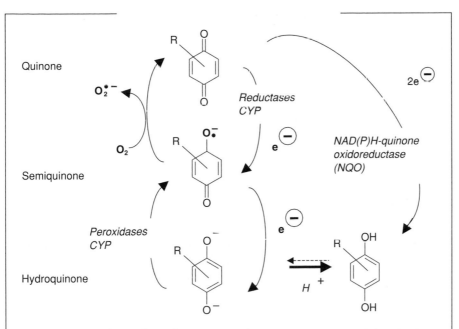

Figure 5.4. Redox cycling of a *p*-quinone/*p*-semiquinone pair and detoxication by NQO-catalyzed two-electron transfer. The structures given are those prevalent at physiological pH.

are electrophilic compounds that can covalently interact with nucleophilic targets (see section 9.1) but also because they can undergo redox cycling and pose oxidoreductive stress in cells. Indeed, in experimental toxicology, many quinones have been selected as model compounds to study cellular and molecular mechanisms underlying the cytotoxicity of xenobiotics.

In mammalian cells, quinones are enzymatically reduced by reductases of the endoplasmic reticulum or mitochondria to the corresponding semiquinone via a one-electron transfer. This partly reduced semiquinone can in turn reduce molecular oxygen and thus undergo redox cycling activity. Semiquinones can also be further reduced by a second one-electron transfer reaction to the corresponding hydroquinone. Unless autoxidation occurs, the hydroquinone is much less reactive than the quinone and thus can be considered a detoxication product, which is conjugated and excreted. To circumvent the potentially dangerous redox cycling via the semiquinone, cells possess an enzyme that is able to reduce quinones by a two-electron transfer reaction directly to the hydroquinone. This enzyme is the NAD(P)H-quinone oxidoreductase (NQO) family (formerly called DT-diaphorase) (see Figure 5.4).

An example of a quinone that produces oxidative stress by redox cycling is the pesticide pentachlorophenol (see section 15.2). Here, it is not the parent compound itself but a metabolite that possesses a quinoid structure (see Figure 5.5).

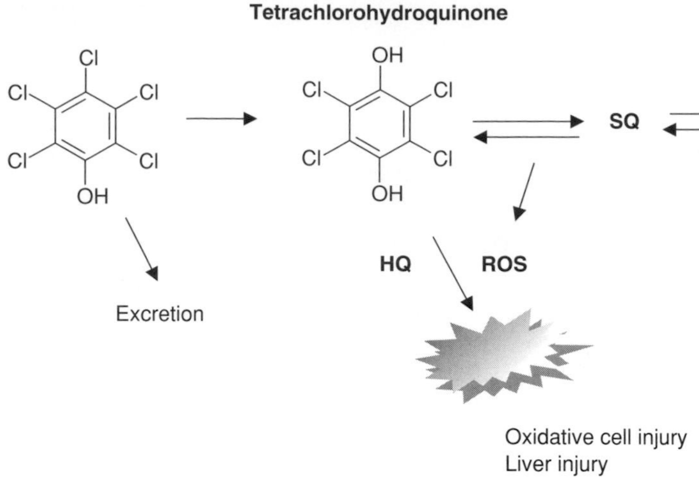

Figure 5.5. Metabolic activation of pentachlorophenol to its major metabolite, TCHQ, leads to oxidative stress via semiquinone (SQ) formation.

Tetrachlorohydroquinone (TCHQ) is the major metabolite of pentachlorophenol, arising from oxidative dechlorination. In liver cell lines, TCHQ is more toxic than the parent compound. There is evidence of oxidative stress associated with TCHQ cell injury, because toxicity can be attenuated by the addition of antioxidants. Therefore, redox cycling is likely to be involved.

Another, more complex, example is the toxicity of benzene. Benzene biotransformation produces, among other metabolites, a hydroquinone that has been implicated in the mechanisms underlying the solvent's toxicity.

Benzene, a small and stable aromatic hydrocarbon, is a widely used industrial product. Its toxic and carcinogenic potential has been recognized for a long time. The most frequently observed toxic effect after chronic exposure both in humans and in animal models is bone marrow toxicity, leading to hypoplastic and aplastic anemia (depletion of erythrocytes and leukocytes), which occurs in an exposure-dependent manner. At even higher or longer exposure, leukemia can occur. Both disorders have been related to benzene-induced damage of the stem cells and progenitor cells in the bone marrow.

To become toxic, benzene must be metabolized to reactive intermediates. The major site of biotransformation is the liver, where benzene is ring-hydroxylated by CYP2E1. In fact, in humans, the monohydroxylated benzene (phenol) is the major metabolite (other biotransformation pathways also occur, such as ring opening). The phenol is then further oxidized to the catechol (1,2-dihydroxy) or 1,4,-benzohydroquinone.

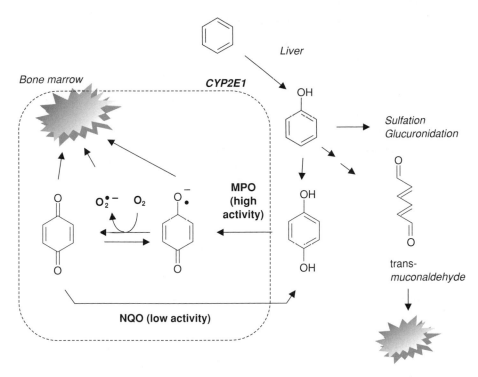

Figure 5.6. Redox cycling from metabolites of benzene produces oxidative stress in the bone marrow. Benzene is metabolized by CYP to *p*-benzohydroquinone, which in the bone marrow is further oxidized by myeloperoxidase (MPO) to the semiquinone and quinone. Another metabolic pathway is ring opening and oxidative metabolism to the reactive muconaldehyde.

Mechanisms of benzene myelotoxicity: Once formed, the hydroquinone accumulates in the bone marrow, which does not express CYP at high levels and is not involved in further biotransformation of benzene metabolites. Instead, the bone marrow is rich in myeloperoxidase activity. Myeloperoxidases are heme-containing enzymes which catalyze the electron transfer from easily oxidizable substrates to hydrogen peroxide, which is then converted to water. Phenols, for example, are excellent electron donors for peroxidases; therefore, the hydroquinone is further oxidized by myeloperoxidases via one-electron oxidations to the corresponding semiquinone and quinone. On the one hand, the resulting *p*-benzoquinone (which is an α,β-unsaturated diketone) has been implicated in the bone marrow toxicity, because it is a protein-reactive species. In addition, redox cycling between the *p*-semihydroquinone and the *p*-hydroquinone may produce superoxide anion radicals and oxidative stress (see Figure 5.6).

What is the biological basis of the bone marrow-selectivity of oxidant-induced stress and toxicity? As already mentioned, bone marrow contains high myeloperoxidase activity. In addition, it features a relatively low expression of NQO, thus rendering the two-electron transfer and inactivation of the *p*-benzoquinone back to

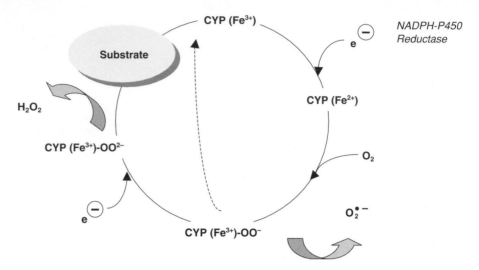

Figure 5.7. Uncoupling of CYP causes release of increased amounts of superoxide anion and/or hydrogen peroxide.

the *p*-hydroquinone inefficient. Finally, the bone marrow contains a high number of rapidly dividing cells where cellular damage is easily manifested.

The targets of these ROS are not known, but they most likely include DNA, DNA and RNA polymerases, tubulin, topoisomerase-II, histones and other DNA-associated proteins. This results in DNA strand breaks and chromosome damage. So, at least in part, oxidative damage from redox cycling of benzene metabolites is a mechanism underlying bone marrow toxicity and carcinogenicity.

Other examples of xenobiotics which undergo redox cycling are nitroaromatic compounds, where the nitro group is reduced by reductases to the nitro anion radical, which in turn can reduce molecular oxygen and thus produce oxidative stress.

ROS can also be produced intracellularly by other mechanisms. One of these pathways is CYP uncoupling. Cytochrome P450 normally is an oxygenase (i.e. it cleaves molecular oxygen, reducing one atom of oxygen to water and inserting the other one into a substrate). However, certain xenobiotics that are poor substrates can cause the electron transfer at the CYP to be uncoupled from substrate oxidation. For example, superoxide anion can be released from one-electron-reduced oxy-CYP, or hydrogen peroxide may be released from two-electron-reduced peroxy-CYP. This shunting of the CYP cycle consumes NADPH and produces large amounts of ROS. Certain CYP forms are more powerful uncouplers than others; for example, human CYP3A4 is the most active one (see Figure 5.7).

5.1.2. The key players: superoxide anion radical, hydrogen peroxide, and hydroxyl radical

Superoxide anion radical is an ROS posing a potential threat to cells, although it is not extremely reactive. It can act both as a reductant and as an oxidant. In cells, superoxide anion is effectively removed by the superoxide dismutases enzymes (see Figure 5.8).

$$O_2^{\bullet-} + O_2^{\bullet-} \xrightarrow[\substack{\textit{Superoxide dismutase} \\ \textit{(SOD)}}]{2H^+} H_2O_2 \; (+O_2)$$

Figure 5.8. Superoxide dismutase catalyzes the conversion of superoxide anion to hydrogen peroxide.

Superoxide dismutase (SOD) is a group of metalloenzymes that have Cu and Zn, Mn, or Fe as the active metal. The form containing Mn is found both in bacteria and in mitochondria of eukaryotic cells. Mn-SOD is inducible upon oxidative stress.

SOD catalyzes the dismutation (i.e. two molecules of the same species react with each other) of superoxide. In this case, one molecule of superoxide is reduced and the other one oxidized, and as a result hydrogen peroxide and molecular oxygen are generated. SOD thus keeps the average amount of cellular superoxide anion on a low level (approximately 10^{-11} M). But now the question arises of whether the removal of superoxide is a real detoxication reaction, because the resulting hydrogen peroxide is also a potentially reactive ROS.

Several lines of evidence support the assumption that removal of superoxide by SOD is indeed a detoxication reaction. For example, practically all aerobic organisms possess SOD. That superoxide accumulation can be harmful is shown in SOD-null mice (generated by knockout techniques). Specifically, Cu,Zn-SOD-null mice are more susceptible to prooxidants, and Mn-SOD-null mice are embryonic lethal. Second, known mutations in the human gene coding for SOD1 (Cu, Zn-SOD) have been associated with the loss of motoneurons resulting in the familial form of amyotrophic lateral sclerosis (Lou Gehrig's disease). It is generally assumed that the functional alterations of SOD in these neurons is responsible for their degeneration (perhaps by some form of uncompensated oxidative stress). Finally, experimental evidence from the toxicity of the model xenobiotic, 1,2-dichlorobenzene, which was greatly reduced in the presence of exogenous SOD, also points to a protective function of SOD against oxidative damage.

1,2-Dichlorobenzene (1,2-DCB) is an industrial solvent that has become toxicologically important as a possible environmental contaminant. It is an acute hepatotoxin in rodents, producing hepatic necrosis in a dose-dependent manner. 1,2-Dichlorobenzene is bioactivated to reactive metabolites (including quinones) and covalently binds to cellular macromolecules. In addition, cells in the liver other than hepatocytes seem to play a crucial role; Kupffer cells and infiltrating macrophages have been implicated in enhancing the oxidative stress.

In rats, administration of SOD largely protected from liver injury induced by 1,2-DCB, as evidenced by the significant decrease in leakage of the hepatic marker enzyme, alanine aminotransferase (ALT), into the blood. This indicates that the production of superoxide anion by DCB is involved in the toxicity

Table 5.1 **Superoxide dismutase (SOD) protects from the hepatic toxicity of 1,2-dichlorobenzene (DCB)**

Treatment	ALT activity (U/L)
Untreated control	41 ± 18
1,2-DCB (in oil)	3,455 ± 584
1,2-DCB + SOD–PEG	770 ± 577*
SOD–PEG (in 0.9% NaCl)	34 ± 4
Oil + NaCl	37 ± 6

Note: Male F344 rats were treated with 1,2-DCB (3.6 mmol/kg, intraperitoneally). SOD (20,000 IU/kg) coupled to polyethyleneglycol (SOD–PEG) was injected intravenously 2 h after 1,2-DCB. Alanine aminotransferase (ALT) activity was determined 24 h later. Data are mean ± SEM (n = 3–8). *$P < 0.05$ vs 1,2-DCB alone.

Source: data are from Gunawardhana, L., Mobley, S.A. and Sipes, I.G. (1993) Modulation of 1,2-dichlorobenzene hepatotoxicity in the Fischer-344 rat by a scavenger of superoxide anions and an inhibitor of Kupffer cells, *Toxicol. Appl. Pharmacol.* 119; 205–213.

of DCB. Because SOD is rapidly degraded in the blood ($t_{1/2}$ approx. 15 min), the enzyme was 'pegylated', i.e. coupled to polyethyleneglycol (PEG), thereby increasing the half-life to approximately 16 h (see Table 5.1).

Aminotransferases ('transaminases') in the serum are widely used (both clinically and experimentally) as markers for hepatic parenchymal injury induced by xenobiotics. The most specific marker is alanine aminotransferase (ALT) activity in serum. Although human ALT isozymes are found in the cytosol and mitochondria of liver, kidney, skeletal and cardiac muscle, the largest pool of ALT is in the cytosol of hepatocytes. In rodents, ALT has been considered liver-specific. In rat liver, ALT is found almost exclusively in periportal hepatocytes, which is consistent with the enzyme's role in gluconeogenesis.

After damage to hepatic parenchymal cells, the enzyme leaks into the serum and peak activities are found 24 to 48 h after a toxic insult. As the half-life of human ALT is >47 h, serum activity measurements are static estimates of the amount of recent damage. Normal serum values of humans (and rodents) are ≤35 U/L. The normal presence of low levels of circulating enzyme reflects normal cell turnover or release from other nonvascular sources.

Another widely used aminotransferase marker in the serum is asparate aminotransferase (AST). In contrast to ALT, AST is more abundantly (<70 percent) expressed in mitochondria, and is also more prevalent in heart muscle, skeletal muscle, brain, kidney and pancreas. Accordingly, serum increases in AST are less specific for liver injury than ALT.

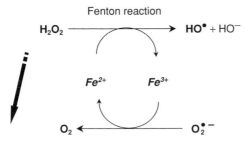

Fenton reaction

$$H_2O_2 \longrightarrow HO^{\bullet} + HO^-$$

Fe^{2+} Fe^{3+}

$$O_2 \longleftarrow O_2^{\bullet -}$$

Degradation by catalase or glutathione peroxidase

Figure 5.9. Metal-catalyzed production of hydroxyl radical from hydrogen peroxide.

The next key player in the ROS cascade is hydrogen peroxide. Hydrogen peroxide is not very reactive *per se*; it can diffuse away from the site of its generation and even cross biological membranes. Nevertheless, it can lead to the formation of much more toxic ROS if not removed. Because H_2O_2 is constantly generated at low levels in mitochondria, the ER, but also in peroxisomes, powerful antioxidant enzyme systems have evolved.

Two major enzymes are involved in enzymatic degradation of hydrogen peroxide: catalase and glutathione peroxidase. The rate constant for degradation of hydrogen peroxide by catalase is several orders of magnitude higher than that for its generation by SOD; therefore H_2O_2 will be rapidly inactivated by catalase. Catalase is especially abundant in the liver, particularly in peroxisomes, which are organelles with a high rate of ROS production. In the cytosol and mitochondria, catalase is not found; therefore, other enzymes are involved to remove H_2O_2. The most important cytosolic enzyme is glutathione peroxidase, a selenium–cysteine-containing enzyme that catalyzes the conversion of hydrogen peroxide to water (see also section 5.3.2).

If hydrogen peroxide escapes degradation of catalase or glutathione peroxidase, it can be converted non-enzymatically to the next ROS, the hydroxyl radical. This reaction is catalyzed by iron or other redox-active transition metals, which reduce H_2O_2, resulting in homolytic cleavage and the generation of an innocuous hydroxyl anion and a highly reactive hydroxyl radical (the so-called Fenton reaction). Superoxide can reduce the oxidized metal back to its divalent state, thus driving this reaction cycle (see Figure 5.9).

The resulting hydroxyl radical is extremely reactive; its $t_{1/2}$ at $37°$ is approximately 10^{-9} sec. This means that the hydroxyl radical will attack any molecule in its immediate vicinity within the cell. Therefore, the presence of even trace amounts of iron or other transition metals is potentially harmful because they can greatly increase the production of hydroxyl radical, the most potent cellular oxidant.

5.1.3. Role of iron and other redox-active transition metals

Redox-active transition metals, notably $Fe^{2+/3+}$ and $Cu^{+/2+}$, have been implicated in catalyzing oxidative stress due to their Fenton activity. Indeed, it has been amply

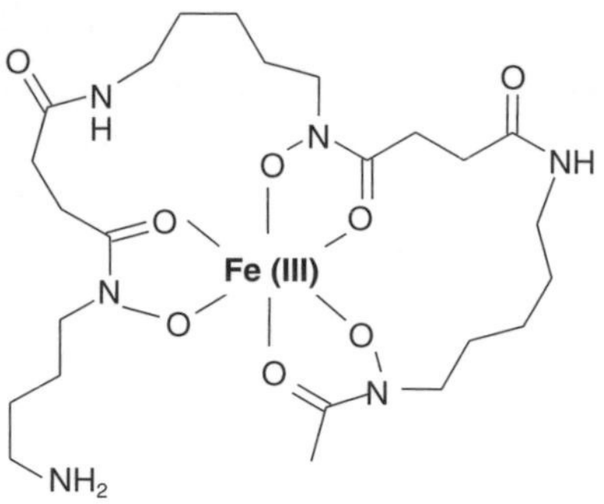

Figure 5.10. Deferoxamine as an Fe(III) chelator.

demonstrated that intracellular, catalytically active iron is causally involved in the toxicity of xenobiotics.

One way to provide the 'proof of concept' for this assumption is to chemically inactivate the intracellular redox-active iron and to see whether the toxic effects inflicted by an oxidative stress-inducing xenobiotic will be reduced. This can be done with some iron-chelating compounds.

Iron chelators: Iron-chelating agents are natural or synthetic compounds with a very high affinity for Fe^{2+} and/or Fe^{3+}. Because iron is essential for cell function, bacteria, fungi, and plants have developed so-called siderophores. These are iron-binding compounds that are secreted (and later taken up when loaded with iron). Higher organisms have developed specific iron transporters in order to recruit the essential element.

One such iron chelator derived from a natural siderophore is deferoxamine (DFO). Deferoxamine features an Fe(III) binding constant of 10^{30} M^{-1} and is therefore an extremely powerful chelator. Importantly, DFO occupies all coordination sites of the ferric ion so that H_2O_2 can no longer bind to iron and the metal can no longer participate in Fenton reactions (other chelators can bind iron or other metals but still produce hydroxyl radicals) (see Figure 5.10).

Deferoxamine has even been clinically used to bind and remove iron from the body in genetically determined or accidental iron overload. It is, however, used with caution because of its low bioavailability in humans and its increasing toxicity at higher doses. Therefore, other compounds are being developed for clinical use which feature better absorption, higher penetration across cell membranes, and lower systemic toxicity.

That the intracellularly available redox-active iron is potentially dangerous can be nicely shown in experiments in which an oxidative stress is provoked by a pro-oxidant xenobiotic in the presence and absence of such an iron chelator, e.g. DFO. Deferoxamine precludes binding of hydrogen peroxide to the catalytically active iron and thus inhibits the formation of hydroxyl radicals (see Table 5.2).

Because intracellular iron and other catalytically active transition metals are potentially dangerous to a cell, they are tightly bound to either proteins or small-molecular ligands and sequestered in specific pools.

Iron in the circulation is bound to transferrin and taken up into cells via the transferrin receptor. Inside the cell (where reducing conditions normally prevail), Fe(III) is readily reduced to Fe(II). Ferrous iron in the cytoplasm is bound to

Table 5.2 The ferric ion chelator deferoxamine (DFO) protects from the hepatotoxic effects of acetaminophen (APAP)

Treatment	Serum ALT activity (U/L)	Mortality (%)
APAP	11,666 ± 4,633	88
APAP + DFO	3,406 ± 894*	38*
APAP + DFO + FeCl₃	10,129 ± 1,685	94
FeCl₃	45 ± 15	0
Untreated control	43 ± 13	0

Note: Rats were treated with APAP (750 mg/kg) with or without prior (−1 h) administration of DFO (200 mg/kg). In some treatment groups, FeCl₃ (125 mg/kg) was given together with APAP. ALT activity was determined in the serum 8 h post-administration. Mean ± SD (n = 5). Mortality was determined after 24 h. *Significant differences vs APAP alone or APAP + DFO + FeCl₃ (P < 0.05).
Source: data are from Sakaida, I., Kayano, K., Wasaki, S., Nagatomi, A., Matsumura, Y. and Okita, K. (1995) Protection against acetaminophen-induced liver injury *in vivo* by an iron chelator, deferoxamine, *Scand. J. Gastroenterol.* 30; 61–67.

small-molecular weight compounds and constitutes the so-called 'free' or labile iron pool (LIP), from where ferrous ions are interchanged with other pools including mitochondria (heme synthesis). The LIP-associated iron is also thought to be the iron fraction that is catalytically active and that can participate in Fenton chemistry. To keep this pool as small as possible, the excess iron is stored (in the form of ferric ions) and sequestered in the major cellular iron-storing protein, ferritin. Ferritin is a hollow globular protein composed of many subunits, which can store in its interior up to 4,500 ferrous ions (see Figure 5.11).

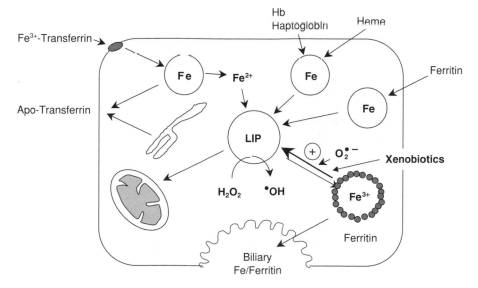

Figure 5.11. The labile iron pool (LIP) is the catalytically active cellular ferrous iron pool, while the bulk of intracellular ferric ions are stored and sequestered in the ferritin molecule.

Not only is xenobiotic-enhanced redox stress in the cell the primary cause for ROS formation, but chemicals or their metabolites featuring a highly negative redox potential are also able to reduce the ferritin-bound Fe(III) and cause the release of Fe(II) into the cytoplasm. This can greatly augment the LIP size and, therefore, increase the production of deleterious hydroxyl radicals.

Although iron is toxicologically the major transition metal involved in catalyzing redox stress, copper can also play a role. For example, under pathophysiological conditions where excess copper is stored in the liver, oxidative stress builds up, and cholestasis and hepatitis can develop. This can occur in humans in Wilson's disease, a genetic defect in the ATP7B gene, which encodes a canalicular transporter (for Cu) in the liver. Similarly, in the LEC (Long-Evans Cinnamon) rat model, excess Cu accumulates in the liver, and these animals develop hepatitis and even liver tumors.

The fact that metal-catalyzed formation of hydroxyl radicals can lead to macromolecular damage in the immediate vicinity of its formation is exemplified by the toxicity caused by bleomycin.

Bleomycin is a group of antimicrobial and antineoplastic glycopeptides, originally derived from *Streptomyces* species, but then semisynthetically modified. The agent is widely used to treat a variety of malignant tumors including squamous cell carcinoma, Hodgkin lymphoma, and testicular tumors. Although bleomycin generally lacks toxicity in normal hematopoietic cells, a serious adverse reaction associated with the drug is pulmonary toxicity. In particular, type I alveolar cells are affected. Chronic use of bleomycin can result in the development of pulmonary fibrosis.

Mechanisms of bleomycin-induced pulmonary toxicity: The bleomycin molecule features two pivotal domains: one is the DNA-binding domain, which allows for interaction with double-stranded DNA and RNA, and which in fact is associated with the underlying and desired cause for DNA damage. The second binding site is a metal-binding domain. Bleomycin is coordinated by copper, iron, and manganese ions (in particular Cu^{2+}, Fe^{2+}, and Fe^{3+}). The coordinating metal is still redox-active and can catalyze the formation of hydroxyl radicals. Indeed, deferoxamine protects from bleomycin-induced oxidative injury (see Figure 5.12).

There are two reasons why the lung is particularly sensitive to the organ-selective toxicity of bleomycin.

1 The lung tissue has a low activity in bleomycin hydrolase (the enzyme which breaks down bleomycin into an inactive form). This enzyme is abundantly expressed in most other tissues except malignant tumors.
2 The lung has a high pO_2, a factor which favors the development of activated ROS.

5.1.4. Mechanisms of xenobiotic-enhanced extracellular ROS production

The extracellular production of ROS differs in a number of ways from the mechanisms of intracellular ROS generation that occur in most metabolically active cells

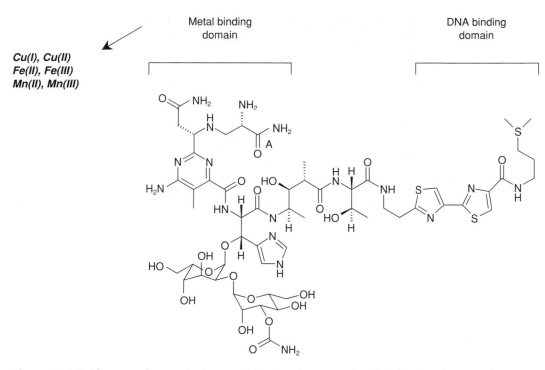

Figure 5.12. Bleomycin features both a metal-binding domain and a DNA-binding domain. The immediate vicinity of Fenton-active iron and the target macromolecule is the underlying cause for the oxidative stress and tissue injury caused by bleomycin.

and are associated with intracellular oxidoreductive stress. For example, it is only a defined group of cells which can produce extracellular ROS. These include phagocytes (macrophages and neutrophils) but also T and B lymphocytes. By virtue of a specific enzyme system located on the plasma membrane, these cells can rapidly produce ROS upon a stimulus (oxidative burst, intended for defense against invading pathogens, but probably also for regulating genes involved in inflammation and immune responses). This enzyme is NADPH oxidase.

> **NADPH oxidase** is a membrane-bound hemoprotein which is normally dormant but which can be activated by a number of stimuli. These stimuli include surface receptor activation by opsonized particles and protein kinase C agonists. By a complexly regulated system, NADPH is oxidized and two electrons transferred to molecular oxygen. Simultaneously, the pentose phosphate pathway is activated to ensure a sustained supply of NADPH. The products are superoxide anion and hydrogen peroxide. The latter is used to oxidize chloride to hypochlorite, a subsequent reaction catalyzed by myeloperoxidase.

A number of xenobiotics can trigger and enhance NADPH oxidase activity of phagocytes and thus induce oxidative stress. A typical example is mineral fibers including asbestos. These fibres are taken up (sometimes incompletely) by phagocytes, where they induce the oxidative burst. If NADPH oxidase activity is sustained, it can induce chronic oxidative stress and tissue damage.

Asbestos is a collective term for anorganic fibers derived from natural silicates. Importantly, the chemical composition and the morphology of asbestos vary greatly. Asbestos has been known since ancient times. It has been used for a variety of industrial applications including insulation and construction. In the 1970s the production of asbestos was at its peak; since the discovery that asbestos fibers can pose a serious risk for human health, production has been declining worldwide.

Inhalation of asbestos fibers can cause lung injury. The size of the fibers is critical for toxicity; if their length is >5 μm, their diameter <3 μm, and the length/diameter ratio approximately 3:1, then the hazard is maximal. Typically, chronic inhalation of asbestos fibers leads to lung fibrosis (asbestosis). In more severe cases, asbestos can cause a typical form of lung tumors, mesotheliomas, i.e. malignant tumors of the pleura or the peritoneum. Because mesotheliomas are rare tumors, their occurrence points to a likely exposure to asbestos fibers. In individuals who smoke, asbestos can also potentiate the formation of bronchial carcinomas. Asbestos fibers can reside in the lung alveoli for a long time ($t_{1/2}$ up to 40 years!). They can even migrate into the pleura, where they have been implicated in mesothelioma formation. Although the production and use of asbestos has been limited, the incidence of such lung tumors is still increasing, due to the long (20–30 years) latency period of cancer development (see Figure 5.13).

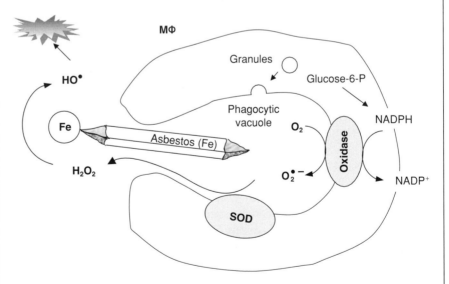

Figure 5.13. Asbestos fibers phagocytosed by macrophages induce NADPH oxidase-catalyzed formation of ROS. The high iron content in asbestos fibers further catalyzes the formation of injurious hydroxyl radicals.

Mechanisms of asbestos-induced lung fibrosis and mesothelioma formation: The mechanisms have not been fully understood, but activation of phagocytes and oxidative stress seem to play a pivotal role. This has been convincingly demonstrated with cultured lung epithelial cells: exposure of such epithelial cells to asbestos fibers does not cause toxicity, while in co-culture with macrophages these fibers readily damage the epithelial cells by oxidative injury. *In vivo*, the situation is more complex. ROS produced by the NADPH-oxidase not only damage the tissue but also are mediators for the release of chemotactic substances (chemokines) including MIP-2 (macrophage inflammatory protein-2) and leukotriene B_4. These chemokines, secreted in part by alveolar cells type II, chemoattract a large number of additional macrophages, lymphocytes, and PMNs, which infiltrate from the vasculature and in turn cause an even greater oxidative stress. Both ROS and proteases, as well as hypochloric acid, directly damage the epithelial cells. Because also a number of growth factors (including tumor necrosis factor-α and transforming growth factor-β) are being released, epithelial cells and fibroblasts proliferate and secrete collagen, which ultimately leads to fibrosis. Both the stimulatory effects of asbestos on cell proliferation and mutagenic activity of asbestos (chromosomal aberrations) are likely to be responsible for its carcinogenic effects (see Figure 5.14).

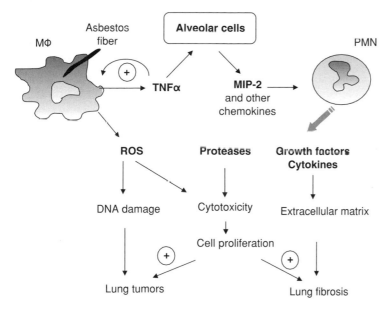

Figure 5.14. Mechanisms of asbestos-induced activation and recruitment of inflammatory cells. Asbestos-activated macrophages secrete TNFα and other mediators which in turn stimulate alveolar cells to produce large amounts of chemoattractants. The infiltrating inflammatory cells produce ROS, which directly damage DNA of target cells, as well as proteases and cytokines/growth factors, which stimulate cell proliferation and the production of extracellular matrix. Thus, asbestos is responsible for directly inducing genotoxicity as well as indirectly stimulating fibrosis and tumor formation (tumor promoter).

5.1.5. Other ROS: ozone and singlet oxygen

Another ROS of high toxicological relevance, which is produced by reactions in the environment and which is a strong prooxidant, is ozone.

Ozone (O_3) is a gas with a slightly blue color and a pungent odor. It is mostly generated from UV activation of molecular oxygen in the stratosphere, where it constitutes a vital layer providing protection from UV irradiation to the earth. In the troposphere, ozone is generated by UV-mediated homolytic cleavage of molecular oxygen, but also by cleavage of NO_2 (car exhausts), which catalyzes the generation of ozone. The resulting oxygen radical reacts with molecular oxygen and forms O_3. Ozone is also generated anthropogenically through UV sources in tanning studios, photocopy machines, etc. Ozone is stable in air ($t_{1/2}$ approximately 7 min) and can thus be shifted away from the site of origin.

Biological targets are eyes (irritation) and airways (bronchia, alveoli). In the latter, the type I alveolar cells are primarily damaged by necrosis, followed by hyperplasia of type II cells. Progressive alveolar edema develops, together with a decrease in lung compliance and hypoxemia from the destruction of cell membranes.

Mechanisms of ozone toxicity: Ozone is a potent oxidant with a reactivity towards biological targets comparable to that of the hydroxyl radical. In other words, ozone will react with macromolecules in the immediate vicinity of exposure to biological tissues. It attacks proteins (in the airways) through reacting with sulfhydryl groups, amino, or hydroxyl groups. Alternatively, ozone can attack fatty acyl carbon–carbon double bonds in lipid biomembranes (see Figure 5.15).

Finally, another ROS that has been implicated in oxidative stress reactions is singlet oxygen. Singlet oxygen ($^1O_2$) is oxygen in an excited energy state, which is much more reactive than the normal, ground-state molecular oxygen (triplet oxygen, $^3O_2$, which is stable). It is generated by UV, for example in the skin during sunbathing. However, singlet oxygen can also be generated enzymatically by at least two systems. First, PMNs and other phagocytes which express myeloperoxidase can generate singlet oxygen during the oxidative burst. Myeloperoxidase can catalyze the oxidation of chloride to hypochlorite (OCl^-), which in turn can react with hydrogen peroxide and transfer the energy to oxygen to generate $^1O_2$. Another reaction where singlet oxygen is produced is the prostaglandin (PG) peroxidase-catalyzed conversion of PGG_2 to PGH_2.

5.1.6. Reactive nitrogen species (RNS) and oxidative stress

The biological role of nitric oxide (NO) has been increasingly recognized. NO, which is a radical, is not only an important biological signal molecule in muscle and vascular physiology but also plays a role in xenobiotic-induced oxidative stress.

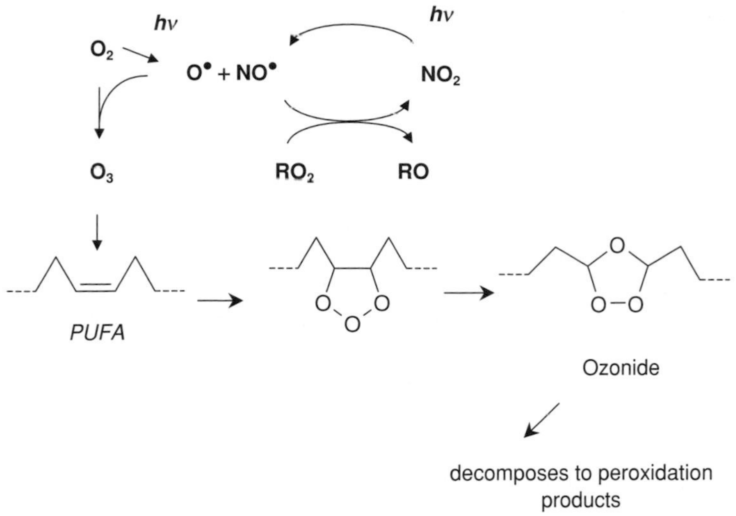

Figure 5.15. Generation of ozone and destruction of biomembranes. UV cleaves both molecular oxygen and NO_2 and generates the monooxygen radical, which in turn reacts with O_2 to ozone. The nitrogen monoxide radical is converted back to NO_2 by peroxides which arise, similarly to NO_2, from VOC (volatile organic compounds) emissions. PUFA, polyunsaturated fatty acid.

Nitric oxide is generated enzymatically by nitric oxide synthetase (NOS) from L-arginine. There are several forms of NOS: constitutive forms, including a mitochondrial form, and an inducible one (iNOS).

The fact that nitric oxide is involved in cell toxicity has often been indirectly demonstrated with the use of specific inhibitors of NOS. For example, aminoguanidine, an inhibitor of the inducible form of NOS (which has minimal activity against the constitutive NOS isoforms), almost fully prevents the hepatic toxicity induced by cocaine (see Table 5.3).

Table 5.3 The iNOS inhibitor aminoguanidine protects from the hepatic toxicity induced by cocaine

Treatment	Serum ALT activity (U/L)
Saline	24 ± 3
Cocaine	$1{,}364 \pm 295$*
Aminoguanidine + cocaine	27 ± 2
Aminoguanidine	22 ± 2

Note: Male ICR mice were treated with a single dose of cocaine (55 mg/kg) or saline. Where indicated, aminoguanidine (300 mg/kg) was administered 1 h prior to cocaine. Serum aminotransferase activity (ALT) was determined 16 h later. Data are mean ± SEM ($n = 3$–5). *$P < 0.05$ vs all other groups.
Source: data from Aoki, K., Ohmori, M., Takimoto, M., Ota, H. and Yoshida, T. (1997) Cocaine-induced liver injury in mice is mediated by nitric oxide and reactive oxygen species, *Eur. J. Pharmacol.* 336; 43–49.

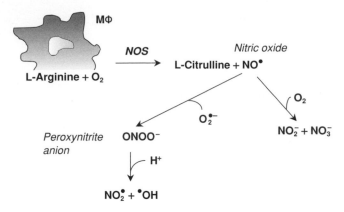

Figure 5.16. Pathways of macrophage-mediated RNS production. A toxicologically important reaction is the generation of peroxynitrite (ONOO⁻) from NO and superoxide, because peroxynitrite can react to the highly toxic hydroxyl radical.

Cocaine is a potent hepatotoxin in mice, and there are reports of cocaine-associated liver injury in humans exposed to high doses of cocaine. The mechanism of cocaine hepatotoxicity is still unclear. One prerequisite is a CYP-catalyzed multistep bioactivation to reactive intermediates (see section 4.2.1) which are protein-reactive.

On the other hand, activation of cocaine is also associated with the production of ROS. For example, the iron chelator deferoxamine protects from cocaine toxicity in cultured hepatocytes. Several lines of evidence indicate that the ROS are not generated in mitochondria but rather are derived from other intracellular sources.

Because *in vivo* both NO-trapping agents and a specific inhibitor of iNOS prevent hepatic toxicity, it is likely that NO is involved in cocaine hepatotoxicity.

Mechanisms of NO-mediated toxicity: Nitric oxide has an intermediate half-life (1–10 s), i.e. it can diffuse away from the site where it was generated. Toxicologically the most relevant feature of NO is its reaction with superoxide anion, which results in the formation of peroxynitrite anion, ONOO⁻. Peroxynitrite is very reactive ($t_{1/2}$ approximately 10^{-3} s) and decays when it becomes protonated to the nitric dioxide radical and the extremely reactive hydroxyl radical. To what extent direct damage by ROS participate in the hepatic toxicity, or how far ROS-mediated signaling and activation of pro-apoptotic pathways are involved, is not known. Redox stress is most likely involved, as cocaine triggers apoptosis in the liver (see Figure 5.16).

5.2. Toxicological consequences of oxidative stress

Oxidoreductive stress can have multiple consequences. If not compensated by antioxidant defense systems, the prooxidants can directly damage cells or tissues. Targets for oxidative damage are nucleic acids, proteins, and lipids, but also small biomolecules (e.g. biogenic amines, ascorbic acid). It has been increasingly recognized, however,

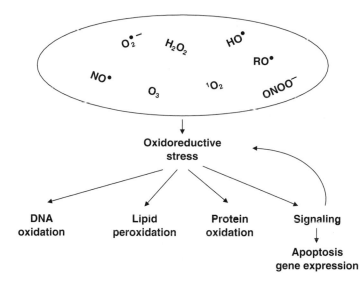

Figure 5.17. Oxidoreductive stress can damage cellular targets either via direct oxidative damage or through redox sensors that transduce signals, which in turn can activate cell-damaging processes.

that the extent of oxidative stress needs to be excessive in order to damage most organs by this direct pathway, as the antioxidant defense is strong and can be regulated or induced by transcriptional activation. Oxidoreductive stress can influence many redox-sensitive processes in cells and thus act as a second messenger that leads to the transactivation of genes. Some of these are involved in promoting apoptosis (see Figure 5.17).

One such signal is a mediator that simply amplifies the primary oxidoreductive stress. For example, in the liver exposed to 1,2-dichlorobenzene (see section 5.1.2), ROS are generated which *per se* are probably insufficient to damage liver cells severely (because their effect would be antagonized by the powerful antioxidant defense system in the liver). Instead, the signal activates chemokines and other activating pathways, which results in the infiltration of extrahepatic macrophages and other immune cells, which flood the liver and produce a second and much stronger wave of oxidative stress (see Figure 5.18).

5.2.1. Oxidative DNA damage

One of the consequences of oxidative stress in cells is oxidation of nucleic acids by ROS. As ROS are physiologically generated all the time, this is a normal process that is counterbalanced by antioxidants and repair mechanisms. In fact, estimates reveal that each day the DNA in a cell of the body is theoretically 'hit' by an oxidative event approximately 1.5×10^5 times, which would culminate as a total of 10^{19} hits per individual. One of the markers to detect oxidative damage to DNA is the measurement of oxidized bases; for example, the presence of 8-hydroxy-deoxyguanosine (8-OH-dG) in urine. Indeed, in nuclear DNA, one out of approximately 130,000 guanine residues is 8-OH-G (see Figure 5.19).

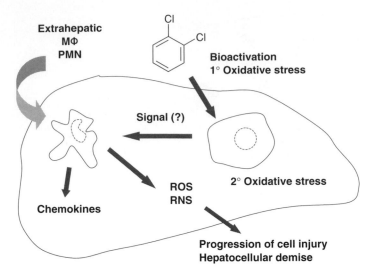

Figure 5.18. Signals released from hepatocytes subjected to a primary oxidative stress, caused by activated 1,2-dichlorobenzene, recruit macrophages and neutrophils, thus amplifying the extent of oxidoreductive stress.

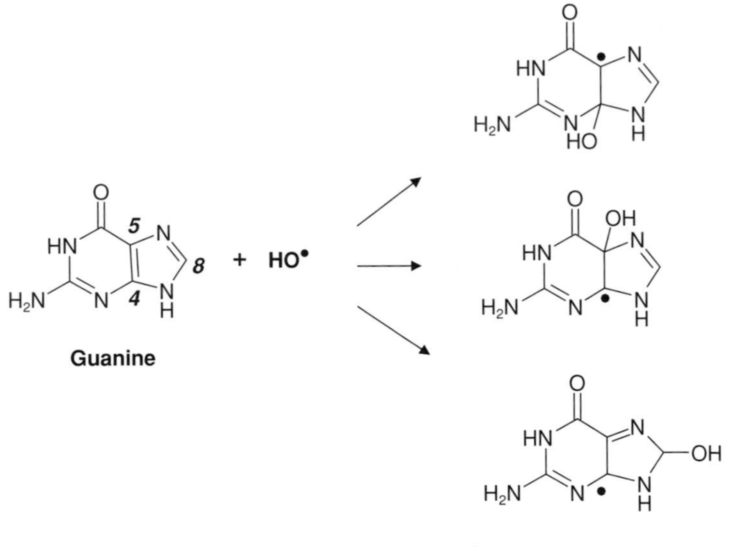

Figure 5.19. Attack of a hydroxyl radical on purine bases.

Mitochondrial DNA is much more prone than nuclear DNA to be hit by an oxidative event and to be permanently damaged. In mitochondrial DNA, one out of approximately 8,000 guanine residues is 8-OH-G. The biological reasons behind this increased susceptibility include the absence of histones (which are protective) in mtDNA, the close proximity to the generation of ROS in mitochondria, and inefficient repair mechanisms, leading to accumulation of oxidatively damaged bases.

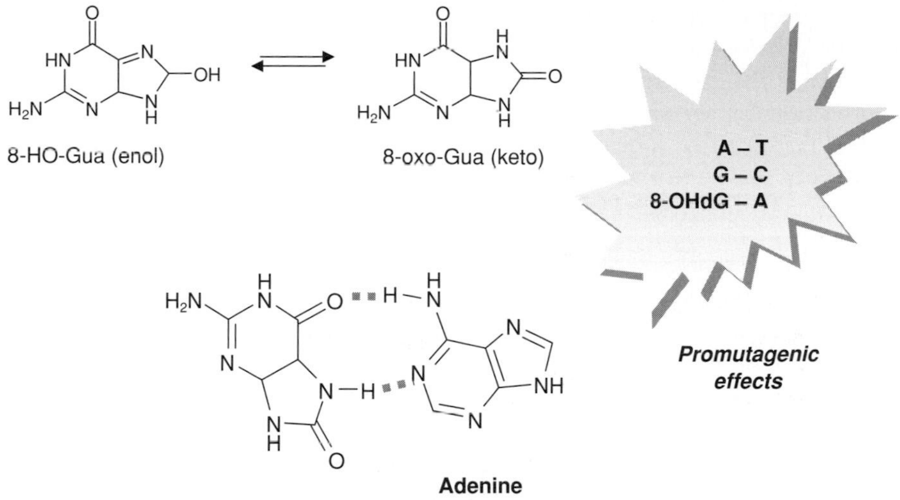

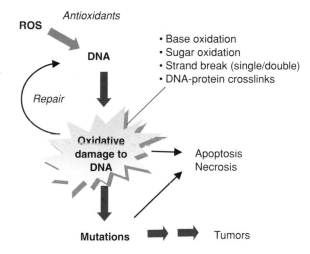

Figure 5.20. DNA base oxidation (at the guanine residue) leads to the insertion of a wrong base (adenine) due to the inability to form hydrogen bonds with cytidine.

Figure 5.21. Oxidative DNA damage can lead to mutations and eventually tumors.

Base oxidation has severe consequences on base pairing: while normally guanine would bind via three hydrogen bonds to cytosine, the oxidized form, 8-oxo-guanine (the keto form), binds now to adenine via two hydrogen bonds. If not repaired by base excision, this mismatch will lead to a base pair transformation in the next cycle of DNA synthesis (see Figure 5.20).

If these changes persist during the next replication cycle, a mutation is generated. In most cases such damage will be repaired, or mutated cells will undergo cell death by apoptosis or necrosis. However, DNA oxidation can also be the basis for tumor formation (see Figure 5.21).

One group of xenobiotics that have clearly been associated with eliciting oxidative DNA damage and cancer are metals. One of the reasons for this carcinogenic potential is the catalytic activity of redox-active metals, including iron or copper (see section 5.1.3), which may entail the production of hydroxyl radicals. The second reason is the inherent DNA-binding properties of these metals, bringing the freshly generated and highly reactive hydroxyl radicals in close proximity to the molecular target, the DNA.

Oxidative DNA damage has been implicated in the **carcinogenic activity of many metals**. For most metals (except beryllium) oxidized bases have indeed been identified after exposure. Examples are Cr(VII) and Ni(II), but also indium, all of which induce tumors in lung and nose.

The propensity of the airway systems to develop tumors has a number of biological causes. Among these is the obvious fact that lungs are constantly exposed to air that might contain toxic particles including metal dust and/or volatile RNS (NO radical) or ROS (ozone). In addition, the perfusion rate of lungs is high, exposing them to xenobiotics in the bloodstream. Finally, the cells lining the airway are exposed to high oxygen tension, facilitating the production of ROS.

For example, **nickel** sulfides and other nickel compounds pose an increased risk of respiratory cancer. Nickel sulfides can enter the nucleus and induce DNA damage *in vivo*. For example, Ni_3S_2 is a highly carcinogenic form of the metal and causes severe DNA lesions and increases in 8-OH-dG levels in the lungs. It also causes an inflammatory response in the lung and greatly enhances NO production by macrophages. Thus, the combined mechanism of ROS release by macrophages during the inflammation and the reaction between Ni^{2+} and H_2O_2 produces an Ni–ROS complex (i.e. an oxo-Ni(IV) complex or an Ni(III)–peroxide complex), which can release OH radicals and hence can damage DNA.

5.2.2. Oxidative protein damage

Xenobiotic-induced production of ROS and oxidative stress can lead to the oxidation of cellular proteins, in particular oxidation of side chains of amino acid residues, formation of protein–protein cross-links, and protein fragmentation due to the oxidation of the peptide backbone. The sulfur-containing amino acids cysteine and methionine are particularly susceptible to oxidation, leading to disulfide bonds or sulfoxide formation respectively. Furthermore, aromatic amino acids are also prone to being attacked by ROS.

Again, the cell harbors a host of antioxidant defense mechanisms to limit the oxidative stress, and there are repair mechanisms to reverse the damage. For example, heat shock proteins (hsp) (see section 4.4.1) are able to renature damaged proteins or to resolubilize aggregates of damaged proteins. Also, oxidatively damaged proteins are recognized and readily degraded by the major cytosolic protease system, the proteasome.

The **proteasome** is a large multi-subunit and multi-catalytic protease. It exists in two major forms (20S and 26S). The proteasomes are found in the cytosol, both free and attached to the ER, and in the nucleus of eukaryotic cells. Proteasomes recognize, unfold and digest protein substrates that have been marked for degradation by the attachment of ubiquitin moieties. The proteasome complex is barrel-shaped, with the proteolytic sites inside the barrel, and features at least five different proteolytic activities.

When oxidized proteins are partially unfolded and expose their hydrophobic sites, they are recognized by the core (20S) proteasome. Importantly, this core proteasome does not require ATP or protein ubiquitinylation. The damaged proteins are then degraded into peptides and amino acids. Undamaged amino acids are recycled for protein biosynthesis.

If oxidation cannot be compensated or repaired, the major consequences for enzymes are loss of catalytic function, or impairment of function for structural proteins. Oxidative modification of proteins also results in increased surface hydrophobicity due to partial unfolding of the protein. One possible consequence is the formation of large protein aggregates, which are often toxic when they accumulate in a cell.

One special example of protein oxidation arising from xenobiotic-induced oxidative damage is the red cell and its major protein, hemoglobin.

Erythrocytes are particularly susceptible to oxidative damage for a number of reasons. The underlying biological causes include the following.

1 A high pO_2 (favoring reduction of molecular oxygen); in fact, hemoglobin-bound oxygen ($Hb-O_2$) is present at concentrations of approximately 25 mM, while the oxygen concentration in other body fluids is <0.2 mM.
2 Xenobiotics are in most cases distributed in blood at high concentrations. Therefore, red cells are readily exposed to these xenobiotics.
3 Erythrocytes feature a relatively long biological $t_{1/2}$ of approximately 120 days. Furthermore, as they do not have a nucleus or ER, they are unable to replace oxidized proteins with newly synthesized proteins.

As the bulk (>90 percent) of the erythrocyte's protein content consists of hemoglobin, this protein is a frequent target for oxidative damage. On one hand, it is the globin chains that are oxidized; on the other hand, it is the heme group that can be affected. Importantly, though, the iron of the oxygen-binding heme moiety does not change its valency upon binding, and the Fe(II) is therefore not involved in catalyzing Fenton-type reactions.

Xenobiotic-induced oxidation of the α- and β-globin chains of hemoglobin in erythrocytes can lead to disulfide bond formation. Such cross-links can also be

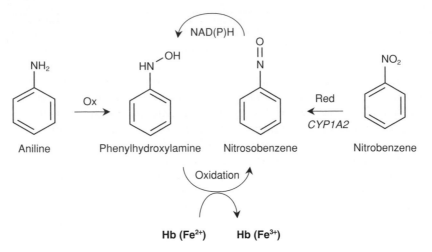

Figure 5.22. The formation of methemoglobin by aromatic amines involves cycling between the hydroxylamine and the nitroso compound and is driven by the redox activity of these intermediates.

formed with spectrin, a component of the erythrocyte's cytoskeleton. The resulting aggregates of denatured hemoglobin in erythrocytes form conspicuous dark bodies attached to the cell membrane and were named 'Heinz bodies'. Erythrocytes with Heinz bodies have impaired function and are removed from the circulation and degraded in the spleen and other organs of the reticulo-histiocyte system.

Under specific conditions, and often concomitant with globin oxidation, it is the heme moiety, containing Fe(II) (ferrous), that can be oxidized by xenobiotics. The resulting Fe(III)- (ferric) hemoglobin, which is termed methemoglobin (MetHb), is no longer able to carry oxygen. Under normal physiological conditions, about 1 percent of hemoglobin is present as MetHb. This is not dangerous as the oxidized Hb is constantly reduced back to normal Hb by a team of reductases (except for some forms of genetic deficiencies). Only under a highly increased prooxidant stress, if the portion of MetHb is increased to approximately 10–20 percent of total Hb, symptoms of toxicity may appear. Oxidation of 60–80 percent of total Hb to MetHb is fatal, due to lack of oxygen supply.

Mechanisms of methemoglobin formation and hemotoxicity: The formation of MetHb is complex and has not been fully elucidated. Methemoglobin can be formed either directly (e.g. by nitrite), or indirectly, i.e. requiring the bioactivation of a xenobiotic to a redox-active intermediate prior to MetHb formation (e.g. by aromatic amines) (see Figure 5.22).

Therefore, MetHb can be formed from both sides, i.e. from reduced aromatic amines (e.g. aniline) or from oxidized aromatic amines (e.g. nitrobenzene). After bioactivation, the resulting intermediates, i.e. the N-hydroxy and the nitroso compounds, drive the formation of hemoglobin oxidation in a futile cycling, until the reducing equivalents are exhausted or other factors limit the production of MetHb. Therefore, even relatively small amounts of strong MetHb-forming compounds can be potentially dangerous, in particular in patients with compromised erythrocytic antioxidant defense systems, as may occur under glucose-6-phosphatate dehydrogenase deficiency (see section 5.3.2).

Oxidative modification of structural protein components of the cytoskeleton is another example where oxidative stress can directly lead to cell injury and necrosis. For example, it has been well known that some cells including hepatocytes or fibroblasts upon exposure to high levels of oxidative stress will form small surface protrusions (blebs). These blebs may rupture, causing a collapse in ion homeostasis and leakage of intracellular components into the extracellular medium, which may lead to necrotic cell death (see section 7.1). What is the nature of these blebs?

Recently, it has become clear that this form of cytotoxicity is a consequence of oxidative modifications of the microfilaments of the cytoskeleton. In particular, the morphological changes are caused by a disruption of the polymerized actin, leading to shortening and/or aggregation of microfilaments. Because these lethal changes can be totally prevented by the addition of thiol-reducing agents (such as dithiothreitol or β-mercaptoethanol), it is logical to assume that oxidation of critical sulfhydryl groups is the basis of the cytoskeletal disruption.

Indeed, actin in both its native state (G-actin) and after polymerization (F-actin) features a thiol group of a cysteine residue (Cys[374]) which is exposed on the surface of the filament. Oxidation of this thiol group leads to the formation of mixed glutathione–actin disulfides (GS-S-actin) or to intermolecular disulfide bridges which cross-link the actin filaments. Sustained oxidative stress can thus lead to irreversible damage of the cytoskeleton. In fact, actin has been shown to be the most sensitive component of the cytoskeleton, prone to readily undergoing oxidative modification.

5.2.3. Oxidative lipid damage

If the microenvironmental conditions favor the generation of ROS in the hydrophobic compartments of a cell, then lipids may be oxidized. As a result, biomembranes may be peroxidized and damaged (see Figure 5.23).

Two important features characterize lipid peroxidation and distinguish it from the oxidation of other cellular compartments.

1 The original radical-induced damage at a particular site in a membrane lipid is readily amplified and propagated in a chain-reaction-like fashion, thus spreading the damage across the biomembrane.
2 The products arising from lipid peroxidation (e.g. alkoxy radicals or toxic aldehydes) may be equally reactive as the original ROS themselves and damage cells by additional mechanisms (see Figure 5.24).

Although membrane lipid peroxidation has been implicated in many instances as a mechanism of xenobiotic-induced tissue injury, it is important to note that lipid peroxidation is not always the causative factor of cell injury. Instead, in many cases lipid peroxidation occurs merely as a non-specific process secondary to initial tissue damage. This can be easily demonstrated by blocking the propagation of membrane lipid peroxidation (e.g. by vitamin E) and observing whether the toxicity is prevented concomitantly. If the markers for lipid peroxidation are reduced or absent

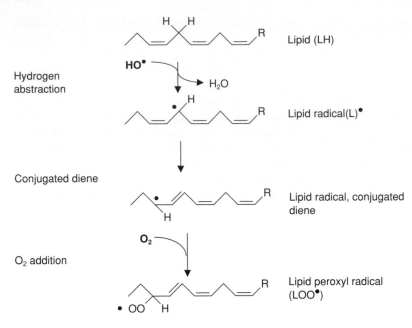

Figure 5.23. Mechanism of lipid peroxidation: oxidation of a fatty acyl carbon and formation of lipid peroxyl radical.

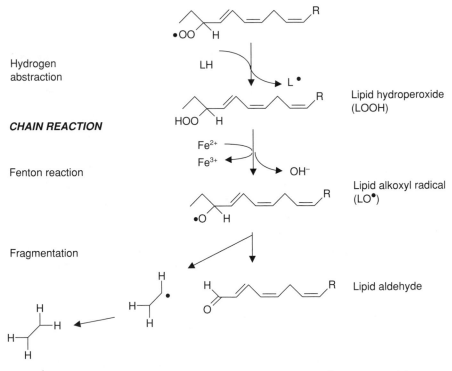

Figure 5.24. Mechanism of lipid peroxidation: propagation of reaction and formation of aldehyde degradation products.

but toxicity remains unchanged, then it is probably is a non-peroxidative process that is responsible for the oxidative cell injury.

However, one typical example where membrane lipid peroxidation is the prime mechanism of tissue injury is the hepatotoxicity induced by carbon tetrachloride.

Carbon tetrachloride is an important and widely used industrial solvent. It was formerly widely used in the household, in fire extinguishers, shampoos, and dry cleaning. Earlier, carbon tetrachloride was even used therapeutically against infections by hook worms, and in the nineteenth century the solvent was used as an anesthetic and analgesic! After the high potential for acute toxicity became evident, all these applications obviously became obsolete. Nevertheless, intoxication with carbon tetrachloride still occurs, e.g. by accidental ingestion.

The major target organs of toxicity are the liver and kidney. In the first few hours after ingestion, slight to severe neurological disorders are prevalent (headache, visual disturbances, CNS depression, coma), but also gastrointestinal irritations (vomiting, diarrhea and bleeding). During the following day(s) liver and kidney toxicity develops. In the liver, toxicity is first manifested as steatosis (fatty change of the liver parenchyma), followed by centrilobular necrosis.

CCl_4 is a small and lipophilic molecule and therefore readily distributes in the lipid compartments of the body. It is metabolized in the liver, and the clue to its toxicity lies in the CYP-mediated bioactivation of CCl_4 and the induction of membrane lipid peroxidation.

Mechanism of carbon tetrachloride-induced hepatotoxicity: CCl_4 undergoes *bioreductive* metabolism catalyzed by CYP2E1 (a rare reaction for CYPs) to the trichloromethyl radical. This CCl_3 radical has been implicated in triggering the membrane lipid peroxidation chain reaction, as it abstracts a hydrogen from a fatty acyl residue, resulting in chloroform and an alkoxy radical formation. This is the major pathway, especially under conditions of low pO_2. In contrast, in the presence of high oxygen tension, the trichloromethyl peroxy radical is formed. This is an extremely reactive species that reacts and inactivates CYP2E1 itself (mechanism-based inactivation, or suicide inactivation of CYP) (see section 4.2.1.2). The consequence is that the remaining CCl_4 can no longer be bioactivated because the CYP form involved is irreversibly damaged (see Figure 5.25).

Carbon tetrachloride toxicity is one of those examples that beautifully illustrate how a detailed understanding of the underlying mechanism of toxicity can help in developing therapeutic strategies in patients. For example, an acute intoxication with CCl_4 can be treated (within the first 24 h, and before necrosis develops) by exposing the patient to hyperbaric oxygen (e.g. 2.5 atm for a short period of <1 h) to prevent further bioactivation and lipid peroxidation.

A general and important consequence of membrane lipid peroxidation is the production of toxic aldehydes stemming from oxidative fatty acyl degradation. Two widely investigated aldehydes are malondialdehyde (MDA) and the α,β-unsaturated aldehyde, 4-hydroxynonenal (4-HNE). Both aldehydes not only are biomarkers to prove that lipid peroxidation has occurred, but have more recently been recognized

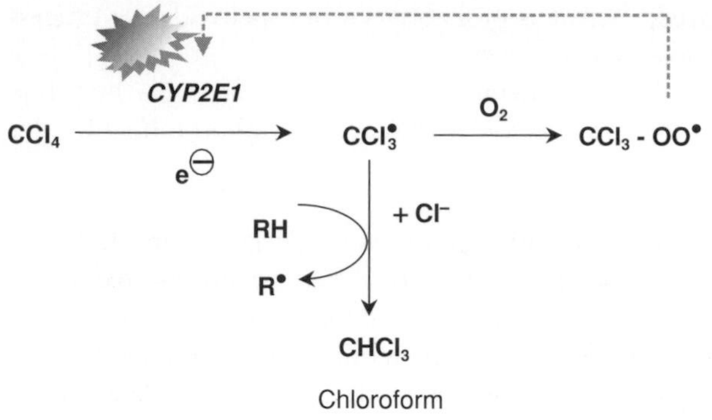

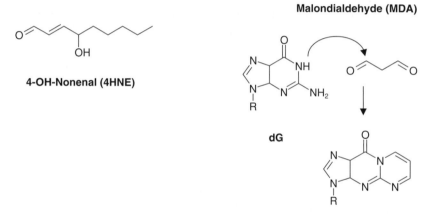

Figure 5.25. Reductive bioactivation of CCl_4 leads to a reactive CCl_3 radical which can react with fatty acyl residues and initiate lipid peroxidation. At high pO_2, the CCl_3-peroxy radical will destroy the bioactivating enzyme, CYP2E1, by suicide inactivation.

Figure 5.26. Aldehydes from lipid peroxidation are protein- and DNA-reactive species. MDA reacts with deoxyguanosine (dG) to form a covalent adduct.

to be reactive electrophilic molecules themselves which can covalently bind to proteins or DNA. Thus, the toxic aldehydes could play a direct role in the toxicity of oxidant xenobiotics, and MDA has even been implicated in cancer formation. Indeed, MDA or 4-HNE adducts to both protein and deoxyguanosine have been found after ethanol or iron overload in human liver. Similar adducts can be found in rat liver after CCl_4 administration (see Figure 5.26).

5.3. Interference with antioxidant defense mechanisms

To prevent the maintenance of mild oxidative stress (which is physiologically required for normal function) from getting out of balance, and to protect from xenobiotic-induced oxidoreductive stress, organisms have evolved a plethora of biological antioxidant systems. Some natural or synthetic antioxidants (enzyme mimics) have even been considered for therapeutic purposes against oxidant stress-induced damage.

The major functions of these antioxidants are:

- to provide scavengers for ROS and RNS
- to keep the cellular thiol redox status in the reduced form
- to prevent and/or repair the oxidation of lipids
- to sequester redox-active metals and to prevent Fenton-type reactions.

It is beyond the scope of this book to give a comprehensive overview of all these antioxidant compounds or enzyme systems. Instead, a few typical and toxicologically relevant examples are selected.

Often, the toxicological relevance of a given antioxidant defense system becomes obvious when it is impaired, either by a xenobiotic or by genetic or environmental factors. Thus, it has become clear that one important mechanism underlying the toxicity of prooxidant compounds is a possible interference with some of these antioxidant defense systems.

The antioxidant enzymes or small molecular compounds are distributed in the body in an organ- or tissue-dependent fashion. Some organs (e.g. the liver and kidney) are endowed with a very high antioxidant arsenal; other organs (e.g. the cardiac and skeletal muscle and the CNS) express low levels of antioxidants. For example, heart tissue expresses catalase at a very low level only (which is compatible with the absence of peroxisomes in cardiomyocytes; catalase is most abundant in peroxisomes). This differential expression is part of the underlying biological causes of organotropic oxidative damage seen with many xenobiotics.

Many antioxidants are tightly regulated and can be induced upon a prooxidant stimulus; their upregulation is part of the 'stress response' (see section 4.4.1). For example, exposure to the anti-cancer drug doxorubicin, which is potentially cardiotoxic (see section 15.4) due to its prooxidant activity in mitochondria, induces a series of antioxidant enzymes or peptides in the heart. This occurs mainly by transcriptional up-regulation. Interestingly, not all of these increased mRNAs are equally translated at the protein level. Some antioxidants remain at unchanged levels or even exhibit decreased activity. This reflects the fact that the enhanced transcriptional activation of antioxidants may simply be a compensatory response to the consumption of antioxidants (e.g. glutathione) during the prooxidant stress posed by the xenobiotic (see Figure 5.27).

5.3.1. Glutathione

Glutathione (GSH), together with its coupled enzyme systems, is one of the most important antioxidant defense lines in the body. Upon need, the levels of GSH can even become up-regulated. The importance of GSH becomes particularly evident when the redox balance is disrupted due to excessive GSH consumption, because this will greatly facilitate the development of toxicity caused by prooxidant xenobiotics.

Glutathione is a ubiquitous tripeptide consisting of glutamate, cysteine, and glycine. A number of characteristics must be recalled for better understanding its biological function.

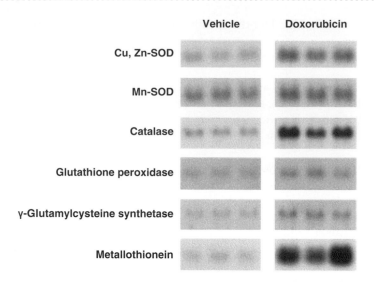

Figure 5.27. Transcriptional activation of antioxidants in mouse heart after doxorubicin. Male FVB mice were treated with doxorubicin (15 mg/kg.day, *i.p.*) or saline for 4 days. mRNA was isolated and analyzed by Northern blotting.
Source: Yin, X., Wu, H., Chen, Y. and Kang, Y.J. (1998) Induction of antioxidants by adriamycin in mouse heart, *Biochem. Pharmacol. 56*; 87–93. With permission of Elsevier Science.

1 GSH has a reactive sulfhydryl group (cysteinyl) which is responsible for its antioxidant acitivities.
2 Glutamate and cysteine are not coupled via a peptide bond at the α-carbon (which would be expected for a regular peptide) but the glutamyl moiety is attached to cysteine via its γ-carboxyl group. This feature protects the tripeptide from protease digestion.
3 In many tissues GSH reaches high (i.e. millimolar) steady state concentrations, and these high levels are maintained.

De novo synthesis of GSH is catalyzed by γ-glutamylcysteine synthetase and glutathione synthetase. These enzymes are often targeted experimentally with selective inhibitors to unravel the role of GSH in xenobiotic toxicity; for example, L-buthionine sulfoximine (BSO) is a selective inhibitor of γ-glutamylcysteine synthetase, the first and rate-limiting enzyme in GSH synthesis.

There are several cellular pools of GSH: the cytosolic pool, the mitochondrial pool, and also, importantly, a large nuclear pool. This distribution reflects the important antioxidant and reactive metabolite-trapping function of this endogenous compound.

GSH is most abundant in hepatocytes, from where it is released into the bloodstream. In addition, GSH is secreted into the hepatobiliary system where it not only protects from oxidative stress but is a major osmotic determinant of bile flow. GSH is produced and released from many other cells too (except erythrocytes).

Mechanisms of GSH-mediated antioxidant activities: GSH has an important function as a co-substrate for GS-transferase-catalyzed conjugation to electrophilic

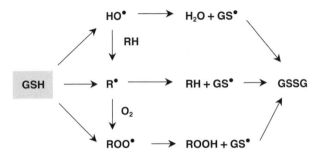

Figure 5.28. Chemical structure of glutathione.

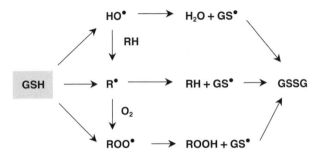

Figure 5.29. GSH is a radical scavenger and becomes oxidized to GSSG.

reactive metabolites (see section 4.2.5). As an antioxidant, GSH fulfills at least three pivotal tasks:

- GSH is a radical scavenger (non-enzymatically)
- GSH is a co-substrate for the enzymatic (GS peroxidase-catalyzed) degradation of H_2O_2
- GSH keeps the cells in a reduced state and is involved in the regeneration of oxidized proteins.

In all three cases, the thiol group of GSH is oxidized to the GS radical which in turn dismutates to glutathione disulfide (GSSG) (these terms are preferable to the frequently used terms, 'reduced' or 'oxidized' glutathione. GSSG is then readily regenerated to GSH by glutathione reductase, a process which is fueled by NADPH. Under normal conditions, the ratio of GSH/GSSG in a cell is >100, i.e. a reducing microenvironment normally prevails in the cytosol (see Figure 5.29).

5.3.1.1. GSH-coupled enzyme systems

GSH is a substrate for glutathione peroxidase (GS-Px, a selenium-containing enzyme) and is involved in the degradation of hydrogen peroxide. In fact, GS-Px is the most important enzyme for the extraperoxisomal inactivation of H_2O_2, especially in the liver (see Figure 5.30).

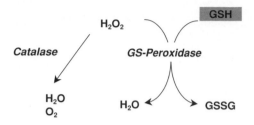

Figure 5.30. Enzymatic degradation of hydrogen peroxide by glutathione peroxidase.

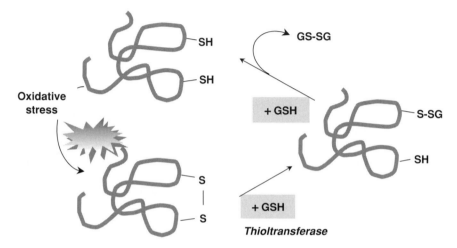

Figure 5.31. Reduction of oxidized sulfhydryl groups in proteins by GSH.

GSH can regenerate oxidized proteins by reducing disulfide bonds back to the sulfhydryls in a two-step reaction catalyzed by thiol reductase (interestingly, in the endoplasmic reticulum, during protein biosynthesis some proteins do need disulfide bonds for their proper folding; the GSH/GSSG ratio in the ER is therefore kept at a much lower level than in the cytosol) (see Figure 5.31).

In spite of the ubiquitous presence of GSH, there are situations where GSH can become depleted. This occurs after extensive conjugation to reactive electrophilic metabolites, but also during exposure to prooxidants and xenobiotic-induced increased oxidative stress. In addition, other factors including the nutritional status and the altered rates of resynthesis may modulate and deplete cellular GSH levels, and this can have severe toxicological consequences.

The availability of reducing equivalents (food!) determines the GSH status. For example, rigorous dieting (with zero calories) for an extended time greatly augments the susceptibility to acetaminophen (APAP) in humans. As APAP is being metabolized to both a prooxidant intermediate and an electrophilic species (see section 9.2.1), its metabolism will consume large amounts of GSH. Because after fasting the GSH levels are low, extreme dieting has even resulted in reported fatal hepatotoxicity after therapeutic doses of APAP.

Table 5.4 Hepatic levels and cytoprotective effects of GSH against acetaminophen toxicity are dependent on the time of day of administration

Time of APAP administration	Plasma ALT activity (U/L)	Hepatic GSH content (µmol/g liver)	
		Before APAP	After APAP (3 h)
8 a.m.	27 + 3	8.7 ± 0.2	4.2 ± 0.6
2 p.m.	70 ± 28	6.8 ± 0.4	2.4 ± 0.5
8 p.m.	3,451 ± 1,036	6.1 ± 0.4	1.5 ± 0.2

Note: Mice were treated with a single dose of APAP (400 mg/kg, i.p.). Plasma ALT activities were determined 24 h post-administration. Mean ± SEM ($n = 6$–13). There were no differences in plasma concentrations of APAP or its metabolites in the different treatment groups.
Source: data are from Kim, Y.C. and Lee, S.J. (1998) Temporal variation in hepatotoxicity and metabolism of acetaminophen in mice, *Toxicology*, 128; 53–61.

Furthermore, the hepatic GSH content is subject to diurnal changes. For example, in mice (which feed during the night and sleep during the day), the GSH levels in the liver and the GSH *de novo* synthesis are lowest at the end of the day. This chronotoxicological characteristic can explain the quite impressive differential toxicity induced by a single dose of APAP given in the morning or early in the night (see Table 5.4).

Another condition where the prooxidant effects of xenobiotics are highly exaggerated due to a compromised function of GSH homeostasis has a genetic background: increased toxicity due to a deficiency of glucose-6-phosphate dehydrogenase.

5.3.1.2. Genetic deficiency in erythrocyte glucose-6-phosphate dehydrogenase

Glucose-6-phosphate dehydrogenase (G6PD) deficiency is apparently the most frequent pharmacogenetic polymorphism in human populations, affecting several hundred million people. The gene is located on the X-chromosome, and the enzymopathy affects only the enzyme of the erythrocytes. The genetic abnormality is particularly frequent among Afro-Americans (~11 percent), and in certain parts of the Mediterranean countries the frequency can be up to 50 percent!

There is a striking overlap between geographical regions with populations that have a high frequency of G6PD deficiency and where malaria is endemic (or used to be endemic, as in the Mediterranean area). The reason is that the G6PD deficiency phenotype protects against infection by the malaria parasite *Plasmodium falciparum*. The plasmodia can invade G6PD-deficient red blood cells, but they cannot mature normally. Such infected erythrocytes are more readily recognized and phagocytosed by macrophages than are parasitized normal erythrocytes. That G6PD deficiency poses a selection advantage by this mechanism is also illustrated by the fact that all the polymorphic gene variants known today (>34) are found in populations in which malaria is frequent.

G6PD deficiency is lethal in mice, but not in humans, because all variants discovered so far are missense mutations or small in-frame deletions that do not result in complete loss of enzyme activity. In the most severe cases the G6PD activity in

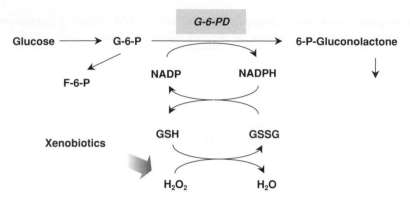

Figure 5.32. Glucose-6-phosphate catalyzes the production of NADPH and thus indirectly drives the reduction of GSSG to GSH.

mutated individuals can be reduced to approximately 10 percent of that in normal individuals.

What are the toxicological consequences of this genetic deficiency, and how is it related to glutathione and oxidative stress?

Key role of G6PD in protecting against oxidative stress: Normally, red cells contain large concentrations of GSH. To this effect, G6PD plays a key role. Because in erythrocytes (which lack mitochondria and ER) the pentose phosphate pathway (in which G6PD is involved) is the only way for the formation of NADPH, deficiency of G6PD activity largely reduces the production of NADPH from $NADP^+$. NADPH, in turn, is required as a reducing equivalent to reduce GSSG back to GSH (see Figure 5.32).

Because not only is GS-Px dependent on GSH, but also catalase requires NADPH to remain in a functional state, hydrogen peroxide can only incompletely be degraded under these conditions. In particular, under xenobiotic-enhanced production of large amounts of ROS, the residual antioxidant system is no longer capable of coping with the oxidoreductive stress, and erythrocyte injury ensues. Such prooxidant xenobiotics include sulfonamides and nitroaromatic drugs. In fact, the G6PD polymorphism was detected and analyzed after the hemotoxicity occurring after ingestion of the anti-malarial drug, primaquine.

Primaquine, an 8-aminoquinoline drug, is an important anti-malarial drug and has been used for more than 40 years. It exhibits unique effectiveness against the exo-erythrocytic forms of the malaria parasite. In fact, primaquine is currently the only drug that is capable of curing the persistent stages of some forms of *Plasmodium* in the liver. However, one of the limiting factors in the use of primaquine has been the hemotoxicity of the drug. This became especially evident in individuals with G6PD deficiency. In these people, the erythrocytes were taken out of circulation prematurely (and degraded in liver and spleen) due to red cell damage. The damage typically consisted of oxidized hemoglobin which was denatured and formed aggregates attached to the inner surface of the red cells (Heinz bodies).

Mechanism of primaquine hemotoxicity: It has been known for a long time that it is a primaquine metabolite that is reactive and that is responsible for the red cell toxicity. In fact, primaquine is extensively metabolized in humans via a number of pathways (ring hydroxylation, alkyl deamination, conjugation). One of these pathways is N-dealkylation to form an 8-amino metabolite. This arylamine is further oxidized to the N-hydroxy derivative. It is therefore possible, although not proven *in vivo*, that the redox cycling between the N-hydroxy and the nitroso form poses an oxidative stress in red cells that could damage the cell if it is uncompensated. Alternatively, the quinone imine formed from 5-hydroxylation of primaquine also forms a potential redox cycling active pair (see Figure 5.33).

Certain natural food constitutents, as they occur in beans, also have a potential prooxidant activity that in individuals with normal G6PD activity is of no further consequence, but in people with G6PD deficiency can cause hemolysis. This condition of food-induced toxicity is named favism.

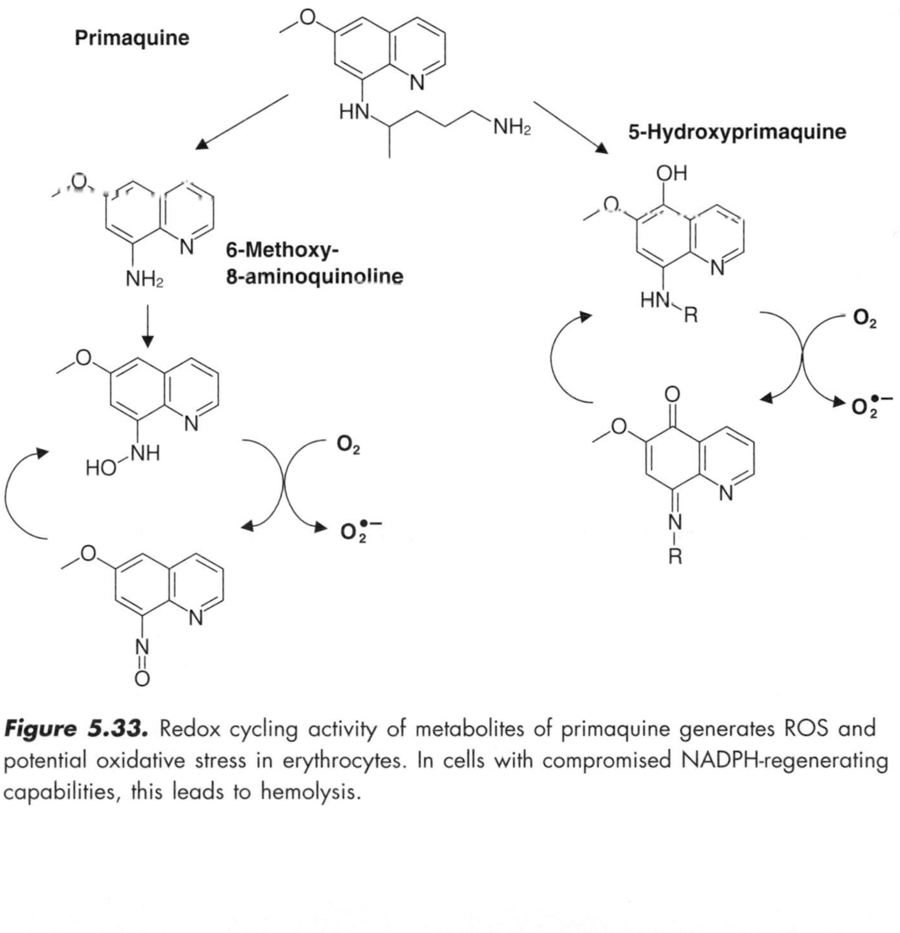

Figure 5.33. Redox cycling activity of metabolites of primaquine generates ROS and potential oxidative stress in erythrocytes. In cells with compromised NADPH-regenerating capabilities, this leads to hemolysis.

Favism is a hemolytic crisis (sometimes life-threatening) that is caused by the ingestion of fava beans (*Vicia faba*) in susceptible individuals with a low activity of G6PD, and it occurs in particular in Mediterranean countries. The two candidate components of the fava beans have been identified as **divicine** and **isouramil**, present as β-glucosides (vicine and convicine). The mechanisms are not entirely clear, but it has been demonstrated that divicine causes a marked oxidative stress, even in normal erythrocytes. Divicine depletes GSH, induces rapid formation of mixed GS-protein disulfides, and activates the hexose monophosphate shunt. It also oxidatively damages the erythrocyte's cytoskeleton by oxidation of sulfhydryl groups.

Besides GSH and its associated enzyme systems, a similar, less famous but equally important enzyme system has gained increasing significance in keeping proteins in a reduced state: thioredoxin.

Thioredoxin: TRX is a small (12 kD) and ubiquitous protein which contains at least two critical thiol groups. It is involved in reducing protein disulfide bonds and also plays a role as an ROS scavenger. It is oxidized to thioredoxin disulfide and regenerated to the thiol by thioredoxin reductase. Thioredoxin plays an important role in cell growth, proliferation, protein folding, and gene activation. Thioredoxin can be upregulated under conditions of oxidative stress. Analogously to GSH, there is also a TRX peroxidase.

The role of TRX is illustrated by the oxidative stress posed by the anticancer drug bleomycin, which has been incriminated in lung toxicity (see section 5.1.3). Murine fibrosarcoma cells which were transfected with human TRX were considerably more resistant to bleomycin-induced cytotoxicity than cells lacking this antioxidant. Furthermore, when mice are exposed to bleomycin, TRX in the lung is strongly induced (and selectively induced *vis-à-vis* other antioxidants, e.g. Mn-SOD, catalase, or GS-Px).

5.3.2. Superoxide dismutase

The pivotal role of SOD has been mentioned in section 5.1.2. Another example which illustrates that SOD plays a paramount and direct role as an antioxidant is ethanol-induced liver injury.

Ethanol is hepatotoxic, but the mechanisms underlying alcohol-induced liver injury are multiple and complex. Alcoholic liver disease is characterized by early fat accumulation and hepatitis, followed by liver fibrosis and cirrhosis. It has been clearly established that oxidative stress is involved as one important factor in the etiology of ethanol injury. One candidate reactive species is the α-hydroxyethyl radical derived from ethanol by CYP2E1 activation, but evidence suggests that this radical (although found in urine and bile) is not the major culprit. Instead, it is now generally believed that Kupffer cell-derived ROS play a major role in ethanol-induced oxidative stress. These resident macrophages produce ROS via NADPH oxidase (see section 5.1.4). Indeed, mice which are genetically deficient in p47[phox], a crucial subunit of NADPH oxidase, are protected from ethanol-induced liver injury in a murine model, and destruction of Kupffer cells with gadolinium chloride (GdCl$_3$ is an agent experimentally used to selectively eliminate Kupffer cells and other hepatic macrophages) also protects from ROS production.

Mechanism of SOD protection against ethanol-induced oxidative stress in the liver: Ethanol ingestion increases the permeability of the intestine for Gram-negative bacterial endotoxin (lipopolysaccharide, LPS). In the blood, LPS binds to LPS-binding protein (LPS-BP), which can activate cells in an LPS-BP-dependent or -independent manner. Specifically, LPS is a potent activator of Kupffer cells in the liver, which release both ROS and proinflammatory cytokines, including tumor necrosis factor-α (TNFα). One of the major ROS produced is superoxide anion radical, which dismutates to hydrogen peroxide. The latter is rapidly inactivated by both catalase and GS-Px, which are both abundant in the liver. In contrast, super-oxide anion, if not eliminated by dismutation, can activate a number of signaling pathways that aggravate the oxidative stress.

The crucial role of SOD can be demonstrated, for example, by overexpressing SOD in the liver (see section 5.1.2). This was experimentally achieved in rats by adenovirus-mediated transfection of both hepatocytes and Kupffer cells with Zn-Cu-SOD, resulting in a two- to three-fold increase in SOD levels over endogenous levels, and which persisted for >3 weeks. This overexpression and enhanced activity of SOD protects from ethanol-induced oxidative stress and development of fatty liver (see Figure 5.34).

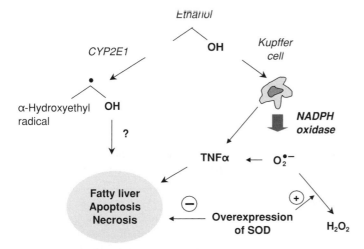

Figure 5.34. Kupffer cell-mediated production of superoxide anion by ethanol. The resulting oxidative stress and early stages of liver injury can be prevented by overexpression of SOD.

The therapeutic use of SOD or GS-Px has also been explored clinically. As these antioxidants are proteins, their therapeutic application poses several obvious problems. One way to circumvent these problems is to use nonpeptidyl SOD mimics (e.g. Mn-TBAP = Mn(III)-tetrakis (5,10,15,20)-benzoic acid). Similarly, a clinically used nonpeptidyl GS-Px mimic is ebselen. So far, the therapeutic success of these enzyme mimics has been rather limited.

Another therapeutically widely used antioxidant is N-acetylcysteine (NAC). The acetylated form of cysteine (cysteine is unstable) acts as a precursor for GSH, a radical scavenger, and has been proven effective as an anti-apoptogen and antioxidant, as it maintains protein thiols in the reduced state. NAC is used successfully in oxidative lung injury, inflammation, AIDS, and reperfusion injury.

5.3.3. Metallothionein

Metals are toxicologically important and notorious oxidants of intracellular thiols. They can even inactivate protein function. Endogenous antioxidants specifically counteract and quench some of these toxic effects. Such endogenous metal scavengers can be induced upon increased oxidative stress. An important group are the metallothioneins which protect from heavy metals, e.g. cadmium.

Metals, including cadmium and mercury (see section 2.1.1), are potentially nephrotoxic, although through different mechanisms. **Cadmium** is especially dangerous because it has a long biological $t_{1/2}$ (20–30 years) and bioaccumulates in tissues. It has, therefore, gained importance not only in workplace safety but also as an environmental pollutant. Because the intestinal absorption of Cd is poor (<8 percent) but on the other hand inhaled Cd readily penetrataes the alveolar epithelia and gets into the bloodstream, the respiratory pathway is an important route of delivery (especially in cigarette smokers). To be taken up into epithelial cells, Cd^{2+} 'mimics' Ca^{2+} and enters the cells via calcium channels.

Cadmium is a typical xenobiotic that exerts its toxicity via slow accumulation. Acute intoxications (in the workplace) are rare; nevertheless, lung injury or mucosal damage of the intestine have been described; at high doses also liver injury. In contrast, chronic toxicity has a clear organotropy; the kidneys are mostly affected, where Cd can accumulate in the cortex. Nephrotoxicity is manifested by increased proteinuria with a progressive damage to proximal tubuli.

Mechanisms of metal-induced thiol oxidation: Cadmium is not a Fenton metal (see section 5.1.2), but it is able to displace other metal ions from protein binding sites. The major characteristic, however, that underlies the toxicity of Cd and Hg is that these metals can avidly bind to and inactivate thiol-containing molecules. Both metals have a great affinity to nucleophilic sites, but in particular to reduced sulfur atoms of endogenous compounds including glutathione, cysteine, homocysteine, metallothionein, and albumin. For example, the affinity constant for mercury binding to thiolate anions is 10^{15} to 10^{20}, whereas the affinity constant for other nucleophilic groups, e.g. carbonyl or amino groups, is approximately ten orders of magnitude lower.

In the presence of high concentrations of such thiol-containing compounds, mercuric ions bind to two partners. In contrast, methylmercury forms 1:1 complexes with thiol-containing molecules. For example, mercuric ions first bind to the sulf-hydryl groups of albumin. However, during the first few hours after initial exposure, the concentrations of albumin-bound mercury decrease, and the content of mercury in the proximal tubular cells increases. Most probably, the mercuric ions are trans-ported in the body by binding to small molecular weight thiols.

In the kidney, it is interesting that dose–response curves associated with mercury are very steep, i.e. toxicity occurs rapidly after a certain threshold has been crossed. This can be best explained by the presence of protective thiols, such as glutathione, in the cells, acting like a buffer. When the capacity of these thiols is exceeded, then toxicity may shoot up. Experimental evidence has revealed that mercury also binds to, and may deplete, thiols within mitochondria. Other targets in cells have not been identified, but membrane proteins can be altered, affecting the permeability of the membrane. Alternatively, due to the depletion of intracellular thiols, the redox balance may be shifted towards increased oxidative stress.

Heavy metal-induced oxidative stress induces specific responses, the most dramatic being the synthesis of metallothionein. Not only does metallothionein inactivate the metal from exerting its thiol-reactivity, but the presence and upregulation of this antioxidant also explain the kidney-selective toxicity of Cd after chronic exposure to Cd.

Role of metallothionein: MT is a ubiquitous low molecular weight (6.5 kD) protein. Its most unique feature is that 30 percent of the amino acid residues of MT are cysteines. Therefore, the protein has a large number of sulfhydryl groups, which can be coordinated by heavy metal ions. In fact, one molecule of MT can bind seven atoms of Cd. The affinity constant for Cd is 10^{16}, which is extremely high and approximately 10^{10} times higher than Cd's affinity for other nucleophilic groups. Thus, MT can sequester heavy metals and prevent oxidation of critical protein or non-protein (GSH) thiol groups. In line with this concept, MT-null (knockout) mice exhibit increased susceptibility to Cd. Besides Cd, MT can also sequester other metal ions (e.g. Zn or Cu), although with lower affinity.

There are two major isoforms of MT in mammalians, MT-I and MT-II, which differ slightly in the amino acid sequence, and which are encoded by two distinct MT genes (other MT isoforms have been identified, but their contribution in mediating nephrotoxicity is minor).

Due to the high –SH content, MT can also protect from non-metal-induced oxidative stress caused by ROS or other prooxidants. Furthermore, MT has been shown to specifically stabilize redox-sensitive processes that are involved in prevent-ing apoptosis. In fact, MT can migrate into the cell nucleus, where it binds to and stabilizes NF-κB (see Chapter 7).

Mechanisms of metallothionein induction and Cd-induced nephrotoxicity: The constitutive levels of MT are low, but MT is readily induced upon a variety of cellular stresses, including exposure to metals, but also other forms of xenobiotic-induced oxidative stress. How are the genes for MT selectively activated? The proximal upstream region of MT genes contains an antioxidative response element and a metal response element, conferring the response to ROS.

Induction of MT is the mechanism that can explain the well-known tolerance phenomenon afforded by a small dose of Cd towards a subsequent higher and normally even lethal dose of Cd. Leading to a similar result, MT-I overexpression in transgenic mice protects against Cd-induced acute toxicity.

However, in contrast to the acute toxic effects, mostly in the liver, nephrotoxicity is a chronic effect. The Cd–MT complex is excreted from the liver and reaches the systemic circulation. Due to the small size of MT, the complex can easily cross the glomerular filter (the cutoff for larger molecules is at approximately 50 kD) and reach the tubular lumen. The Cd–MT complex is then taken up at the apical side of proximal tubular cells and accumulates in the epithelial cells. Upon lysosomal degradation of the protein, the Cd is liberated and, if the concentrations exceed a certain threshold (>300 µg Cd/g cortical tissue), the metal can exert its nephrotoxic effects. These are mediated by oxidation of critical sulfhydryl groups, but also by a displacement of other ions from MT or from metal-dependent enzymes (see Figure 5.35).

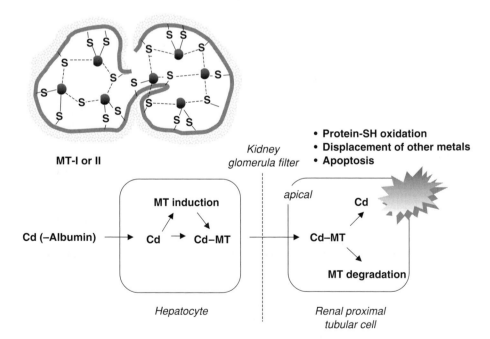

Figure 5.35. Metallothionein (MT) induction by cadmium and Cd-induced nephrotoxicity. Above, structural model of MT (dots = coordinating metal ions).

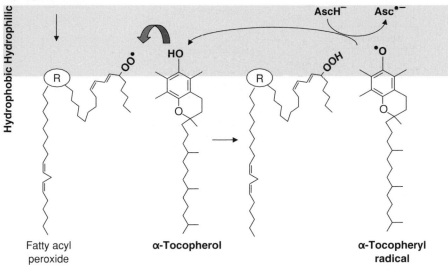

Oxidative stress
Lipid peroxidation

Fatty acyl peroxide

α-Tocopherol

α-Tocopheryl radical

Figure 5.36. α-Tocopherol reduces a lipid peroxide radical and prevents further chain reaction of lipid peroxidation. The oxidized α-tocopherol is regenerated by ascorbate.

5.3.4. α-Tocopherol

To prevent the propagation of lipid peroxidation (see section 5.2.3), there are specific antioxidant defense systems in the cell's hydrophobic environment. The major one is vitamin E, which is actually a mixture of several tocopherols. Among these, α-tocopherol is the most important.

α-Tocopherol consists of a lipophilic phytyl tail and a more hydrophilic chroman head featuring a phenolic group. This phenolic group can reduce radicals (e.g. lipid peroxy radicals) arising from lipid peroxidation processes and is thereby oxidized in turn to the tocopheryl radical. However, this tocopheryl radical is stabilized and relatively unreactive. It is regenerated by ascorbate (vitamin C) which in turn is kept in its reduced state by GSH (see Figure 5.36).

5.4. Intracellular signaling and gene regulation by oxidative stress

Earlier concepts had always put much emphasis on the direct macromolecule-damaging effects of ROS. Thus, xenobiotics had been implicated in causing cell injury by direct oxidation of lipids, proteins, and nucleic acids, which would lead to their loss of function and/or structure. This is certainly true in some cases, in particular when the initial oxidative stress in a cell, triggered by a xenobiotic, is amplified, e.g. by infiltrating macrophages and/or PMNs. However, in many instances, the phalanx of antioxidant defense systems is so strong that the cell can resist a modest oxidoreductive challenge.

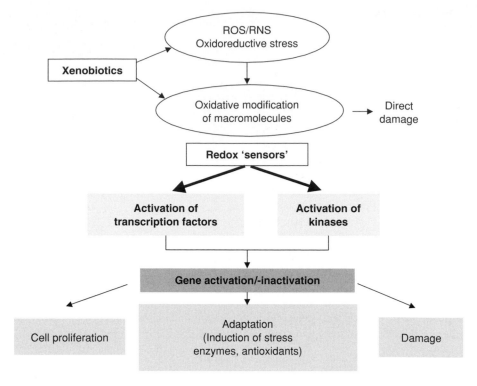

Figure 5.37. Oxidative stress-induced signaling pathways via transcription factors or kinase cascades mediate selective gene activation.

More recently, newer concepts have gained broad acceptance. These concepts imply that oxidoreductive stress in a cell not only modifies target macromolecules but also alerts a number of 'redox sensors' (mostly via thiol oxidation), and that these redox sensors alter cell signaling, which ultimately leads to specific gene activation. There are several levels of oxidative stress; a low level is required for normal tissue homeostasis (e.g. is involved in cell proliferation). Intermediate levels of oxidative stress cause selective gene activation and protein expression which can be considered an adaptive response to this increased oxidative stress (e.g. antioxidants, stress proteins). It is only in these cases when there is a high level of oxidative stress that the signaling pathways cause cell demise by apoptosis or necrosis (see Figure 5.37).

Mechanisms of oxidative stress-mediated gene activation: An example that illustrates how the production of oxidative stress in a cell can activate a number of genes involved in an antioxidant or stress response is polycyclic aromatic hydrocarbons (PAHs). These compounds exert multiple effects in a cell and trigger multiple pathways that lead to downstream biological effects (including covalent binding to DNA (see section 9.3) and activation of the AH receptor (see section 12.1)). However, one important feature of bioactivated PAHs is that they generate oxidative stress. For example, benzo[a]pyrene is subject to redox cycling following metabolic activation.

Benzo[a]pyrene (BaP) is a prototype xenobiotic and toxicologically one of the best studied PAH. It is a ubiquitous environmental contaminant that is produced by various combustion processes and occurs in cigarette smoke and charbroiled food.

Due to its lipophilicity, BaP is readily taken up by cells. BaP is extensively metabolized by CYP1A1 and subsequent phase II enzymes. One of the major metabolites is BaP-1,6-hydroquinone. This hydroquinone can be autoxidized to the BaP-1,6-semiquinone and finally to the BaP-1,6-quinone. During the redox cycling of these intermediates, ROS are generated that are involved in the activation of a stress response (see Figure 5.38).

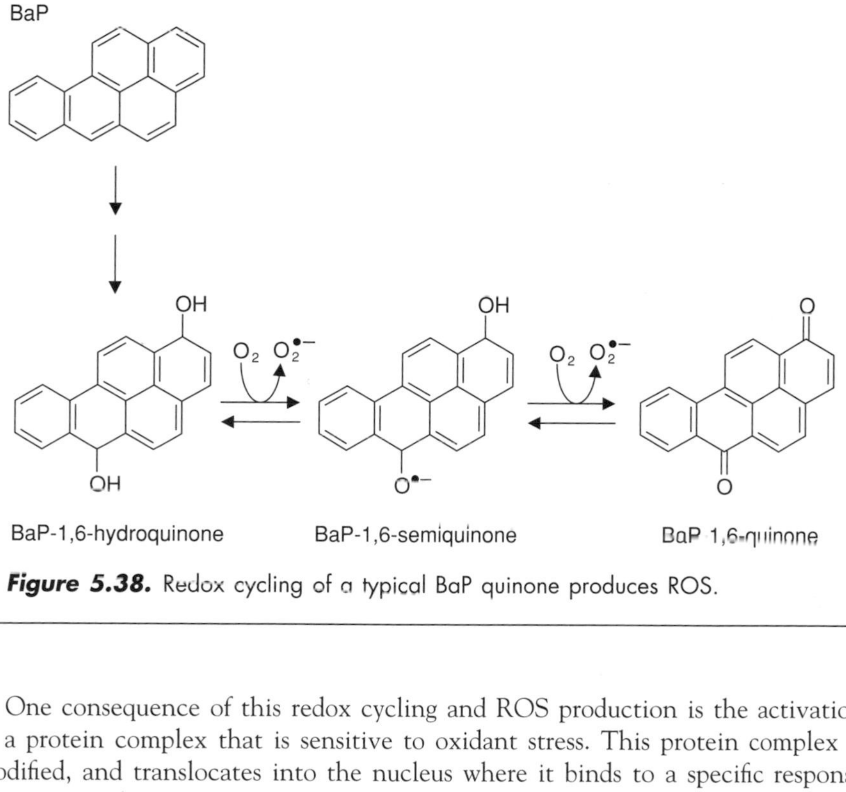

BaP

BaP-1,6-hydroquinone   BaP-1,6-semiquinone   BaP 1,6-quinone

Figure 5.38. Redox cycling of a typical BaP quinone produces ROS.

One consequence of this redox cycling and ROS production is the activation of a protein complex that is sensitive to oxidant stress. This protein complex is modified, and translocates into the nucleus where it binds to a specific response element in the promoter region of specific genes involved in an antioxidant response. The response is pleiotropic (causing multiple phenotypic effects from a single cause).

This particular protein complex is found in many different cell types and responds to a number of different activators. The details of the signaling process have only slowly been emerging. It is known that the complex can bind to and transactivate the 'antioxidant response element' (ARE) (sometimes referred to as the 'electrophilic response element', EpRE). The ARE is located in the 5′ region of critical target genes (stress genes). It is a regulatory sequence involved in basal and inducible expression of several genes involved in detoxication and antioxidant

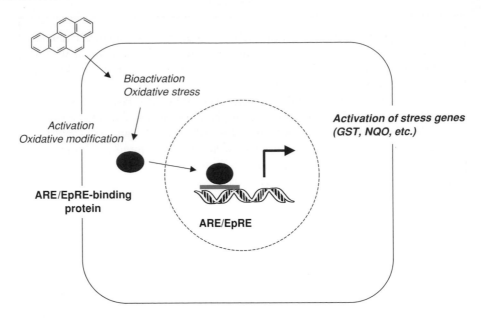

Figure 5.39. Oxidative stress (and electrophilic metabolites) of benzo[a]pyrene can modify and thus activate a protein complex in the cell, the ARE/EpRE-binding protein. This ARE/EpRE-binding protein translocates into the nucleus where it binds to the ARE/EpRE (antioxidant/electrophilic response element), located in the promoter region of genes involved in antioxidant and stress response.

defense. For example, it activates certain isoforms of GST, NQO, ALDH, enzymes involved in GSH synthesis, and c-Ha-ras (an oncogene). The ARE not only binds PAH-modified binding protein complexes but also responds in the same way to other prooxidants, including hydrogen peroxide or t-butylhydroperoxide. Thus, it appears as though it is a general response to a potential oxidative threat to the cell (activation of 'cellular bodyguards'). If the oxidant stress is moderate, these cellular reactions to the potential insult can be compensated or antagonized. Therefore, the mere presence of the upregulated genes does not necessarily indicate toxicity. Instead, this upregulation can be ideally used as a marker indicative of oxidant stress. However, if high oxidant stress levels are maintained or if repeated exposure to high doses occurs, then the cell may succumb to the insult (see Figure 5.39).

A typical antioxidant enzyme which is up-regulated via ARE as a response to oxidative stress and as a cytoprotective mechanism is heme oxygenase. In the promoter region of the heme oxygenase-1 (HO-1) gene, there are multiple copies of the ARE, which makes it a powerful sensor. Exposure of cells to a variety of prooxidant xenobiotics, including cadmium and other metals, H_2O_2 and other ROS, quinones, but also diesel exhaust particles, readily induces HO-1. The findings that HO-1-deficient mice (and humans!) exhibit a greatly attenuated defense against xenobiotic-induced oxidative stress underline the current belief that HO-1 is a powerful antioxidant.

Heme oxygenase-1 (HO-1) is the rate-limiting enzyme in the degradation of heme, converting it to biliverdin. Biliverdin in turn is degraded by biliverdin reductase to bilirubin. Induction of HO-1 results in a decrease in the cell's heme and heme-containing protein pool, which is a way to limit potential prooxidants (i.e. Fenton-reactive iron). In addition, the resulting bilirubin acts as an anti-oxidant (it is a scavenger of oxygen radicals). The constitutive form of heme oxygenase, HO-2, is also an antioxidant but acts via different mechanisms.

Because of its sensitivity, induction of HO-1 is also frequently used as a marker for oxidative stress in a cell.

Oxidant sensors in a cell are mainly cysteinyl residues whose redox status determines their activities. In fact, many transcription factors are regulated by one or several oxidant-dependent mechanisms. A toxicologically relevant example is the NF-κB pathway.

NF-κB (nuclear factor-κB): This is a transcription factor that is activated by a number of stimuli including oxidative stress. It plays a central role in the regulation of many genes involved in antioxidant defense, anti-apoptosis, immunological responses, cytokine production, and others. In the promoter region of all these NF-κB-responsive genes there is a functional NF-κB-binding site. The active NF-κB protein is a dimer of two subunits, named by their molecular mass, p50 and p65. The inactive form of NF-κB is found in the cytoplasm and is kept in its inactive form by an inhibitor protein, I-κB. Upon stimulation, I-κB is phosphorylated, ubiquitinated and rapidly degraded. The free NF-κB then rapidly translocates into the nucleus, where it binds to the DNA.

Practically all stimuli that can activate NF-κB can be blocked by antioxidants. In fact, even the phosphorylation of I-κB can be blocked by antioxidants, strongly suggesting that the I-κB kinases are activated by oxidative stress or directly by ROS (see Figure 5.40).

Another redox-sensitive transcription factor is AP-1. This oxidative stress-activated signaling and transcription pathway is involved in the response to asbestos and other particles. This results in cell proliferative activity in the lung.

AP-1 (activator protein-1): This is a family of transcription factors which specifically bind to and transactivate genes containing the TPA (12-O-tetradecanoyl phorbol-13-acetate)-response element (TRE). The transcription factor is a heterodimer or homodimer formed by the subunits Fos–Jun or Jun–Jun (Fos and Jun are gene products of the immediate–early response gene families). AP-1 binds to the TREs in the promoter region of many genes including cytokines but also cyclins (involved in the cell cycle).

Oxidative stress readily induces transcription of c-jun and c-fos, so-called protooncogenes (because they are also involved in cell proliferation and cell cycle and play a role in carcinogenesis). These protooncogenes encode the transcription factor AP-1. This leads to activation of AP-1, binding to the regulatory DNA elements, and increase in transcription of genes involved in cell proliferation. However, other genes involved in antioxidative defense are also controlled by AP-1 (for example, Mn-SOD).

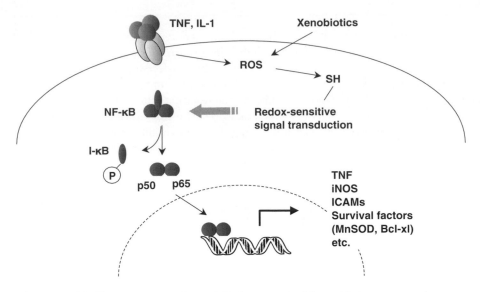

Figure 5.40. The transcription factor NF-κB is activated by oxidative stress and induces the transcription of target genes.

It is unlikely that AP-1 transactivates through the antioxidant response element, ARE (see above), because, with a few exceptions, AREs have no perfect TRE, and binding of AP-1 to ARE is poor.

The presence of prooxidants, or other xenobiotic-induced alterations in the cellular redox status, contributes to the activation of these transcription factors. For example, transactivation is greatly decreased by pretreating cells with the antioxidant and GSH precursor, N-acetylcysteine. Alternatively, exposing cells to buthionine sulfoximine, a specific inhibitor of γ-glutamylcysteine synthetase, greatly stimulates DNA binding and transactivation, because the cellular GSH pool is depleted and oxidative stress has increased.

Mechanisms of oxidative stress-mediated signal transduction: Xenobiotic-induced oxidative stress not only induces the transcription of many genes but also regulates the activity of preexisting proteins. In particular, prooxidant xenobiotics can be involved in many forms of signal transduction. Signal transduction is the transmission of a molecular signal triggered by hormones, growth factors, cytokines, etc. at a cell surface receptor and/or via second messengers all the way down to a final metabolic target or to a genetic target in the nucleus. These signaling pathways often proceed via self-amplifying cascades of protein kinases and phosphatases. Interestingly, but perhaps not surprisingly, ROS and increased oxidative stress can mimic some of these pathways and induce cell proliferation in many cells.

ROS can regulate the signal transduction because many of the proteins involved in transmitting these signals exhibit critical and reactive cysteinyl residues, the redox status of which is crucial for their activity. For example, redox cycling xenobiotics can activate protein kinase C through oxidation of the enzyme's thiol groups. Other serine/threonine protein kinases, and the mitogen-activated protein (MAP) kinase pathway, are also activated by ROS which alter the redox status of these kinases.

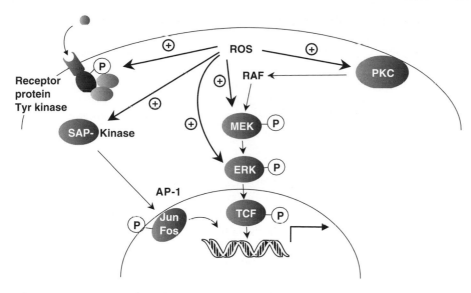

Figure 5.41. ROS and oxidative stress activate the protein kinase cascade by oxidizing (and thus activating) the kinases' thiol groups. Mitogen-activated protein (MAP) kinase pathways include extracellular signal-regulated kinase (ERK) and the stress-activated protein (SAP) kinases, as well as upstream and downstream kinases.

In addition, oxidative stress not only activates kinase activity but also inhibits protein phosphatases, thus amplifying the activating effects. In maintaining the redox homeostasis, intracellular glutathione is a key regulator (see Figure 5.41).

In addition, oxidative stress can also modulate other major systems involved in cellular signaling. For example, ROS can affect the thiol status at receptors that are involved in Ca^{2+} signaling, as well as possibly activate the arachidonic acid pathway and the cAMP pathway. Thus, the same signals that trigger cellular events, e.g. proliferation, are also related to inducing an adaptive response against increased oxidative stress. However, while the physiological signals that are modulated by redox events are usually transient, of short duration, and quantitatively minor, those xenobiotic-induced oxidative stress signals that cause major damage or even cell demise are often sustained, of longer duration, and quantitatively of greater impact.

Learning points

- Oxidative stress not only is involved in direct cell injury but, importantly, mediates signal transduction and regulates gene expression.
- Enzymatic or non-enzymatic multistep reduction of molecular oxygen leads to partially reduced oxygen intermediates.
- ROS are generated intracellularly by redox cycling xenobiotics (e.g. quinones), by uncouplers of monooxygenases, or by compounds which divert electrons from the electron transport chain in mitochondria.
- Redox-active transition metals (Fe, Cu) are critical because they can catalyze the Fenton reaction, which leads to the generation of the ultra-reactive hydroxyl

radical. The distribution of these metals thus largely determines the site of oxidative damage.

- ROS can be generated extracellularly by the activation of the plasma membrane-bound NADPH oxidase, which is a hallmark of phagocytes. Therefore, macrophages and PMNs, recruited to sites of primary injury, can cause extensive oxidative stress and enhance the damage.

- Nitric oxide is an RNS which can condense with superoxide anion to peroxynitrite, an intermediate that has been implicated in the toxicity of some NO-generating xenobiotics.

- DNA, in particular dG, is a frequent target of highly reactive ROS. Oxidation can change the base pairing behavior, leading to mismatch and, if not repaired, introduction of a point mutation upon DNA replication.

- Membrane lipid peroxidation is dangerous not only because it is a self-progagating chain reaction destroying lipid bilayers, but also because reaction products include reactive aldehydes which can augment the toxicity.

- Upon oxidative stress there is an adaptive antioxodative response. Major biological antioxidants are GSH, a radical scavenger, thiol reductant, and electrophile scavenger, and α-tocopherol, a chain-breaking antioxidant in the lipid phase.

- Metallothionein is a cysteine-rich small protein which can bind and sequester cadmium and other heavy metals.

- Redox sensors in the cell are modified by prooxidant xenobiotics. They can in turn activate transcription factors such as NF-κB and AP-1, or activate redox-sensitive kinase cascades, and thus activate specific sets of genes.

Further reading

ROS and oxidoreductive stress

Davies, K.J.A. (2000) Oxidative stress, antioxidant defenses, and damage removal, repair, and replacement systems, *IUBMB Life* 50: 279–289.

Kehrer, J.P. (1993) Free radicals as mediators of tissue injury and disease, *Crit. Rev. Toxicol.* 23: 21–48.

Xenobiotic-induced intracellular ROS production

Bolton, J.L., Trush, M.A., Penning, T.M., Dryhurst, G. and Monks, T.J. (2000) Role of quinones in toxicology, *Chem. Res. Toxicol.* 13: 135–160.

Dinkowa-Kostova, A.T. and Talalay, P. (2000) Persuasive evidence that quinone reductase type 1 (DT diaphorase) protects cells against the toxicity of electrophiles and reactive forms of oxygen, *Free Radic. Biol. Med.* 29: 231–240.

Gut, I., Nedelcheva, V., Soucek, P., Stopka, P., Vodicka, P., Gelboin, H.V. and Ingelmansundberg, M. (1996) The role of CYP2E1 and 2B1 in metabolic activation of benzene derivatives, *Arch. Toxicol.* 71: 45–56.

Monks, T.J., Hanzlik, R.P., Cohen, G.M., Ross, D. and Graham, D.G. (1992) Quinone chemistry and toxicity, *Toxicol. Appl. Pharmacol.* 112: 2–16.

O'Brien, P.J. (1991) Molecular mechanisms of quinone cytotoxicity, *Chem.-Biol. Interact.* 80: 1–41.

Puntarulo, S. and Cederbaum, A.I. (1998) Production of reactive oxygen species by microsomes enriched in specific human cytochrome P450 enzymes, *Free Radic. Biol. Med.* 24: 1324–1330.

Snyder, R., Witz, G. and Goldstein, B.D. (1993) The toxicology of benzene, *Environ. Health Perspect.* 100: 293–306.

Subrahmanyam, V. and Smith, M.T. (1997) Free-radical-mediated hematopoietic toxicity by drugs, environmental pollutants, and ionizing radiation, *Free Radical Toxicology*, Wallace, K.B. (ed.), Taylor & Francis, Washington, DC, pp. 249–278.

Wang, Y.J., Lee, C.C., Chang, W.C., Liou, H.B. and Ho, Y.S. (2001) Oxidative stress and liver toxicity in rats and human hepatoma cell line induced by pentachlorophenol and its major metabolite tetrachlorohydroquinone, *Toxicol. Lett.* 122: 157–169.

Aminotransferases

Amacher, D.E. (1998) Serum transaminase elevations as indicators of hepatic injury following the administration of drugs, *Reg. Toxicol. Pharmacol.* 27: 119–130.

Matsuzawa, T., Kobayashi, T., Ogawa, H. and Kasahara, M. (1997) Microheterogeneity and intrahepatic localization of human and rat liver cytosolic alanine aminotransferase, *Biochim. Biophys. Acta* 1340: 115–122.

Iron chelators

Barbouti, A., Doulias, P.T., Zhu, B.Z., Frei, B. and Galaris, D. (2001) Intracellular iron, but not copper, plays a critical role in hydrogen peroxide-induced DNA damage, *Free Radic. Biol. Med.* 31: 490–498.

Epsztejn, S., Kakhlon, O., Glickstein, H., Breuer, W. and Cabantchik, Z.I. (1997) Fluorescence analysis of the labile iron pool of mammalian cells, *Anal. Biochem.* 248: 31–40.

Hider, R.C. (1995) Potential protection from toxicity by oral iron chelators, *Toxicol Lett.* 82–83: 961–967.

Kontoghiorghes, G.H. (1995) Comparative efficacy and toxicity of desferrioxamine, deferiprone and other iron and aluminium chelating drugs, *Toxicol. Lett.* 80: 1–18.

Rothman, R.J., Serroni, A. and Farber, J.L. (1992) Cellular pool of transient ferric iron, chelatable by deferoxamine and distinct from ferritin, that is involved in oxidative cell injury, *Mol. Pharmacol.* 42: 703–710.

Stäubli, A. and Boelsterli, U.A. (1998) The labile iron pool in hepatocytes: prooxidant-induced increase in free iron precedes oxidative cell injury, *Am. J. Physiol (Gastrointest. Liver Physiol.)* 274: G1031–G1037.

Zanninelli, G., Glickstein, H., Breuer, W., Milgram, P., Brissot, P., Hider, R.C., Konijn, A.M., Libman, J., Shanzer, A. and Cabantchik, Z.I. (1997) Chelation and mobilization of cellular iron by different classes of chelators, *Mol. Pharmacol.* 51: 842–852.

Bleomycin-induced pulmonary toxicity

Gon, Y., Sasada, T., Matsui, M., Hashimoto, S., Takagi, Y., Iwata, S., Wada, H., Horie, T. and Yodoi, J. (2001) Expression of thioredoxin in bleomycin-injured airway epithelium. Possible role of protection against bleomycin induced epithelial injury, *Life Sci.* 68: 1877–1888.

NADPH oxidase

Segal, A.W. and Abo, A. (1993) The biochemical basis of the NADPH oxidase of phagocytes, *Trends Biochem. Sci.* 18: 43–47.

Asbestos-induced lung fibrosis

Kamp, D.W. and Weitzman, S.A. (1997) Asbestosis: clinical spectrum and pathogenic mechanisms, *Proc. Soc. Exp. Biol. Med.* 214: 12–26.

Moyer, V.D., Cistulli, C.A., Vaslet, C.A. and Kane, A.B. (1994) Oxygen radicals and asbestos carcinogenesis, *Environ. Health Perspect.* 102: 131–136.

Vallyathan, V. and Shi, X. (1997) The role of oxygen free radicals in occupational and environmental lung diseases, *Environ. Health Perspect.* 105 (Suppl. 1): 165–177.

Varani, J. and Ward, P.A. (1997) Activation of the inflammatory responses by asbestos and silicate mineral dusts, *Free Radical Toxicology*, Wallace, K.B. (ed.), Taylor & Francis, Washington, DC, pp. 295–322.

Ozone toxicity

Paterson, J.F., Hammond, M.D., Montgomery, M.R., Sharp, J.T., Farrier, S.E. and Balis, J.U. (1992) Acute ozone-induced lung injury in rats: Structural–functional relationship of developing alveolar edema, *Toxicol. Appl. Pharmacol.* 117: 37–45.

RNS and oxidative stress

Aoki, K., Ohmori, M., Takimoto, M., Ota, H. and Yoshida, T. (1997) Cocaine-induced liver injury in mice is mediated by nitric oxide and reactive oxygen species, *Eur. J. Pharmacol.* 336: 43–49.

Ghafourifar, P., Schenk, U., Klein, S.D. and Richter, C. (1999) Mitochondrial nitric-oxide synthase stimulation causes cytochrome *c* release from isolated mitochondria, *J. Biol. Chem.* 274: 31185–31188.

Cocaine and oxidative stress

Boelsterli, U.A., Wolf, A. and Göldlin, C. (1993) Oxygen free radical production mediated by cocaine and its ethanol-derived metabolite, cocaethylene, in rat hepatocytes, *Hepatology* 18: 1154–1161.

Devi, B.G. and Chan, A.W.K. (1996) Cocaine-induced peroxidative stress in rat liver: antioxidant enzymes and mitochondria, *J. Pharmacol. Exp. Ther.* 279: 359–366.

Devi, B.G. and Chan, A.W.K. (1997) Cocaine-induced increase of Mn-SOD in adult rat liver cells, *Life Sci.* 61: 1245–1251.

Diez-Fernandez, C., Zaragoza, A., Alvarez, A.M. and Cascales, M. (1999) Cocaine cytotoxicity in hepatocyte cultures from phenobarbital-induced rats: Involvement of reactive oxygen species and expression of antioxidant defense system, *Biochem. Pharmacol.* 58: 797–805.

Toxicological consequences of oxidative stress

Hoglen, N.C., Younis, H.S., Hartley, D.P., Gunawardhana, L., Lantz, R.C. and Sipes, I.G. (1998) 1,2-Dichlorobenzene-induced lipid peroxidation in male Fischer 344 rats is Kupffer cell dependent, *Toxicol. Sci.* 46: 376–385.

Younis, H.S., Hoglen, N.C., Kuester, R.K., Gunawardhana, L. and Sipes, I.G. (2000) 1,2-Dichlorobenzene-mediated hepatocellular oxidative stress in Fischer-344 and Sprague-Dawley rats, *Toxicol. Appl. Pharmacol.* 163: 141–148.

Oxidative DNA damage

Gottschling, B.C., Maronpot, R.R., Hailey, J.R., Peddada, S., Moomaw, C.R., Klaunig, J.E. and Nyska, A. (2001) The role of oxidative stress in indium phosphide-induced lung carcinogenesis in rats, *Toxicol. Sci.* 64: 28–40.

Kawanishi, S., Inoue, S., Oikawa, S., Yamashita, N., Toyokuni, S., Kawanishi, M. and Nishino, K. (2001) Oxidative DNA damage in cultured cells and rat lungs by carcinogenic nickel compounds, *Free Radic. Biol. Med.* 31: 108–116.

Richter, C. (1997) Free-radical-mediated DNA oxidation, *Free Radical Toxicology*, Wallace, K.B. (ed.), Taylor & Francis, Washington, DC, 89–113.

Waalkes, M.P. (1995) Metal carcinogenesis, *Metal Toxicology*, Goyer, R.A., Klaassen, C.D. and Waalkes, M.P. (eds), Academic Press, San Diego, CA, pp. 47–69.

Oxidative protein damage
Shacter, E. (2000) Quantification and significance of protein oxidation in biological samples, *Drug Metab. Rev.* 32: 307–326.
Shringarpure, R., Grune, T. and Davies, K.J.A. (2001) Protein oxidation and 20S proteasome-dependent proteolysis in mammalian cells, *Cell. Mol. Life Sci.* 58: 1442–1450.

Methemoglobin formation and hemotoxicity
Bolchoz, L.J.C., Budinsky, R.A., McMillan, D.C. and Jollow, D.J. (2001) Primaquine-induced hemolytic anemia: Formation and hemotoxicity of the arylhydroxylamine metabolite 6-methoxy-8-hydroxylaminoquinoline, *J. Pharmacol. Exp. Ther.* 297: 509–515.
Dalle-Donne, I., Rossi, R., Milzani, A., Di Simplicio, P. and Colombo, R. (2002) The actin cytoskeleton response to oxidants: From small heat shock protein phosphorylation to changes in the redox state of actin itself, *Free Radic. Biol. Med.* 31: 1624–1632.
Donnelly, G.B. and Randlett, D. (2000) Methemoglobinemia, *New Engl. J. Med.* 343: 337.

Oxidative lipid damage
Chaudhary, A.K., Nokubo, M., Reddy, G.R., Yeola, S.N., Morrow, J.D., Blair, I.A. and Marnett, L.J. (1994) Detection of endogenous malondialdehyde–deoxyguanosine adducts in human liver, *Science* 265: 1580–1582.
Farber, J.L. (1994) Mechanisms of cell injury by activated oxygen species, *Environ. Health Perspect.* 102: 17–24.
Göldlin, C. and Boelsterli, U.A. (1991) Reactive oxygen species and non-peroxidative mechanisms of cocaine-induced cytotoxicity in rat hepatocyte cultures, *Toxicology* 69: 79–91.
Scott, M.D. and Eaton, J.W. (1997) Markers of free-radical-mediated tissue injury: Tales of caution and woe, *Free Radical Toxicology*, Wallace, K.B. (ed.), Taylor & Francis, Washington, DC, 401–420.
Sevanian, A. and McLeod, L. (1997) Formation and biological reactivity of lipid peroxidation products, *Free Radical Toxicology*, Wallace, K.B. (ed.), Taylor & Francis, Washington, DC, 47–70.

Carbon tetrachloride-induced hepatotoxicity
Dai, Y. and Cederbaum, A.I. (1995) Inactivation and degradation of human cytochrome P4502E1 by CCl4 in a transfected HepG2 cell line, *J. Pharmacol. Exp. Ther.* 275: 1614–1622.
Hartley, D.P., Kolaja, K.L., Reichard, J. and Petersen, D.R. (1999) 4-Hydroxynonenal and malondialdehyde hepatic protein adducts in rats treated with carbon tetrachloride: Immunochemical detection and lobular localization, *Toxicol. Appl. Pharmacol.* 161: 23–33.

Interference with antioxidant defense mechanisms
Yin, X., Wu, H., Chen, Y. and Kang, Y.J. (1998) Induction of antioxidants by adriamycin in mouse heart, *Biochem. Pharmacol.* 56: 87–93.

Glutathione

Bellomo, G., Vairetti, M., Stivala, L., Mirabelli, F., Richelmi, P. and Orrenius, S. (1992) Demonstration of nuclear compartmentalization of glutathione in hepatocytes, *Proc. Natl Acad. Sci. USA* 89: 4412–4416.

DeLeve, L.D. and Kaplowitz, N. (1991) Glutathione metabolism and its role in hepatotoxicity, *Pharmac. Ther.* 52: 287–305.

Kaplowitz, N., Fernandezcheca, J.C., Kannan, R., Garciaruiz, C., Ookhtens, M. and Yi, J.R. (1996) GSH transporters: molecular characterization and role in GSH homeostasis, *Biol. Chem. Hoppe Seyler* 377: 267–273.

Reed, D.J. (1990) Glutathione: Toxicological implications, *Annu. Rev. Pharmacol. Toxicol.* 30: 603–631.

Genetic deficiency in erythrocyte G6PD

Luzzatto, L. and Notaro, R. (2001) Protecting against bad air, *Science* 293: 442–443.

Primaquine hemotoxicity

Bolchoz, L.J.C., Budinsky, R.A., McMillan, D.C. and Jollow, D.J. (2001) Primaquine-induced hemolytic anemia: Formation and hemotoxicity of the arylhydroxylamine metabolite 6-methoxy-8-hydroxylaminoquinoline, *J. Pharmacol. Exp. Ther.* 297: 509–515.

Favism

McMillan, D.C., Bolchoz, L.J.C. and Jollow, D.J. (2001) Favism: Effect of divicine on rat erythrocyte sulfhydryl status, hexose monophosphate shunt activity, morphology, and membrane skeletal proteins, *Toxicol. Sci.* 62: 353–359.

Thioredoxin

Arner, E.S.J. and Holmgren, A. (2000) Physiological functions of thioredoxin and thioredoxin reductase, *Eur. J. Biochem.* 267: 6102–6109.

Gon, Y., Sasada, T., Matsui, M., Hashimoto, S., Takagi, Y., Iwata, S., Wada, H., Horie, T. and Yodoi, J. (2001) Expression of thioredoxin in bleomycin-injured airway epithelium. Possible role of protection against bleomycin induced epithelial injury, *Life Sci.* 68: 1877–1888.

Powis, G. and Montfort, W.R. (2001) Properties and biological activities of thioredoxins, *Annu. Rev. Pharmacol. Toxicol.* 41: 261–295.

SOD protection in the liver

Kono, H., Rusyn, I., Yin, M., Gäbele, E., Yamashina, S., Dikalova, A., Kaduska, M.B., Connor, H.D., Mason, R.P., Segal, B.H., Bradford, B.U., Holland, S.M. and Thurman, R.G. (2000) NADPH oxidase-derived free radicals are key oxidants in alcohol-induced liver disease, *J. Clin. Invest.* 106: 867–872.

Wheeler, M.D., Kono, H., Yin, M., Rusyn, I., Froh, M., Connor, H.D., Mason, R.P., Samulski, R.J. and Thurman, R.G. (2001) Delivery of the Cu/Zn-superoxide dismutase gene with adenovirus reduces early alcohol-induced liver injury in rats, *Gastroenterology* 120: 1241–1250.

Metal-induced thiol oxidation

Zalups, R.K. (2000) Molecular interactions with mercury in the kidney, *Pharmacol. Rev.* 52: 113–143.

Metallothionein
Dalton, T., Palmiter, R.D. and Andrews, G.K. (1994) Transcriptional induction of the mouse metallothionein-I gene in hydrogen peroxide-treated HeLa cells involves a composite major late transcription factor/antioxidant response element and metal response promoter elements, *Nucleic Acids Res.* 22: 5016–5023.
Vasak, M. and Hasler, D.W. (2000) Metallothioneins: New functional and structural insights, *Curr. Opinion Chem. Biol.* 4: 177–183.

Metallothionein induction and Cd-induced nephrotoxicity
Klaassen, C.D. and Liu, J. (1997) Role of metallothionein in cadmium-induced hepatotoxicity and nephrotoxicity, *Drug Metab. Rev.* 29: 79–102.
Park, J.D., Liu, Y. and Klaassen, C.D. (2001) Protective effects of metallothionein against the toxicity of cadmium and other metals, *Toxicology* 163: 93–100.

α-Tocopherol
Buettner, G.R. (1993) The pecking order of free radicals and antioxidants: Lipid peroxidation, α-tocopherol, and ascorbate, *Arch. Biochem. Biophys.* 300: 535–543.

Oxidative stress-mediated gene activation
Dalton, T.P., Shertzer, H.G. and Puga, A. (1999) Regulation of gene expression by reactive oxygen, *Annu. Rev. Pharmacol. Toxicol.* 39: 67–101.
Kass, G.E.N. (1997) Free-radical-induced changes in cell signal transduction, *Free Radical Toxicology*, Wallace, K.B. (ed.), Taylor & Francis, Washington, DC, 349–374.
Li, N., Venkatesan, M.I., Miguel, A., Kaplan, R., Gujuluva, C., Alam, J. and Nel, A. (2000) Induction of heme oxygenase-1 expression in macrophages by diesel exhaust particle chemicals and quinones via the antioxidant-responsive element, *J. Immunol.* 165: 3393–3401.
Miller, K.P. and Ramos, K.S. (2001) Impact of cellular metabolism on the biological effects of benzo[a]pyrene and related hydrocarbons, *Drug Metab. Rev.* 33: 1–35.
Sreerama, L. and Sladek, N.E. (2001) Three different stable human breast adenocarcinoma sublines that overexpress ALDH3A1 and certain other enzymes, apparently as a conseqence of constitutively upregulated gene transcription mediated by transactivated EpREs (electrophilic responsive elements) present in the 5′-upstream regions of these genes, *Chem.-Biol. Interact.* 130–132: 247–260.
Suzuki, Y.J., Forman, H.J. and Sevanian, A. (1997) Oxidants as stimulators of signal transduction, *Free Radic. Biol. Med.* 22: 269–285.
Timblin, C.R., Janssen, Y.M.W. and Mossman, B.T. (1997) Free-radical-mediated alterations of gene expression by xenobiotics, *Free Radical Toxicology*, Wallace, K.B. (ed.), Taylor & Francis, Washington, DC, 325–348.

Nuclear factor κ-B
Ginn-Pease, M.E. and Whisler, R.L. (1998) Redox signals and NF-κB activation in T cells, *Free Radic. Biol. Med.* 25: 346–361.

Chapter 6

Disruption of cellular calcium homeostasis

Contents

6.1. Xenobiotic-induced alterations in intracellular Ca^{2+} distribution

6.2. Toxicological consequences of increased intracellular Ca^{2+} concentrations

Calcium-dependent processes have been implicated in a number of molecular mechanisms underlying the toxicity of many xenobiotics. Unlike the metals discussed in the preceding chapter, Ca^{2+} is not redox-active itself and is therefore not involved in the generation of oxidative stress. Cellular oxidative stress can, however, dramatically alter calcium homeostasis, and this can have severe consequences for a cell.

The reason lies in calcium's pivotal physiological role in regulating cellular metabolism, in activating many enzymes and other proteins, and in acting as a second messenger. In fact, Ca^{2+} controls a vast array of cellular processes due to the versatility of the signaling mechanisms. It seems logical that cells have acquired rigorous control mechanisms to fine-tune the distribution and availability of intracellular calcium and to regulate its concentration and compartmentation in cells.

It is exactly this central role of calcium, however, that makes a cell vulnerable to potentially harmful chemicals which target this Achilles' heel. For example, if xenobiotics activate some of the calcium-dependent processes by abruptly altering calcium homeostasis, and if they interfere at one or several sites with the compensatory and regulatory processes, a cascade of events may be triggered that may even culminate in the precipitation of cell death.

6.1. Xenobiotic-induced alterations in intracellular Ca²⁺ distribution

Because of its pivotal role in regulating many cellular processes, intracellular 'free' Ca^{2+} concentrations are kept at a very low level. This is accomplished by a number of mechanisms.

The bulk of the body's **calcium** (99 percent) is stored in the skeleton. However, calcium ions are also dissolved in body fluids, and these extracellular concentrations are high (approximately 1 mM). In sharp contrast, intracellular concentrations of calcium are about four orders of magnitude lower and kept in the range of 100 nM. This enormous concentration gradient constantly causes Ca^{2+} to leak from extracellular compartments into the cytosol. However, the intracellular concentrations of Ca^{2+} are rigorously maintained at low levels by both calcium-binding proteins and calcium pumps, i.e. ATP-dependent transporters present in both the plasma membrane and the membranes of the endoplasmic reticulum. These pumps effectively transport Ca^{2+} either out of the cell or into the ER lumen. Indeed, the ER has compartmentalized Ca^{2+} at high concentrations (>100 μM), i.e. approximately 1,000-fold higher than in the cytosol.

In contrast, mitochondria play only a minor role in storing large amounts of intracellular Ca^{2+} (although they constantly cycle small amounts of Ca^{2+} in and out during the normal physiological process). The mitochondrial Ca^{2+} transporter has a lower affinity and is ten-fold less efficient in transporting Ca^{2+} into mitochondria than the other pumps. Therefore, mitochondria become important only if the cell is flooded with high concentrations of calcium and may then act as a 'safety valve'.

Certain xenobiotics can interfere with these Ca^{2+}-sequestering mechanisms. They can do so by attacking the cell at a number of targets and in different ways. For example, a nonspecific increase in the permeability of the plasma membrane leads to a rapid influx of Ca^{2+} ions. Alternatively, xenobiotics can modify the calcium pumps of the plasma membrane or the ER either by oxidative damage or by covalently binding to these structures. This invariably leads to an increase in $[Ca^{2+}]_i$ which, if not immediately compensated for, can lead to irreversible damage.

An example of a group of xenobiotics that specifically damage the calcium-sequestering mechanisms and hence increase the intracellular free calcium concentrations is organotin (and other organometal) compounds.

Tri-*n*-butyltin (TBT) and other organotin compounds have frequently been used as pesticides with a variety of applications. For example, TBT has found application as a molluscicide and antifoulant on boats, ships, and fish nets, and as a biocide in cooling systems, paper mills, breweries, etc. Due to this widespread use, TBT is now found ubiquitously in the environment and poses a potential hazard to many species including mammals. The most important targets of toxicity are the immune system (thymus), neurons, the liver, and skin.

Tri-*n*-butyltin has a variety of adverse cellular effects including a direct action on energy homeostasis in mitochondria. However, one of its best-studied effects is damage to the endoplasmic reticulum with subsequent release of Ca^{2+}.

Other organotin compounds have similar effects on cells. For example, increasing the alkyl chain length from triethyltin to tripropyltin up to TBT is associated with increasing potency of the compounds to release Ca^{2+}. This may be due to a combination of the hydrophobic interactions of the side chain and specific effects of the central tin atom.

Mechanisms of TBT-induced cell injury: Tri-*n*-butyltin chloride (or a metabolite of it) has been implicated in relasing Ca^{2+} from intracelluar stores including the ER and causing sharp increases in $[Ca^{2+}]_i$. The current hypothesis holds that organotin compounds directly interact with thiol groups of the calcium pump. This is inferred from the observations that TBT induces a rapid depletion of thiols, and that several TBT-induced effects can be prevented by thiol-reducing agents. The major consequence of calcium pump damage is the rapidly increasing intracellular calcium levels to approximately 500 or 600 nM (depending on the dose of TBT), which is sufficient to trigger a cascade of cellular effects which result in either necrotic or apoptotic cell death (Figure 6.1) (see Chapter 7).

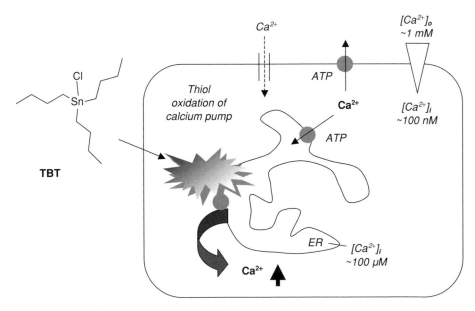

Figure 6.1. Tri-*n*-butyltin (TBT) chloride causes mobilization of Ca^{2+} from the endoplasmic reticulum and results in a rapid increase of $[Ca^{2+}]_i$. The filled circles on the plasma membrane and ER membrane represent ATP-dependent calcium transporters.

6.2. Toxicological consequences of increased intracellular Ca^{2+} concentrations

A fundamental question that has been discussed over and over again is whether the pathological increases in intracellular calcium might be the actual *cause* of toxicity, or whether high $[Ca^{2+}]_i$ is rather a *consequence* of irreversibly damaged cells and thus only a biomarker of a preceding injury. Such a debate perhaps seems obsolete because both cases might be true. While it is true that calcium levels are invariably increased in lethally damaged and necrotic cells as a logical consequence of membrane permeability alterations and the great concentration gradients between intra- and extracellular compartments, and while there are examples showing that cells can be injured without a causative role of calcium, there are many paradigms in which sustained increases in intracellular Ca^{2+} concentrations indeed represent the primary trigger for a self-amplifying reaction leading to irreversible tissue damage.

To provide a proof of concept that calcium is indeed causally involved in cell injury, at least two prerequisites have to be fulfilled: first, the increases in $[Ca^{2+}]_i$ must precede cell injury, and second, prevention of these increases in $[Ca^{2+}]_i$ should prevent cell injury. Both issues have been resolved.

The consequences of xenobiotic-induced increases in $[Ca^{2+}]_i$ are manifold, and this initial rise in calcium is a point of convergence among many downstream mechanisms. For example, low concentrations of calcium-disrupting xenobiotics (e.g. tri-*n*-butyltin) cause moderate increases in calcium and lead to Ca^{2+}-dependent caspase activation and apoptosis (see Chapter 7). Alternatively, higher concentrations of such xenobiotics can cause many additional effects; excessive Ca^{2+} release from intracellular stores causes activation of a number of calcium-dependent proteins. Among these are Ca^{2+}-dependent proteases, endonucleases, and lipases, all of which can contribute to lethal cell injury.

First, one of the major effects of increased $[Ca^{2+}]_i$ is activation of calpains (calcium-dependent cysteine proteases). These proteases have become well-known because they have been implicated in disrupting protein components of the cytoskeleton.

Calpains are non-lysosomal, Ca^{2+}-dependent proteolytic enzymes. About 15 mammalial calpain forms have been described, the m- and the μ-forms being ubiquitous. Calpains exist as zymogen heterodimers; upon activation by Ca^{2+} they are processed autolytically and form heterodimers. Because activation might become dangerous for the cell, calpains are also regulated by an endogenous inhibitor, calpastatin. Once activated, calpains cleave preferentially at valine, leucine, or isoleucine residues at the next-to-terminal positions of a target protein.

If calpains are over-activated, e.g. by sudden and extensive increases in $[Ca^{2+}]_i$, they can cleave intracellular critical proteins. However, not all proteins are equally vulnerable; in fact, most of them are resistant against calpains. Among the most sensitive protein targets are cytoskeletal proteins, including spectrin, vimentin,

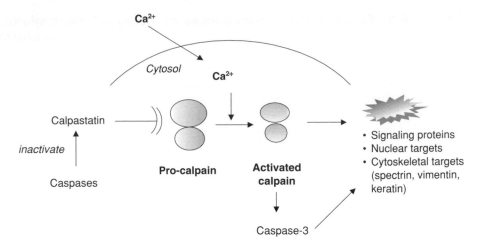

Figure 6.2. Increased cytosolic Ca^{2+} levels activate calpains. These proteases selectively attack protein targets which they share as substrates with some caspases. Some calpain-sensitive proteins are components of the cytoskeleton.

and keratin, but also plasma membrane-associated proteins (e.g. growth factor receptors). In addition, calpains can also cleave proteins involved in signal transduction pathways and transcription factors. If calpain activation remains modest, then this can result in non-lethal signaling; if, on the other hand, calpains are over-activated, then their proteolytic activity might culminate in cell death. Calpains actually can facilitate apoptosis by assisting certain caspases in the proteolytic process because they share a number of substrates (e.g. the cytoskeletal proteins) with caspases (see Figure 6.2).

The second consequence of increases in $[Ca^{2+}]_i$ affects the nucleus. Calcium-dependent endonucleases can be activated and result in DNA single- and double-strand breaks and apoptotic or necrotic cell death. Perhaps the most compelling evidence for a direct and causal role of Ca^{2+} in activation of endonucleases, DNA damage, and necrotic (and/or apoptotic) cell death stems from experiments with cytotoxic concentrations of acetaminophen (APAP). Acetaminophen is bioactivated to a reactive metabolite which is both an oxidizing species and a protein-arylating intermediate (see section 9.2.1). This reactive intermediate causes an increase in $[Ca^{2+}]_i$, which has a pleiotropic response but in which endonuclease activation plays a key role. Specifically, APAP damages double-stranded intact DNA and causes disruption of genomic integrity. Sequestration and inactivation of Ca^{2+} with the calcium chelator, EGTA (ethylene glycol-bis(b-aminoethyl ether) N′, N′, N′, N′-tetraacetic acid) completely protects cells from DNA damage and subsequent cell death induced by APAP in cultured hepatocytes. One might argue that such chelators are not specific for a single ion species and that EGTA can also coordinate other metals including Fe^{3+}/Fe^{2+} ions. However, the selectivity for Ca^{2+} is very high, and, importantly, EGTA–Fe complexes are still highly redox active, thus minimizing the possibility that the protection from cytotoxicity might be due to inhibition of Fenton-type reactions. Taken together, the fact that the changes in Ca^{2+} levels and the DNA

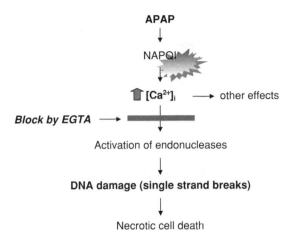

Figure 6.3. Intracellular free calcium is directly involved in activation of endonucleases, DNA damage, and cell death. Chelation of Ca^{2+} by EGTA blocks all downstream events. APAP, acetaminophen; NAPQI, *N*-acetyl-*p*-benzoquinoneimine.

damage precede cell injury and the fact that inactivation of the available 'free' Ca^{2+} by a chelating agent prevents toxicity clearly demonstrate a pivotal mechanistic role of calcium (see Figure 6.3).

The third consequence of increased $[Ca^{2+}]_i$ is activation of calcium-dependent phospholipases. In particular, phospholipase A_2 activation can cause liberation of arachidonic acid and disruption of membrane integrity, leading to necrotic cell death. Besides these changes of the plasma membrane, phospholipase activation has also been implicated in mitochondria. Here, increases in Ca^{2+} would lead to activation of phospholipase A_2 in the inner mitochondrial membrane, leading to an accumulation of lysophospholipids and non-esterified fatty acids. Indeed, high concentrations of these latter have been implicated in the induction of the mitochondrial membrane permeability transition and the opening of the pore, which could culminate in lethal cell death (see sections 7.2.4 and 15.5).

A fourth and related consequence of increased $[Ca^{2+}]_i$ affects another mitochondrial function. As stated above, mitochondria can transiently take up small amounts of Ca^{2+} from the cytosol, but they have to release it again in order not to become permanently damaged. This 'calcium cycling' is achieved through an antiport system which exports calcium in exchange for Na^+ (in heart, muscle, and brain mitochondria) or H^+ (in liver and kidney mitochondria). In the latter case, transporter function is regulated by ADP-ribosylation of an acceptor protein of the inner mitochondrial membrane, which is derived from degradation of NAD^+. Excessive cycling (due to calcium overload in the cell) not only causes depletion of NAD^+ but also results in a collapse of the mitochondrial membrane potential (see section 15.1) and a severe energy crisis due to ATP depletion. This invariably leads to cell death.

Finally, increased intracellular Ca^{2+} concentrations can activate gene expression; for example, immediate-early genes (including MAP kinases and c-*fos*, c-*myc*, and

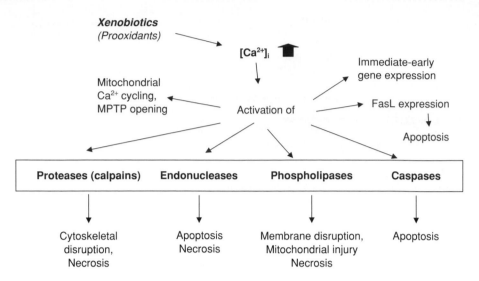

Figure 6.4. Multiple consequences of prooxidant-induced increases in intracellular Ca²⁺ concentrations.

c-jun, which are involved in cell replication) become activated. In addition, calcium mediates the expression of ligands that activate the Fas death receptor pathway which induces apoptosis (see Figure 6.4).

To make things more complex, all these pathways that are activated by xenobiotic-induced increases in intracellular calcium levels, and many of those not mentioned here, are interdependent, and a cross-talk exists between them. We are far from understanding the complex regulatory mechanisms, but undoubtedly it has become clear that calcium is an important mediator of cell death in xenobiotic-induced cell injury.

Learning points

- Intracellular Ca^{2+} concentrations are finely regulated and kept to a low level because free calcium is a second messenger and activator of many pathways involved in critical cellular processes. Xenobiotics which disrupt the Ca^{2+}-sequestration in the ER or extracellular space therefore greatly increase $[Ca^{2+}]_i$ levels and disrupt this homeostasis.
- Moderately increased Ca^{2+} leads to caspase activation and increased FasL expression and can thus initiate apoptosis. In contrast, higher levels of cytosolic Ca^{2+} can activate calpains, endonucleases, and phospholipases A_2, all of which have been implicated in necrotic cell death.
- Sustained increases in Ca^{2+} concentrations in mitochondria can cause opening of the membrane permeability transition pore and result in ATP depletion. Furthermore, extended calcium cycling in mitochondria disrupts mitochondrial function.
- Ca^{2+} can induce the expression of immediate-early genes.

Further reading

Alterations in intracellular Ca²⁺ distribution

Berridge, M.J., Lipp, P. and Bootman, M.D. (2000) The versatility and universality of calcium signalling, *Nature Rev. Mol. Cell Biol.* 1: 11–21.

Kass, G.E.N. and Orrenius, S. (1999) Calcium signaling and cytotoxicity, *Environ. Health Perspect.* 107 (Suppl. 1): 25–35.

Trump, B.F. and Berezesky, I.K. (1995) Calcium-mediated cell injury and cell death, *FASEB J,* 9: 219–228.

TBT-induced cell injury

Kawanishi, T., Kiuchi, T., Asoh, H., Shibayama, R., Kawai, H., Ohata, H., Momose, K. and Hayakawa, T. (2001) Effect of tributyltin chloride on the release of calcium ion from intracellular calcium stores in rat hepatocytes, *Biochem. Pharmacol.* 62: 863–872.

Stridh, H., Gigliotti, D., Orrenius, S. and Cotgreave, I. (1999) The role of calcium in pre- and postmitochondrial events in tributyltin-induced T-cell apoptosis, *Biochem. Biophys. Res. Commun.* 266: 460–465.

Zaucke, F., Zöltzer, H. and Krug, H.F. (1998) Dose-dependent induction of apoptosis or necrosis in human cells by organotin compounds, *Fresenius J. Anal. Chem.* 361: 386–392.

Calpains

Huang, Y. and Wang, K.K.W. (2001) The calpain family and human disease, *Trends Molec. Med.* 7: 355–362.

Wang, K.K.W. (2000) Calpain and caspase: Can you tell the difference?, *Trends Neurosci.* 23: 20–26.

DNA damage and cell death

Ray, S.D., Kamendulis, L.M., Gurule, M.W., Yorkin, R.D. and Corcoran, G.B. (1993) Ca²⁺ antagonists inhibit DNA fragmentation and toxic cell death induced by acetaminophen, *FASEB J.* 7: 453–463.

Salas, V.M. and Corcoran, G.B. (1997) Calcium-dependent DNA damage and adenosine 3′,5′-cyclic monophosphate-independent glycogen phosphorylase activation in an *in vitro* model of acetaminophen-induced liver injury, *Hepatology* 25: 1432–1438.

Chapter 7

Mechanisms of necrotic and apoptotic cell death

Contents

Cell death by necrosis or apoptosis is the ultimate endpoint of lethal cell injury induced by xenobiotics. This multistep process is executed through different upstream mechanisms. Initiating events triggering these processes include the production of reactive metabolites, excessive oxidative stress, covalent binding, and direct signaling from receptor activation.

The mechanisms leading to the induction of cell death, in particular apoptosis, are extremely complex. From a biological point of view, it also 'makes sense' that these processes are tightly regulated and that there are a number of control mechanisms upstream to the 'point of no return'. In fact, there are a number of checkpoints where decisions are made as to whether a cell is further pushed towards demise or whether the process comes to a stop and the cell is rescued.

Although necrosis and apoptosis are two mutually exclusive ways of cell demise, either option is present in a cell. Importantly, the same exogenous trigger (including xenobiotics, but also other factors) can induce either the apoptotic or the necrotic pathway. However, depending on the cellular energy status and the duration and extent of the insult, both modes of cell demise can occur in the same tissue.

7.1. Mechanisms of necrosis

Many reactive metabolites, but also direct membrane-damaging xenobiotics, cause acute lethal cell injury leading to necrosis. This pathway of cell demise, which often occurs in a number of adjacent cells or even large tissue areas, is particularly frequent if cells are exposed to high concentrations of a toxic xenobiotic and if the duration of exposure is prolonged.

Necrosis, historically, is a morphological term that describes the consequences of acute cell death. These include cell swelling and rupture, usually followed by an inflammatory response. Necrosis has also been termed 'accidental cell death', underlining that this mode of cell demise is a passive event and an unscheduled process. Lethal cell injury is first characterized by swollen organelles, pyknotic nuclei (fragmentation, condensation, then lysis), and the formation of small 'blebs' (small protruding bubble-like plasma membrane projections). When the cell membrane finally ruptures and the cell undergoes lysis, cytosolic constituents are released into the extracellular space (highly increased levels of cell-specific markers are therefore found in the peripheral blood).

Mechanisms of necrotic cell death: Necrosis is the result of damage to a number of cellular constituents including the plasma membrane. Several mechanisms alone or in combination can initiate and promote necrotic cell death. These include plasma membrane permeability changes, which lead to a collapse of ion homeostasis, followed by cell and organelle swelling and culminating in rupture of the cell membrane. Necrosis-promoting mechanisms are oxidative stress, mitochondrial damage and ATP depletion, or activation of Ca^{2+}-dependent proteases, phospholipases, and endonucleases (see Chapter 6.)

For a given xenobiotic, the exact mechanisms leading to necrosis are not always known because the sequence of events is complex and because many of these molecular events are causally interrelated with other mechanisms. Cause and effect cannot always be dissected from each other. Nevertheless, a common early hallmark of the processes that accompany necrosis is a disassembly of the cytoskeleton and loss of plasma membrane–cytoskeleton attachment. Furthermore, cellular ATP pools are depleted, which can lead to inactivation of ATP-dependent ion pumps in the plasma membrane and ER, causing a rapid alteration of Na^+, K^+, Mg^{2+}, and Ca^{2+} homeostasis. Alternatively, these ion pumps can also be directly damaged by, for example, oxidative modification or by modification through reactive metabolites. The execution of necrosis does not require ATP and is a passive process. In contrast to apoptosis, DNA fragmentation is a late event, and it occurs by random digestion (see Figure 7.1).

7.2. Apoptosis

Unraveling of the mechanisms of xenobiotic-induced apoptosis has seen enormous progress in recent years. Although many issues are still unresolved, the resolution of many underlying molecular events and their control mechanisms has given us more insight into these complex mechanisms of cell death.

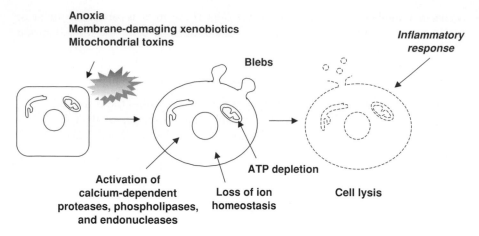

Figure 7.1. General mechanisms of necrosis.

7.2.1. Molecular mechanisms and pathways of apoptosis

In contrast to necrotic cell death, apoptosis is a highly organized mode of cell demise, following tightly regulated pathways and involving both transcriptional and post-transcriptional gene activation. Furthermore, and again distinct from necrotic cell death, apoptosis is tightly linked (through oncogenes and tumor suppressor genes) with the machinery that controls cell proliferation and DNA repair.

Apoptosis, like necrosis, was also first characterized entirely on morphological criteria. Apoptosis, however, was detected much later than necrosis and is still a relatively young area of research. It is likely to have escaped for a long time from becoming recognized as a highly important mechanism of cell demise because apoptosis is a discrete process, occurring rapidly, and often, but not always, involving single cells rather than large areas of tissue. Because apoptosis is involved in many physiological processes (e.g. during ontogenesis, tissue modeling, and cell turnover) it has also been termed 'programmed cell death', underlining that the initiation and progression of cell demise is genetically determined. Meanwhile it has become general knowledge that this inherent 'suicide' program is present in all cells and that it can be activated by a chemical insult. In other words, in contrast to the physiological role of apoptosis, where the time of onset of apoptosis is also programmed, apoptosis can also be triggered anytime by xenobiotics.

Molecular mechanisms of apoptotic cell death (I): Apoptosis, in contrast to necrosis, is an active, energy-consuming process. The sequence of events, at the morphological and biochemical level, reflects the fact that the initiation and progression of cell demise is a concerted action, surgically dissecting intracellular critical constituents and targets rather than randomly destroying the cell.

One of the earliest events, after the cell has received a signal which starts the process of apoptosis, is the activation of specific proteases, the caspases (aspartate-specific cysteine proteases). There are basically two types of caspases; one type act as activators of other caspases, thus amplifying the initial effects. The second type of caspases are the real executors of cell demise, as these proteolytic enzymes break down critical cellular constituents. During this entire process, the plasma membrane remains intact, preventing intracellular components from leaking into the extra-cellular space (which is one of the reasons why there is no inflammatory response during apoptosis).

The first morphological changes are seen in the nucleus, where the chromatin is condensed. At the molecular level, DNA is fragmented by caspase-activated endonu-cleases. Typically, this cleavage of the DNA occurs between histone octamers (not at specific restriction sites; in other words, DNA cleavage is not dependent on the sequence). This internucleosomal DNA cleavage generates a variety of fragments which are multitudes of 200 base pairs and which in agarose gels therefore lead to the typical 'ladder' pattern. Besides caspase-activated endonucleases, another endonuclease has recently been discovered. Endonuclease G (endoG), a mitochondrion-specific nuclease, translocates to the nucleus during apoptosis. Once released from mitochondria, endoG cleaves chromatin DNA into nucleosomal fragments independently of caspases.

Besides DNA and nuclear proteins, other cellular proteins are also degraded by caspases, and this leads to a rapid and global collapse of the cell. The cell body (still with the intact plasma membrane) forms small extrusions which can become detached from the remaining cell (apoptotic bodies), and the entire cell shrinks. This can occur within minutes. Macrophages and other cells then clean up and phagocytose the apoptotic bodies, a process which occurs rapidly (in the liver, for example, in approximately 3 h).

How do phagocytes recognize a cell doomed to undergo apoptosis? It is widely accepted that this is brought about by phosphatidylserine, a phospholipid normally strictly confined to the inner leaflet of the plasma membrane by active processes, now appearing at the outside of the plasma membrane. Whether this is a specific 'eat me' signal, tagging the cell for being phagocytosed by neighboring cells, or just a consequence of altered phospholipid sorting, is not known (see Figure 7.2).

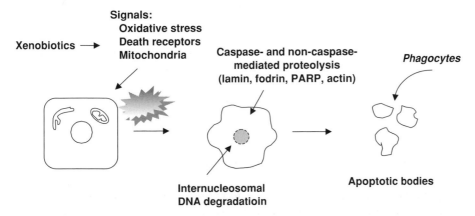

Figure 7.2. General mechanisms of apoptosis.

A variety of xenobiotics have the potential to induce apoptosis in different tissues, and they can trigger cell demise by different initiating mechanisms. Among these, excessive oxidative stress and its downstream signaling cascades are a major and critical initiator of apoptosis. A typical and toxicologically important example is heavy metals that are present naturally or as contaminants in the environment. Here, arsenic and its well-known neurotoxic effects, which have been attributed in part to apoptosis, will be highlighted as a paradigm.

Arsenic is an environmental toxicant produced from industrial use but which is also naturally present in ground water. The chemistry and metabolism of arsenicals is complex. Inorganic As^{3+} (arsenite) is the most toxic form. *In vivo*, the major biotransformation product of inorganic arsenite is the (pentavalent) dimethylarsenic acid, which can be found as an excretory product in the urine. Further reduction of the metal to the trivalent state yields mono- or dimethylated As(III) species which have been implicated in chronic toxic effects and even carcinogenesis.

Besides other forms of toxicity, arsenic has been primarily implicated in causing neurotoxic effects, manifested as polyneuropathy with prolonged sensory and motor deficits. Again, inorganic arsenite ($NaAsO_2$) is approximately 1,000-fold more potent than dimethylarsenic acid in producing these neurotoxic effects.

Mechanisms of arsenic-induced neurotoxicity: Multiple mechanisms have been implicated in the toxicity of arsenic, and one of them is apoptosis. In fact, arsenite induces a significant increase in the number of apoptotic cerebellar neurons. This sensitivity to undergo apoptosis seems to be specific for CNS neurons, as non-neuronal cells are much less susceptible to the toxic effects of arsenite. Indeed, arsenite activates neuron-specific kinases (e.g. JNK3 and p38 MAP kinase). This activation is critical for the induction of apoptosis, as inhibition of these kinases by chemical inhibitors greatly reduces the extent of apoptosis. The fact that redox-sensitive kinases are involved points to the possibility that oxidative stress might be involved in triggering arsenic-induced apoptosis (see section 5.4).

Indeed, arsenite, arsenic trioxide, and arsenate (As^V) all produce ROS both *in vivo* and *in vitro* (while the role of methylated arsenicals in producing oxidative stress is less clear). The resulting oxidative stress activates redox-sensitive transcription factors and signaling molecules. Thus, although not the only pathway, apoptosis triggered by oxidative stress is likely to be one of the major mechanisms underlying the neurotoxic effects of arsenic in human brain.

Molecular mechanisms of apoptotic cell death (II): Oxidative stress is just one of the triggering events that activate apoptosis. In addition, there are a number of cellular key players which all have an important role in xenobiotic-induced apoptosis.

1 There are specific plasma membrane receptors, called 'death receptors', which receive the 'suicide' signal and which are involved in the downstream transduction of the signal.

2 Mitochondria play a pivotal role because they can release factors which activate downstream events. These mitochondrial factors can be released following death receptor activation (acting as a transformer of the signal received by the death receptor) or by death receptor-independent stimuli.

3 As already mentioned, there is a group of specific proteases, the caspases, that are involved in initiating, propagating, and executing apoptotic cell death by activating mediators and damaging the final intracellular targets.

4 There are a number of checkpoints where the apoptotic process can be controlled; one of these checkpoints is the Bcl-2 protein family. All these key players will be discussed in more detail below.

Importantly, apoptosis can proceed via two distinct pathways, depending both on the initiating signal and the type of cell that will undergo apoptosis. In the first case, death receptor activation leads to direct activation of caspases that execute cell death. Cells undergoing this direct way of demise are called Type I cells. Here, mitochondria play a secondary role; up-regulation (or direct addition) of the mitochondria-protective protein Bcl-2 does not prevent apoptosis (because mitochondria are circumvented). This mechanism is prevalent, for example, in T cells. The second pathway is a process involving mitochondria in the first place. In this case, mitochondria activate the caspase cascade, either as initiators or following activation through a death receptor signal. Cells using (and exclusively using) this alternative pathway are called Type II cells. Here, Bcl-2 can indeed protect from apoptosis, because this protective protein acts at a proximal site of the cascade. An example for Type II cells is hepatocytes (see Figure 7.3).

7.2.2. Signaling through death receptors

One way by which xenobiotics can trigger apoptosis is by sending signals which cause activation (and sometimes even transcriptional up-regulation) of death receptors (and/or their ligands).

Apoptosis can be initiated by plasma membrane-associated receptors, called **death receptors**. These death receptors belong to the nerve growth factor gene superfamily (also called TNF receptor superfamily, with a growing number of members being identified). Among these, important members are Fas, the TNF receptors, and DR-3, -4 and -5. These receptors all possess an extracellular cysteine-rich domain, a membrane-spanning domain, and an intracellular domain with a common sequence called the 'death domain'. The plasma membrane receptors can trimerize through extracellular interactions. Binding of trimerized receptors with their respective ligands then triggers activation. This happens by recruiting other accessory proteins, forming the DISC (death inducing signal complex). The DISC initiates apoptosis by directly activating the effector caspases 2, 8, and 10 (signaling caspases), which in turn will activate other caspases, e.g. caspases 3, 6, and 7 (effector caspases) which execute the cell death program.

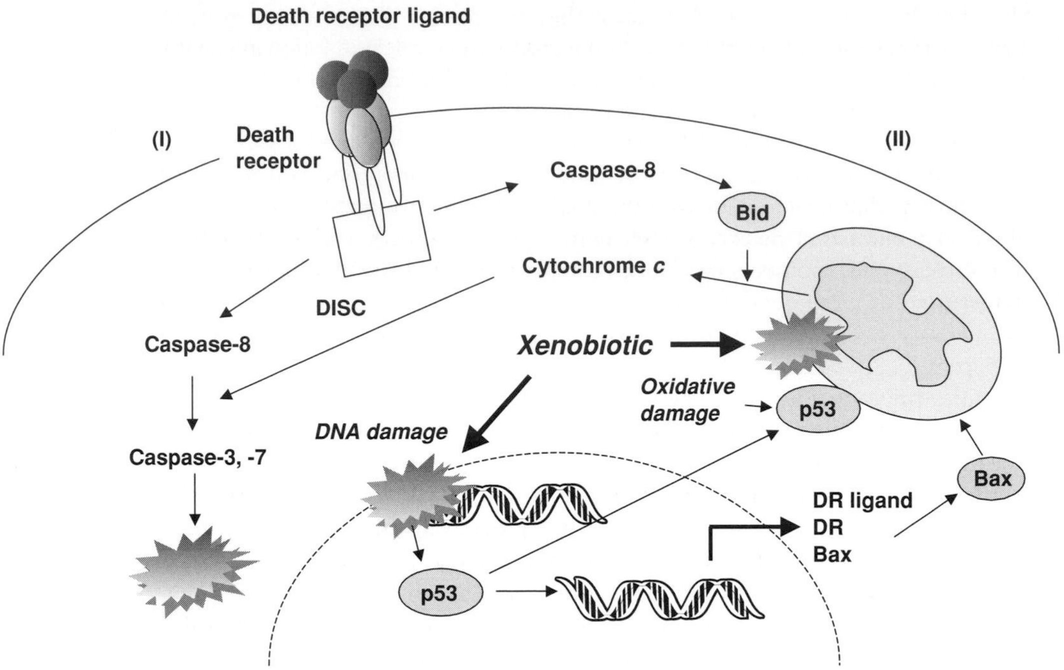

Figure 7.3. The two independent pathways of xenobiotic-induced apoptosis and the role of the key players. (I) Xenobiotic-induced binding of ligands to death receptors causes activation of the death-inducing signal complex (DISC) and direct activation of caspases, resulting in apoptosis. (II) Alternatively, a death receptor-activated caspase can activate Bid, which causes release of cytochrome c from mitochondria. Cytochrome c in turn activates other caspases. Another initial event by which xenobiotics induce apoptosis is by directly damaging DNA or by producing oxidative injury to mitochondria. In response, p53 is activated and induces up-regulation of pro-apoptotic proteins including death receptors (DR) and their ligands, as well as Bax. Alternatively, p53 directly targets mitochondria, initiating cytochrome c release.

One of these death receptors that has been implicated in mediating xenobiotic-induced apoptosis is Fas.

Fas (**CD95**, also called APO-1) is a transmembrane protein and death receptor expressed in many cells. Upon aggregation and trimerization, Fas signals a caspase-mediated cell death cascade. Normally, this reaction is triggered by the Fas ligand (FasL, CD95L).

A number of xenobiotics can promote apoptosis by inducing the synthesis of both Fas and FasL. However, interestingly, receptor trimerization and activation of the death domain can also occur in the absence of the ligand if Fas is overexpressed and abundant in a cell. Because this is potentially dangerous for a cell, Fas is normally sequestered within intracellular pools. Upon need, the receptor is shuttled to the plasma membrane by vesicle transport. Hence, any increase in the density of Fas on the cell surface will increase the propensity to aggregate and cause apoptosis.

One condition under which this mechanism can become effective is xenobiotic-induced cholestasis. This will result in retention and accumulation of toxic bile salts, some of which can trigger the Fas-mediated apoptosis machinery.

One of the most important and toxic bile acids in cholestasis is glycochenodeoxycholate (see section 15.5).

Mechanisms of toxic bile salt-induced Fas activation: Toxic concentrations of glycochenodeoxycholate cause increases in the cell surface expression of Fas. This occurs by accelerating the shuttling of Fas receptor protein from intracellular stores to the plasma membrane. The resulting highly increased receptor density facilitates the oligomerization of Fas on the cell surface and hence results in triggering of the apoptosis cascade (see Figure 7.4).

The second crucial death receptor involved in mediating apoptosis is the TNF receptor.

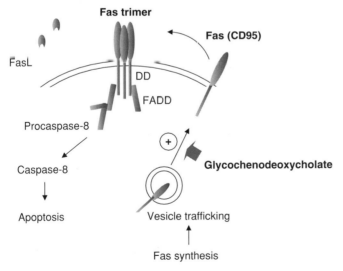

Figure 7.4. Induction of cell surface expression of Fas by toxic bile salts (e.g. glycochenodeoxycholate). Toxic bile salts increase the vesicle trafficking of *de novo* synthesized Fas to the plasma membrane, where Fas trimerizes and triggers apoptosis. DD, death domain; FADD, Fas-associated death domain.

The **tumor necrosis factor receptor (TNF-R)** family is the second important death receptor and consists of TNF-R1 and TNF-R2. They have differential roles; both types, however, are activated by TNFα or TNFβ (also called lymphotoxin-α). The ligands have multiple roles in inflammation, immunology, but also in tissue regeneration (see section 11.1).

Xenobiotics can induce the production and release of TNF, and thus trigger TNF-R activation, in a number of ways. One way is by stimulating macrophages which release large amounts of the proinflammatory cytokine, TNF. This can result in apoptosis; however, an opposite rescue pathway is simultaneously activated by the same mechanism.

Activation of the TNF receptor mediates both cell death and cell survival – at first thought a paradoxical situation. How is this accomplished? Our current concept implies that the TNF receptor recruits a number of intracellular adaptor proteins which couple the receptor to intracellular signaling pathways. Two opposite pathways are involved: the JNK and the NF-κB pathway, both of which involve protein kinase cascades (see section 5.4). JNK belongs to the family of mitogen-activated protein kinases (MAPKs). These kinases translocate into the nucleus and phosphorylate other kinases, ultimately resulting in cell death. On the other hand, NF-κB is kept in a dormant state by the inactivator protein, I-κB. TNF signaling triggers a chain of events that leads to the phosphorylation of I-κB, causing release of NF-κB. The free NF-κB next moves into the nucleus and transactivates genes which are part of an anti-apoptosis program. These proteins include Gadd45β (a protein involved in cell cycle control) and XIAP, both of which *inhibit* the JNK pathway. Exactly how this process occurs is still unclear (see Figure 7.5).

7.2.3. Caspases – the executors

The **caspase** (cysteine-aspartate-proteases) protein family plays a crucial role in executing apoptosis. Caspases are the only proteases which cleave after an aspartate residue, while cysteine is used for catalyzing the cleavage. Pre-caspases are present as zymogens in an inactive state and, in order to become active catalytically, the pre-caspases need to be cleaved by other caspases, whereupon they form oligomers.

Because caspases execute the cell death program, they have also been termed 'killer proteases'. In fact, they cause cell death so specifically and so rapidly that one can compare the caspase-mediated cell killing with an erected tent whose supporting strings are being cut and which instantly collapses. On the one hand, there are initiator caspases, e.g. caspase-8 (whose function is to activate other caspases, thus initiating a cascade). On the other hand, there are executor caspases, e.g. caspase-3 or -7, which do the job. Recently, a new caspase

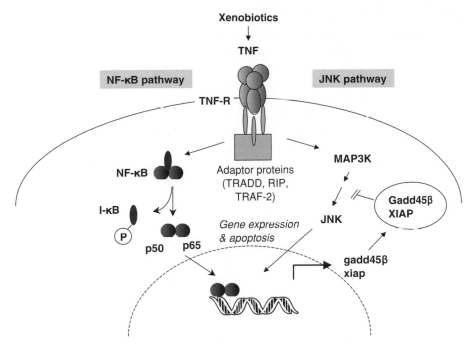

Figure 7.5. The dual pathways of the TNF receptor-mediated signaling. The JNK pathway transactivates genes that induce apoptotic cell death, while the NF-κB pathway transactivates anti-apoptotic genes. This is accomplished by the transcription and *de novo* synthesis of proteins which inhibit the MAP kinase pathways.

(caspase-12) has been identified; this enzyme is activated by Ca^{2+} resulting from damage to the endoplasmic reticulum. The downstream consequences of caspase catalytic activity include activation of kinases and inactivation of Bcl-2 and DNA polymerases. Through the specific inactivation of these rescue pathways and repair machineries, the cell no longer wastes energy on inefficient rescue once the final and irreversible death countdown has started. Also, the caspases selectively degrade the nuclear envelope proteins including lamin, actin and fodrin, which results in the collapse of the nuclear organization.

Many apoptogenic xenobiotics have indeed been shown to cause activation of the caspase cascade, and this seems to be a general and commonly used pathway. However, it is also both toxicologically interesting and therapeutically relevant that the caspases themselves can be prone to undergoing oxidative damage and inactivation by xenobiotics. Consequently, although there is a compound-induced signal to execute apoptosis, the cell does not die under certain conditions. One such example is compounds which produce excessive oxidative stress in liver cells through redox cycling.

Menadione (2-methyl-1, 4-naphthoquinone; vitamin K_3) is under consideration as an anticancer drug and is a widely used model compound to investigate the mechanisms of oxidative stress and apoptosis. As a typical quinone (see section 5.1.1), menadione can undergo either one- or two-electron reduction. In the first case, menadione is reduced to the semiquinone radical which can in turn reduce molecular oxygen, thereby being oxidized back to the parent compound and producing superoxide anion radical. In the presence of high concentrations of menadione, extensive amounts of ROS are thus being formed, which results in a general oxidative stress entailing GSH depletion, NAD(P)H oxidation, oxidative protein modification, and ultimately cell death.

Although menadione typically produces oxidoreductive stress (even extensive oxidative stress), and although exposure of cells to menadione results in mitochondrial release of cytochrome c (which would normally mediate caspase activation), the major mode of cell death is necrotic cell death rather than apoptosis.

Mechanisms of menadione-induced cell death: Although menadione exposure and metabolism pose a massive oxidative stress in liver cells, the compound does not activate caspases. In fact, the addition of menadione to cells undergoing apoptosis quenches caspase activity and switches the mode of cell death to necrosis. Why? The answer, as so often in toxicology, is based on the quantitative aspect. High levels of ROS not only can modify a number of different cellular targets but can oxidize, and thus inactivate, the caspases themselves. This is reasonable, since caspases possess an active cysteine residue (which is the catalytic site) which is sensitive to oxidation or alkylation by an electrophile. Therefore, under highly oxidizing conditions, caspase activity is inhibited. This effect can be mimicked by H_2O_2 or by a number of other prooxidants. Whether a cell exposed to a xenobiotic that has the potential to produce oxidative stress will undergo oxidant stress-induced apoptosis or whether it will be driven into necrosis due to caspase inactivation largely depends on the differential rates of prooxidant production, which is cell-type dependent (see Figure 7.6).

7.2.4. Role of mitochondria

Mitochondria play a pivotal role in apoptosis. They sequester a potent arsenal of pro-apoptotic proteins (including AIF and Smac/DIABLO). Among these proteins, cytochrome c has recently gained increased attention. Once released into the cytosol, cytochrome c can directly activate caspases. But how can a large molecule like cytochrome c, which is attached to the inner membrane and is part of the normal electron transport chain, cross the mitochondrial outer membrane? One attractive hypothesis is the role of the mitochondrial permeability transition pore (MPTP, see section 15.5). This is a megachannel formed by the outer and inner mitochondrial membrane, composed of a number of protein complexes. Opening of the MPTP complex, thus promoting efflux of cytochrome c, can be achieved by a number of triggering factors. One of them is the pro-apoptotic protein Bax, which interferes with the protein complex. Another is Bid, a protein present in an inactive state in the cytosol and which is cleaved (and thus activated) by caspase-8 to a truncated

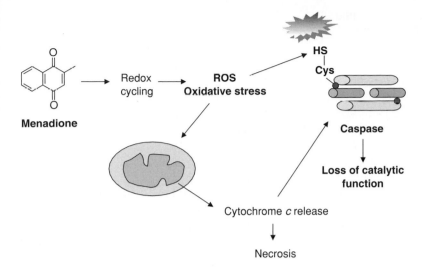

Figure 7.6. Menadione-induced oxidative modification of caspases and inhibition of caspase activity pushes the cell into necrosis. One factor that decides whether a cell will die via apoptosis or necrosis is the extent of oxidative stress.

form (tBid), which in turn can cause opening of the pore. Finally, the pore is also redox-sensitive, and sustained oxidative stress (in part mediated by intramitochondrial NO radical and peroxynitrite formation) can cause opening of the MPTP and release of cytochrome c. Because this is obviously a very dangerous process, it is tightly regulated by modulating proteins of the Bcl-2 family.

Many xenobiotics can interfere with the MPTP and either promote or inhibit the release of cytochrome c. One example is cyclosporin A.

Cyclosporin A (CsA) is an immunosuppressive drug widely used in organ transplantation and autoimmune disease, but it is also therapeutically applied in cancer chemotherapy.

CsA is often used as an experimental tool in apoptosis research. At low concentrations (nanomolar range) CsA can effectively *block* apoptosis in Type II cells (i.e. in cells in which the major pathway of apoptosis induction proceeds via mitochondria, e.g. in hepatocytes). The mechanistic basis for the apoptosis-preventing effect is a specific inhibition of the opening of the mitochondrial permeability transition pore (MPTP) mediated by CsA. The exact mechanisms are not known, but most likely specific interactions of CsA with one or several of the proteins that are part of the MPTP (cyclophilin) are involved.

On the other hand, CsA has been shown to *induce* apoptosis of renal tubular and intestinal cells, as well as thymocytes, both *in vitro* and *in vivo*. This apparent paradox can best be explained by a dual effect of CsA: at low concentrations and when used for short periods of time (e.g. 1 h), it blocks apoptosis, but at high concentrations (micromolar range), and if exposure is maintained for extended periods of time, it can actually induce apoptosis.

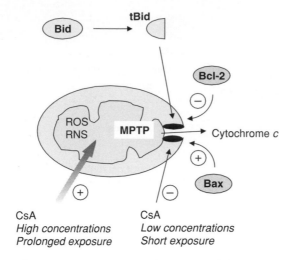

Figure 7.7. Activation and opening of the mitochondrial membrane permeability transition pore by reactive oxygen and nitrogen species (ROS, RNS), activated Bid, Bax, or high concentrations of cyclosporin A. In contrast, Bcl-2 or low concentrations of CsA keep the MPTP closed and protect from apoptosis.

Mechanisms of cyclosporin A-induced apoptosis: In hepatocytes, both CsA (≥ 1 µM) and its congener, IMM 125, cause opening of the MPTP and induce a decrease of the mitochondrial membrane potential. This is followed by cytochrome c release and activation of caspases (in particular caspase-3), followed by DNA fragmentation, as would be expected from a compound that can induce apoptosis in Type II cells. How can this apparently opposite effect to the above described inhibition of MPTP-mediated apoptosis be explained? Most probably, the cause lies in CsA's ability to cause oxidative stress and/or disruption of intracellular Ca^{2+} homeostasis when used at high concentrations (see Figure 7.7).

7.2.5. Checkpoints – the Bcl-2 proteins

The Bcl-2 protein family comprises a number of positive or negative regulators of apoptotic cell death, which play a key role in molecular toxicology: the regulatory proteins can be activated by xenobiotics and thus form a crucial decision point where a cell is pushed either into cell death or rescue pathways.

The **Bcl-2 proteins** include both inhibitors of apoptosis (Bcl-2, Bcl-xL, Mcl-1, and A1) and promoters of apoptosis (Bax, Bad, Bid, and Bcl-XS). All members form dimers (homodimers or heterodimers). For example, a Bcl-2/Bcl-2 dimer protects, while a Bax/Bax dimer pushes the cell further into apoptosis. Bcl-2/Bax heterodimers also exist; however, it is the overall prevalence of Bcl-2 or Bax in a cell that will ultimately decide whether a cell will die or be rescued.

Bcl-2, the rescue molecule, is present in mitochondria as the 'gatekeeper', keeping the MPTP in a closed state and thus preventing cytochrome c from leaking out. In contrast, Bax leads to an opening of the megachannel, thus promoting apoptosis. Bcl-2 is transcriptionally induced by oxidative stress and transported into mitochondria, where it exerts its protective role.

Normally, a cell can defend itself against a potential pro-apoptotic threat by up-regulating the anti-apoptotic protein Bcl-2. However, some xenobiotics can prevent this induction and thus indirectly act as pro-apoptotic compounds. One example is COX-2 inhibitors.

COX-2 inhibitors are a novel group of isoform-selective cyclooxygenase inhibitors mainly used to treat pain and inflammatory conditions. This therapeutic group includes the coxibs, but also nimesulide. COX-2 inhibitors inhibit the enzyme cyclooxygenase (also called prostaglandin endoperoxide synthase), which catalyzes the conversion of prostaglandins from arachidonic acid. COX-2 is the inducible isoform of this enzyme and can be increased by cytokines and other factors. As a result, prostaglandin production is inhibited (a desired effect in inflammation).

One side-effect of these COX-2 inhibitors (which will undoubtedly be further explored with a view to a potential therapeutic indication) is their proven ability to push certain cells into apoptosis. This may at first sight look like an undesired effect, but it can turn very beneficial if, for example, the target cells are cancer cells. Indeed, colon cancer cell growth can be stopped by COX-2 inhibitors, and, similarly, cells of a human prostate cancer cell line are killed by these compounds. In all these cases, the increased propensity of cancer cells to die was related to their decreased expression of Bcl-2.

This complex regulation can be nicely demonstrated in hepatocytes, which under normal conditions do not express Bcl-2. Stress signals can change the picture; stress can up-regulate COX-2 in the hepatic resident macrophages, the Kupffer cells, which results in increased production and release of prostaglandins. These in turn mediate the up-regulation of Bcl-2 in hepatocytes. This protects hepatocytes from an increased oxidative stress. Indeed, prostanoids have been shown to be hepatoprotective against liver injury in animal models and in humans. Conversely, exposure to COX-2 inhibitors blocks the production of prostaglandins and hence prevents the induction of the cytoprotective Bcl-2. While this may be beneficial in cancer cells, COX-2 inhibitors may push other cells such as hepatocytes, when exposed to an increased oxidative stress, into apoptosis (see Figure 7.8).

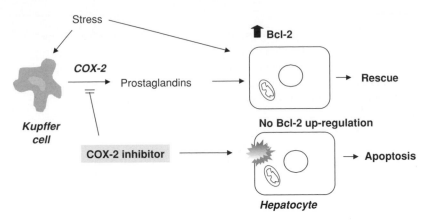

Figure 7.8. Prostaglandins as mediators of Bcl-2 induction in hepatocytes. COX-2 inhibitors block prostaglandin production and prevent induction of Bcl-2.

7.2.6. Suppression of apoptosis – toxicological consequences

Although a host of xenobiotics are known potentially to cause apoptosis, there are other compounds which *inhibit* apoptosis. This is not always beneficial, as the process of apoptosis has an important physiological function: it is involved in regulating tissue mass homeostasis. If such xenobiotics inhibit cell elimination by apoptosis, then the mitotic generation of new cells may add to an increase in tissue mass and result in hyperplasia of the organ. An example of such a drug is phenobarbital.

Phenobarbital is a barbiturate drug used therapeutically as an anticonvulsant, antihypnotic and depressant. When given to mice or rats, phenobarbital causes a massive increase in liver mass and cell number (and also induction of a number of drug-metabolizing enzymes). In addition, mitoses, which normally occur in very few hepatocytes only, are highly stimulated in the liver after phenobarbital.

Phenobarbital in rodents has also been shown to increase the number of liver tumors. As phenobarbital does not damage the DNA, it must exert its tumor-promoting role by non-genotoxic mechanims. It should be emphasized, however, that these effects are most likely rodent-specific. There is no evidence for phenobarbital-related increases in the incidence of liver tumors in humans taking the drug.

What is the mechanism underlying these liver growth-stimulating and tumor-promoting effects?

Mechanisms of phenobarbital-induced increases in liver cell mass: If the balance between cell proliferation and cell death (by apoptosis) is disturbed by an

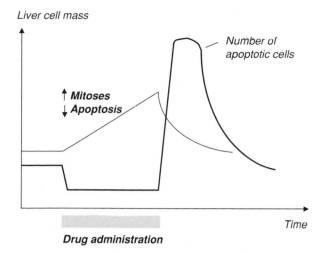

Liver cell mass

Number of apoptotic cells

↑ Mitoses
↓ Apoptosis

Time

Drug administration

Figure 7.9. Inhibition of apoptosis by phenobarbital causes an imbalance between cell replication and cell removal and leads to a massive increase in liver cell mass. Upon cessation of drug treatment, the cell number is restored by a sharp and transient increase in apoptotic cell death.

exogenous factor, such as a xenobiotic, then the cell mass homeostasis can be massively disturbed. Indeed, phenobarbital inhibits hepatocellular apoptosis. The exact mechanism is unknown, but Bcl-2 is involved: phenobarbital up-regulates Bcl-2 and thus stimulates the anti-apoptotic signals. As a result of prolonged phenobarbital exposure, the liver cell mass rapidly increases. This is a reversible effect, though; upon discontinuation of the drug, the liver cell mass is readily restored to its normal dimensions, and this is achieved by removing the excess cells by apoptosis. Accordingly, shortly after cessation of phenobarbital and similar drugs, the number of apoptotic cells in the liver sharply increases but later subsides to normal values (see Figure 7.9).

Mechanisms of tumor promotion by xenobiotics which inhibit apoptosis: Following a genotoxic insult, DNA-damaged cells are recognized and usually eliminated by apoptosis. This involves a cell cycle (see Chapter 8). If the damaged cell escapes this control mechanism, it can still be eliminated later. However, once the DNA alterations become established and are fixed and passed on during cell divisions (mutation), such DNA-altered cells form foci (clusters of daughter cells). In particular if such pre-neoplastic cells have acquired a growth selection advantage over non-initiated cells, they can further proliferate and set the stage for eventual development into a tumor. Xenobiotics which reduce or prevent the apoptotic removal of these intially damaged cells indirectly stimulate their proliferation. One downstream consequence of the administration of such compounds can be an increased risk of tumor formation. Indeed, there are xenobiotics which promote tumor formation through this mechanism (tumor promoters). Typical examples are phenobarbital and some peroxisome proliferators (e.g. nafenopin). Other xenobiotics, e.g. Pb salts, exert their effects through direct stimulation of cell proliferation: they are direct mitogens. The result, however, is similar (see Figure 7.10).

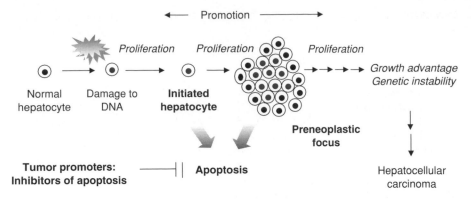

Figure 7.10. Xenobiotics (tumor promoters) can shift the equilibrium between cell proliferation and apoptosis towards increased proliferation. This has consequences on the survival and growth of initiated cells and populations of preneoplastic cells.

Learning points

- Xenobiotics can induce both apoptotic and necrotic cell death, depending on the concentration, the duration of exposure, and the specific tissue or cell type. The initial signals include oxidative stress, reactive metabolites, covalent protein modification, and DNA damage.
- Necrosis is the endpoint of accidental lethal cell injury. It is a passive process and not ATP-dependent. Plasma membrane injury leads to a collapse of ion homeostasis, swelling and ultimately rupture of cells.
- Apoptosis is a complex, genetically programmed sequence of events and energy-requiring process that leads to cell demise. This multistep process is tightly regulated and involves a number of checkpoints. The key players are (i) plasma membrane death receptors, triggering signaling cascades; (ii) the caspases (both activating and executing proteases); (iii) mitochondria which release cytochrome *c* (proximal to caspase activation in type II cells); and (iv) Bcl-2 proteins (anti-apoptotic or pro-apoptotic regulators).
- Excessive oxidative stress can inactivate caspases, thus preventing apoptosis, and shift the mode of cell death to necrosis.
- Stress can induce opening of the mitochondrial membrane permeability transition pore with subsequent release of cytochrome *c* and activation of caspases.
- Bcl-2 is an important anti-apoptotic protein, which can be up-regulated by prostaglandins.
- Suppression of apoptosis is not always beneficial; it can prevent normal cell turnover and increase the cell mass in a tissue. Apoptosis-inhibiting agents can be tumor promoters.

Further reading

Necrotic cell death
Pessayre, D., Haouzi, D., Fau, D., Robin, M.A., Mansouri, A. and Berson, A. (1999) Withdrawal of life support, altruistic suicide, fratricidal killing and euthanasia by lymphocytes: Different forms of drug-induced hepatic apoptosis, *J. Hepatol.* 31: 760–770.

Rosser, B.G. and Gores, G.J. (1995) Liver cell necrosis: Cellular mechanisms and clinical implications, *Gastroenterology* 108: 252–275.

Molecular mechanisms of apoptotic cell death
Blatt, N.B. and Glick, G.D. (2001) Signaling pathways and effector mechanisms. Pre-programmed cell death, *Bioorg. Med. Chem.* 9: 1371–1384.
Daniel, P.T. (2000) Dissecting the pathways to death, *Leukemia* 14: 2035–2044.
Darzynkiewicz, Z., Bedner, E., Traganos, F. and Murakami, T. (1998) Critical aspects in the analysis of apoptosis and necrosis, *Human Cell* 11: 3–12.
Hengartner, M.O. (2000) The biochemistry of apoptosis, *Nature* 407: 770–776.
Li, L.Y., Luo, X. and Wang, X. (2001) Endonuclease G is an apoptotic DNase when released from mitochondria, *Nature* 412: 95–99.
Malassagne, B., Ferret, P.J., Hammoud, R., Tulliez, M., Bedda, S., Trébéden, H., Jaffray, P., Calmus, Y., Weill, B. and Batteux, F. (2001) The superoxide dismutase mimetic MnTBAP prevents Fas-induced acute liver failure in the mouse, *Gastroenterology* 121: 1451–1459.

Arsenic-induced neurotoxicity
Namgung, U. and Xia, Z. (2001) Arsenic induces apoptosis in rat cerebellar neurons via activation of JNK3 and p38 MAP kinases, *Toxicol. Appl. Pharmacol.* 174: 130–138.
Thomas, D.J., Styblo, M. and Lin, S. (2001) The cellular metabolism and systemic toxicity of arsenic, *Toxicol. Appl. Pharmacol.* 176: 127–144.

Death receptors
Bratton, S.B. and Cohen, G.M. (2001) Apoptotic death sensor: An organelle's alter ego?, *Trends Pharmacol. Sci.* 22: 306–315.
Denecker, G., Vercammen, D., Declercq, W. and Vandenabeele, P. (2001) Apoptotic and necrotic cell death induced by death domain receptors, *Cell. Mol. Life Sci.* 58: 356–370.
Kyriakis, J.M. (2001) Life-or-death decisions, *Nature* 414: 265–266.

Toxic bile salt-induced Fas activation
Sodeman, T., Bronk, S.F., Roberts, P.J., Miyoshi, H. and Gores, G.J. (2000) Bile salts mediate hepatocyte apoptosis by increasing cell surface trafficking of Fas, *Am. J. Physiol. (Gastrointest. Liver Physiol.)* 278: G992–G999.

Menadione-induced cell death
Samali, A., Nordgren, H., Zhivotovsky, B., Peterson, E. and Orrenius, S. (1999) A comparative study of apoptosis and necrosis in HepG2 cells: Oxidant-induced caspase inactivation leads to necrosis, *Biochem. Biophys. Res. Commun.* 255: 6–11.

Role of mitochondria
Ghafourifar, P., Schenk, U., Klein, S.D. and Richter, C. (1999) Mitochondrial nitric-oxide synthase stimulation causes cytochrome *c* release from isolated mitochondria, *J. Biol. Chem.* 274: 31185–31188.
Lemasters, J.J. (1998) The mitochondrial permeability transition: From biochemical curiosity to pathophysiological mechanism, *Gastroenterology* 115: 783–786.
Lemasters, J.J. (1999) Mechanisms of hepatic toxicity. V. Necrapoptosis and the mitochondrial permeability transition: Shared pathways to necrosis and apoptosis, *Am. J. Physiol. (Gastrointest. Liver Physiol.)* 39: G1–G6.

Cyclosporin A-induced apoptosis

Grub, S., Pehrson, E., Trommer, W.E. and Wolf, A. (2000) Mechanisms of cyclosporin A-induced apoptosis in rat hepatocyte primary cultures, *Toxicol. Appl. Pharmacol.* 163: 209–220.

Wolf, A., Trendelenburg, C., Diez-Fernandez, C., Prieto, P., Houy, S., Trommer, W.E. and Cordier, A. (1997) Cyclosporine A-induced oxidative stress in rat hepatocytes, *J. Pharmacol. Exp. Ther.* 280: 1328–1334.

The Bcl-2 proteins

Souto, E.O., Miyoshi, H., Dubois, R.N. and Gores, G.J. (2001) Kupffer cell-derived cyclooxygenase-2 regulates hepatocyte Bcl-2 expression in choledocho-venous fistula rats, *Am. J. Physiol. (Gastrointest. Liver Physiol.)* 280: G805–G811.

Voehringer, D.W. (1999) BCL-2 and glutathione: Alterations in cellular redox state that regulate apoptosis sensitivity, *Free Radic. Biol. Med.* 27: 945–950.

Phenobarbital-induced increases in liver cell mass

Hasmal, S.C. and Roberts, R.A. (1999) The perturbation of apoptosis and mitosis by drugs and xenobiotics, *Pharmacol. Ther.* 82: 63–70.

Tumor promotion by xenobiotics which inhibit apoptosis

Goldsworthy, T.L., Conolly, R.B. and Fransson-Steen, R. (1996) Apoptosis and cancer risk assessment, *Mut. Res. Rev. Gen. Toxicol.* 365 (S1): 71–90.

White, M.K. and McCubrey, J.A. (2001) Suppression of apoptosis: Role in cell growth and neoplasia, *Leukemia* 15: 1011–1021.

Chapter 8

Impairment of cell proliferation and tissue repair

Contents

Mitotic cell division and proliferation are essential for the homeostasis of most tissues or organs. These processes fulfill two basic functions:

1 Continuous mitogenesis replaces lost cells which are eliminated by apoptosis as part of the normal physiological turnover, thus keeping the cell mass homeostasis in balance.
2 Cell proliferation is activated after a mechanical or chemical insult to an organ in order to replace the lost cell mass so that a tissue can regain its normal dimensions and structures. This transient process is involved in repair and regeneration.

Xenobiotics can interfere with both processes. They can not only inhibit DNA synthesis and cell proliferation, but also stimulate DNA synthesis. Both effects can have potentially dangerous consequences. The key to these effects is the cell cycle, which is closely linked to apoptosis.

8.1. The cell cycle

The cell cycle is defined as the entire process by which a cell undergoes cell division. Thus, the cell cycle not only involves processes in the nucleus but also encompasses signaling pathways from plasma membrane receptors (receptor tyrosine kinases) to the cytoplasm and from there to the nucleus (via distinct mitogen-activated protein (MAP) kinases), where specific cell cycle-related genes are activated. The nuclear cell cycle is tightly controlled by cyclin-dependent kinases (Cdks), an enzyme family of constitutively expressed proteins which play a pivotal role. Cdks in turn are tightly controlled by cyclins, which are regulatory units that are synthesized on demand and rapidly degraded if no longer required. To make things even more complex, the Cdks/cyclins are further regulated by additional fine-tuning mechanisms.

The cell cycle is a highly complex but also a potentially 'dangerous' process as cells are extremely vulnerable during this phase. The reason is that if a cell is once committed to go through the cell cycle, there is no way back – either it undergoes cell division or it dies. Therefore, if a xenobiotic blocks the cell cycle at one or several points, the cell is doomed to undergo apoptosis.

The cell cycle is subdivided into distinct phases: the G_1 phase ('G' stands for 'gap'), where cells prepare for DNA synthesis; the S phase, where DNA is synthesized; the G_2 phase, where cells prepare for mitosis; and finally the M phase, during which two daughter cells are produced. This order is highly regulated, and one stage has to be successfully completed before the next one can begin. Often cells remain in a quiescent stage (the so-called G_0 phase), and they need growth factors (mitogens) to enter into the G_1 phase. After having passed across a certain restriction point ('point of no return'), the cells are no longer dependent on growth factors and take off to undergo the cycle.

The cell cycle process is controlled at distinct levels and involves specific checkpoints (which are decision points). If there is an 'alarm' (due to, for example, DNA damage, or if a preceding step has not been completed) at one or another checkpoint, cell cycle progression is inhibited. Often apoptosis ensues (see Figure 8.1).

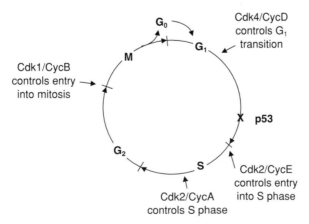

Figure 8.1. The four phases of the cell cycle and control of phase transitions by cyclin-dependent kinases (Cdk) and cyclins (Cyc).

8.2. Stimulation of DNA synthesis and cell proliferation: xenobiotics as mitogens

Direct mitogens are xenobiotics which can push cells into the mitotic cycle without prior tissue injury that would require compensatory proliferation. Hence, the ratio of cell division/cell demise gets out of balance, and the tissue mass will increase. An example is inorganic lead.

Inorganic lead is a widespread environmental pollutant which has been implicated in developmental neurotoxicity and carcinogenicity. The mechanisms of lead toxicity are not fully understood at the molecular level. Evidence indicates that Pb interferes with cellular signal transduction pathways, in particular with members of the calcium-dependent protein kinase C (PKC) family. These kinases play an important role in cell proliferation.

Lead has also been implicated in carcinogenesis. Specifically, Pb produces renal adenocarcinomas and lung adenomas, but also gliomas in the brain of experimental animals. Excess incidences of renal, lung and brain tumors have also been found in epidemiological studies of lead-exposed workers. Therefore, lead has been classified as a possible human carcinogen.

Mechanisms of lead-induced stimulation of cell proliferation: Lead induces DNA synthesis in a number of cells, including astrocytoma cells, liver cells, and renal cells. The mechanism is not entirely clear, but evidence suggests that Pb^{2+} causes activation of PKC-mediated pathways by facilitating the translocation of PKC from the cytosol to the plasma membrane (perhaps by mimicking Ca^{2+}). This kinase activation greatly stimulates cell cycle progression, pushing an increased number of cells into the S/G_2 phase. Inorganic lead is therefore a powerful mitogen that causes cell replication without causing tissue damage. In other words, the cell replication is not a compensatory response but a primary mitogenic effect (see Figure 8.2).

The consequence of this stimulated cell proliferation is the development of hyperplasia in a given organ. Similarly to apoptosis-inhibiting xenobiotics, direct mitogens are also likely to act as tumor promoters. Indeed, lead has been implicated in playing a role in tumor promotion through enhancing cell division.

However, besides causing increased proliferation of cells, another mechanism can be involved in promoting tumor formation. If a cell loses its ability to recognize and repair a potentially harmful DNA damage, it will no longer eliminate this DNA-altered cell through apoptotic cell death. The basic control mechanism for this damage-recognizing function is maintained by the protein p53.

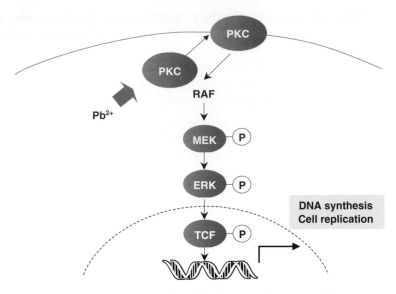

Figure 8.2. Direct activation by Pb^{2+} of protein kinase C induces DNA synthesis and cell proliferation.

p53 is a short-lived phosphoprotein which is expressed at low levels in the nucleus of most cells. It is, however, readily induced by a variety of cellular stress signals. p53 is a sequence-specific transcription factor which in turn induces the expression of a number of target genes.

The p53 protein has multiple functions. For example, p53 has also been called the 'guardian of the genome' because it can monitor and check the cell's health status and initiate repair, or else push the severely damaged cell into apoptosis. In other words, p53 is a single decision-making point which controls whether a cell should really enter the S phase.

p53 is also a so-called tumor suppressor gene because its normal function is to induce cellular growth arrest in cases of suspected genotoxicity. However, if its function is lost, e.g. by mutations in the gene coding for p53, it can no longer fulfill this task, and cells, even when exhibiting damaged DNA, can propagate in an uncontrolled manner. In cells with abnormal p53, damaged sequences in the genome may be inherited by the daughter cells. Therefore, p53 has been implicated in cancer formation. Indeed, p53 is one of the most commonly mutated genes in human cancer (see Figure 8.3).

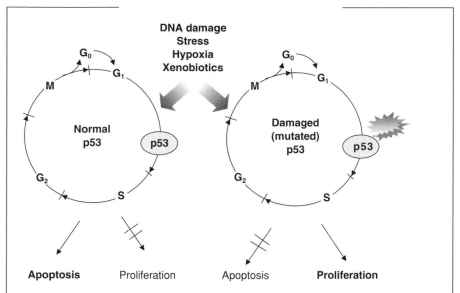

Figure 8.3. Role of p53 in controlling the cell cycle and protecting cells from undergoing cell proliferation after different forms of stress. In normal cells, the damage can be repaired, or the cell is pushed into apoptosis (left). However, in cells with mutated p53 (right), resulting in lack of p53 function, this control mechanism is no longer operating, and the cell undergoes uncontrolled proliferation.

p53 is transcriptionally activated by different forms of stress including hypoxia, thermal and mechanical stress, and UV radiation. Importantly, however, xenobiotic-induced stress can also induce p53. For example, chemicals producing oxidative stress (e.g. doxorubicin) can readily transactivate p53. It should be noted that the response to these various forms of stress is not uniform; it is highly stimulus-specific and cell type-specific.

8.3. Inhibition of cell proliferation by xenobiotics

In contrast to chemicals acting as mitogens, other xenobiotics can induce the opposite effect: they can inhibit the cell cycle and thus block the normal proliferation. In fact, many anti-tumor agents are specially designed to inhibit cell proliferation. However, while this effect is desired and aimed at eliminating cancer cells, it can become dangerous for normal cells. For example, tissues which feature a high cell turnover or proliferation rate, e.g. intestinal epithelia, male germ cells, skin, and the hematopoietic system, are particularly prone to becoming severely damaged by such compounds. One example of a group of drugs that are toxic via anti-mitotic activity is the taxoids.

Paclitaxel (Taxol®) is one of the most important anti-cancer drugs recently introduced. It is a taxoid, belonging to a group of naturally occurring compounds derived from the bark of the Western yew, *Taxus brevifolia*. Paclitaxel has excellent clinical acitivity against various cancers including ovarian and breast cancer. The proliferation of these cancer cells is effectively reduced by the cytotoxic action of paclitaxel.

However, paclitaxel has also serious toxic side-effects. These include myelosuppression (neutropenia, i.e. suppression in the bone marrow of neutrophil precursor proliferation and differentiation, and depletion of peripheral neutrophils), alopecia (hair loss), gastrointestinal effects, and skin toxicity. This toxicity reflects injury to rapidly dividing cells.

Mechanisms of taxoid-mediated inhibition of cell proliferation: Paclitaxel interrupts the cell cycle by specifically disrupting mitosis. The compound interacts with the microtubules that are important in forming the spindle apparatus during the M phase of the cell cycle. However, in contrast to other spindle poisons (e.g. colchicine, which prevents the molecular assembly of microtubules), paclitaxel promotes the polymerization of microtubules and disrupts the dynamic equilibrium between the soluble dimers (α- and β-tubulin) and the assembled tubulin polymer. Specifically, paclitaxel binds to the β-subunit of tubulin in a stochiometric fashion (1 mol paclitaxel per mol tubulin dimer) and promotes the polymerization of the dimers to the polymer, even in the absence of energy-providing GPT, which is normally required to assemble the tubulin polymers. As a consequence, the disassembly of tubulin polymers is prevented, and the process of mitosis is disrupted. This arrest in cell cycle progression invariably pushes the cell into apoptosis (see Figure 8.4).

Other mechanisms may also be involved in paclitaxel-induced pro-apoptotic activities (for example, hyperphosphorylation of Bcl-2 and loss of Bcl-2's anti-apoptotic function). However, it is a matter of dispute whether this is a direct effect of paclitaxel or just a consequence of cell cycle arrest.

Microtubules are hollow filaments (~24 nm in diameter) composed of a backbone of tubulin dimers and microtubule-associated proteins. The dimers are composed of α- and β-tubulin. Chaperones are involved in proper folding and are important in keeping the subunits in a functional form. In mammals, many tubulin isotypes have been identified, featuring posttranslational modification including phosphorylation and glutamylation. The α,β-tubulin dimers polymerize to large polymeric tubulin structures, being part of the microtubule. Microtubules are involved in a number of cellular functions, including mitosis, but also in intracellular transport and axon dynamics (see section 9.2.2.2); they are also part of the cytoskeleton.

Because tubulin is abundant in neurons, tubulin-binding agents such as the taxoids are often neurotoxic.

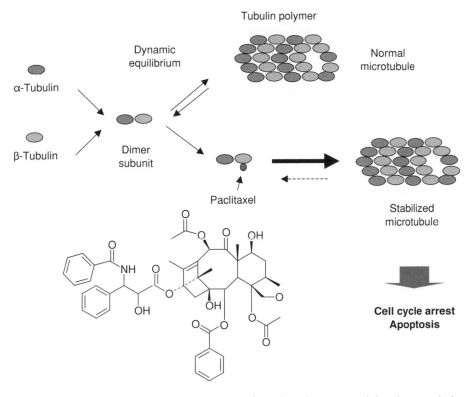

Figure 8.4. Taxol-stimulated polymerization of tubulin subunits to stabilized microtubule structures, preventing the dynamic assembly–disassembly equilibrium and disrupting normal mitosis.

8.4. Inhibition of tissue repair

Xenobiotics can specifically interfere with the cell proliferation involved in compensatory tissue repair processes. Tissue repair normally occurs after tissue injury in those organs that have phylogenetically retained a certain regenerative capacity (liver, kidney, skin, etc.). Following loss of cell mass by lethal damage, the surviving cells start to enter the cell cycle and undergo mitosis to replace the lost tissue. In particular, one major organ that has an enormous regenerative capacity is the liver.

> **Liver regeneration.** Although the vast majority of the parenchymal cells in the liver are in the G_0 (resting) phase of the cell cycle, the liver has retained its capacity to respond readily with a regenerative burst when part of the hepatocellular mass is lost. This can occur, for example, by removal of part of the liver (in fact, a 2/3 hepatectomy causes regeneration and full restoration of the entire liver mass in about a week). Alternatively, liver regeneration

is triggered by necrosis of large areas of liver tissues caused by viruses or hepatoxic xenobiotics.

At the molecular level, a number of genes are activated after such a loss of liver cell mass. This occurs in several phases. A very early response of hepatocytes to the initial mitogenic stimulus is activation of a set of primary response genes (approximately 70 distinct genes, called 'immediate–early genes'). These gene products include transcription factors, receptors for growth factors, JNK kinase, and others. One consequence is that the cells leave the G_0 phase and are pushed into the cell cycle. The next step is the activation of 'delayed early genes' (e.g. Bcl-X_L, an anti-apoptotic gene). Subsequently, cell cycle genes (e.g. p53, cyclins, cyclin-dependent kinases) and genes involved in DNA replication and mitosis are activated.

This whole process is extremely complex, and it is essential to know how this starts, how it is regulated, and how it stops (with a view to possible therapeutic applications). Initiators include signaling molecules such as TNFα and IL-6, which are multifunctional cytokines. For example, in TNF receptor 2-null mice, the lack of signaling after liver injury or partial hepatectomy precludes DNA replication and causes mortality. In short, TNF primes hepatocytes for proliferation and makes them responsive to growth factors, including hepatocyte growth factor (HGF). DNA synthesis is completed after 72 h. It is assumed that another multifunctional growth factor, the transforming growth factor TGFβ1, is involved in the cessation of regenerative activity.

In normal liver, the bulk of hepatocytes are in the resting state, the G_0 phase. A small proportion (6–7 percent) are in the G_2 phase. Only a small percentage of hepatocytes at a given time actually undergo mitosis. This quiescent state can, however, rapidly change when regeneration of lost tissue mass is required. Many hepatocytes rapidly enter the M phase of the cycle. For example, after chemical injury to liver tissue, increased numbers of mitoses can already be seen after 2 h, indicating that cells in the G_2 phase have entered the M phase. The peak of the mitotic activity, however, is attained much later (at 36 to 48 h post-injury), again indicating that the quiescent cells which have been in the G_0 phase have gone through the whole cycle of DNA replication and mitosis.

During this broad onset of cell division, genes involved in the replication process are active, while other genes, less important in this phase, are down-regulated. For example, CYP becomes expressed at low levels only. This can have implications on metabolism and bioactivation of xenobiotics; as the dividing cells no longer bioactivate compounds to reactive metabolites; they are temporarily resilient against the toxic effects of the parent compounds. Furthermore, anti-apoptotic genes (such as Bcl-2) are over-expressed, while pro-apoptotic genes (such as myc or p53) are downregulated.

The pivotal role of a normally functioning repair process after a chemical insult is illustrated with the example of carbon tetrachloride.

Carbon tetrachloride (see section 5.2.3) is a dose-dependent hepatotoxin. In laboratory rodents, the potential toxicity inflicted by apparently 'non-toxic' doses, or the reversible mild toxicity caused by intermediate doses of CCl_4, from which the animals recover, is actually kept to a minimum by many defense mechanisms of the body. One of these defense mechanisms is **compensatory proliferation and tissue repair** of the remaining hepatic parenchymal cell mass, which will make up for the damaged and lost hepatocytes. For example, if rats are administered a single dose of CCl_4 (100 µl/kg), there is a massive stimulation of hepatocellular mitosis. This occurs in two waves. First, the small proportion of hepatocytes which are already in the G_2 phase will start dividing after approximately 6 h. Second, the bulk of hepatocytes, which are in the G_0 phase of the cell cycle, will enter the cycle and undergo mitosis approximately 48 h post-injury.

As a consequence, this will progressively lead to tissue healing and restoration of the liver architecture and function.

The real significance of compensatory proliferative response mechanisms in chemically-induced tissue injury becomes apparent under conditions where these tissue repair processes become disturbed by a second xenobiotic. In the presence of such repair-inhibiting compounds, a small (normally non-toxic) dose of a first xenobiotic (e.g. CCl_4) can lead to severe toxicity because the compensatory repair mechanism is blocked or eliminated by the second xenobiotic. An example of an agent that inhibits tissue repair is chlordecone.

Chlordecone is an organochlorine insecticide. The production and use of chlordecone, and that of related organochlorine compounds, has been greatly reduced due to the environmental toxicity and bioaccumulation associated with these chemicals. A tragic accident in the USA in 1975, where the James River in Virginia was heavily contaminated with chlordecone, caused severe toxicity to aqueous organisms. In addition, workers of the plant exhibited symptoms of toxicity including reproductive toxicity, hepatic changes, neurotoxicity, and spleen dysfunction.

Although deplorable, such acute effects are rare and limited. Of much greater concern are low concentrations of organochlorine compounds which slowly accumulate in the environment. These xenobiotics may not be acutely toxic *per se*, but they can modulate the toxicity of other xenobiotics, such as organic halomethane solvents.

The toxicity of halomethanes, such as carbon tetrachloride, chloroform, or $BrCCl_3$, can be greatly potentiated by concomitant exposure to chlordecone. For example, if rats are pretreated with 10 ppm chlordecone in the diet for 2 weeks (a dose that does not cause any detectable adverse effects), and then administered a subtoxic dose of CCl_4 (100 µl/kg body weight), all rats will die of acute hepatic failure! What is the underlying reason for this potentiation of the toxicity of CCl_4?

Mechanisms of potentiation of CCl_4-induced liver injury and lethality by chlordecone: After the possibility that chlordecone was an inducer of the CYP forms that bioactivate CCl_4 was ruled out and the possibility that chlordecone potentiated lipid peroxidation (the major mechanism by which CCl_4 damages the hepatic parenchyma) was eliminated, two observations were made regarding the mechanism of potentiation: first, there was no recovery from the initial injury, and second, there was an acceleration of injury. The clue to the combination effect of the two compounds lies in the fact that chlordecone renders the liver unable to overcome tissue injury and to stimulate regeneration.

Two major events are responsible for this effect. First, the initial wave of cell proliferation (i.e. the small number of hepatocytes waiting in the G_2 phase and rapidly entering mitosis upon a stimulus) was completely ablated. Second, the follow-up wave of proliferation (i.e. the bulk of hepatocytes being in G_0) was greatly diminished. The underlying reasons for the inability to respond to a mitogenic stimulus is not known at the molecular level, but one factor is an early depletion of ATP (see Figure 8.5).

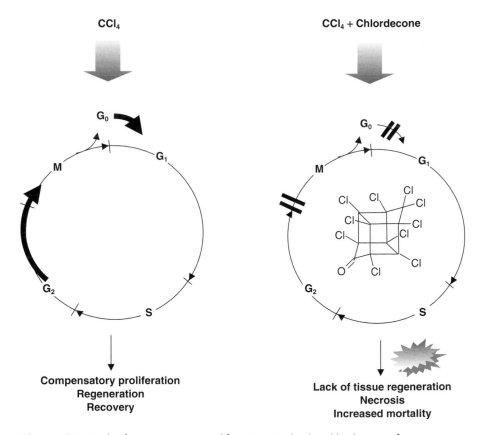

Figure 8.5. Lack of response to a proliferative stimulus by chlordecone after a subtoxic dose of CCl_4 results in an inhibition of the $G_2{\rightarrow}M$ and $G_0{\rightarrow}G_1,S,G_2$ cell cycle progression.

Similar principles may be applicable if a single potentially toxic xenobiotic is given as a large dose. Again, tissue repair may be inhibited and this may contribute to the overall extent of injury and mortality. Thus, insufficient or delayed tissue repair may contribute to the toxicity. The net outcome of the balance of dose-related tissue injury and dose-related tissue repair ultimately determines the extent of recovery and survival.

Learning points

- Xenobiotics can disrupt the cell cycle and block the pathways of both normal and compensatory (regenerative) cell division.
- The cell cycle is tightly regulated at several levels and involves a number of checkpoints. Once started, a cell has to go through the whole cycle or else enter apoptosis.
- Directly mitogenic xenobiotics (e.g. lead) induce cell proliferation via protein kinase C-mediated pathways. Such mitogens are often tumor promoters.
- p53 is a nuclear protein and tumor suppressor gene product. Its major function is to stop cell division in case of suspected DNA damage and to push cells into apoptosis. Mutations in p53 (leading to inactivation) are associated with the formation of cancer.
- Xenobiotics can inhibit the cell cycle. The anticancer agent paclitaxel inhibits mitosis by preventing tubulin disassembly, which leads to cell cycle arrest and apoptosis.
- Xenobiotics such as organochlorine pesticides can inhibit tissue regeneration following a mild toxic insult. This can cause aggravation of the initial damage and potentiation of the toxicity induced by other compounds.

Further reading

The cell cycle

Flatt, P.M. and Pietenpol, J.A. (2000) Mechanisms of cell-cycle checkpoints: At the crossroads of carcinogenesis and drug discovery, *Drug Metab. Rev.* 32: 283–305.

Schafer, K.A. (1998) The cell cycle: A review, *Vet. Pathol.* 35: 461–478.

Stewart, Z.A. and Pietenpol, J.A. (2001) p53 Signaling and cell cycle checkpoints, *Chem. Res. Toxicol.* 14: 243–263.

Lead-induced stimulation of cell proliferation

Kubo, Y., Yasunaga, M., Masuhara, M., Terai, S., Nakamura, T. and Okita, K. (1996) Hepatocyte proliferation induced in rats by lead nitrate is suppressed by several tumor necrosis factor alpha inhibitors, *Hepatology* 23: 104–114.

Lu, H., Guizzetti, M. and Costa, L.G. (2001) Inorganic lead stimulates DNA synthesis in human astrocytoma cells: Role of protein kinase Cα, *J. Neurochem.* 78: 590–599.

p53

Fisher, D.E. (2001) The p53 tumor suppressor: Critical regulator of life and death in cancer, *Apoptosis* 6: 7–15.

Taxoid-mediated inhibition of cell proliferation

Altmann, K.H. (2001) Microtubule-stabilizing agents: A growing class of important anticancer drugs, *Curr. Opinion Chem. Biol.* 5: 424–431.

Blagosklonny, M.V. and Fojo, T. (1999) Molecular effects of paclitaxel: Myths and reality (a critical review), *Int. J. Cancer* 83: 151–156.

Dumontet, C. and Sikic, B.I. (1999) Mechanisms of action of and resistance to anti-tubulin agents: Microtubule dynamics, drug transport, and cell death, *J. Clin. Oncol.* 17: 1061–1070.

Eisenhauer, E.A. and Vermorken, J.B. (1998) The taxoids. Comparative clinical pharmacology and therapeutic potential, *Drugs* 55: 5–30.

Kingston, D.G.I. (2001) Taxol, a molecule for all seasons, *Chem. Commun.* 10: 867–880.

Liver regeneration

Fausto, N. (2000) Liver regeneration, *J. Hepatol.* 32 (Suppl.): 19–31.

Mehendale, H.M. (1991) Role of hepatocellular regeneration and hepatolobular healing in the final outcome of liver injury – A two-stage model of toxicity, *Biochem. Pharmacol.* 42: 1155–1162.

Mehendale, H.M. and Thakore, K.N. (1997) Hepatic defenses against toxicity: Regeneration, *Hepat. Gastrointest. Toxicol.* 9: 209–231.

Michalopoulos, G.K. and DeFrances, M.C. (1997) Liver regeneration, *Science* 276: 60–66.

Chapter 9

Covalent binding of reactive metabolites to cellular macromolecules

Contents

In contrast to the frequent binding of many xenobiotics to plasma proteins or intracellular macromolecules, which is a non-covalent and reversible effect (see section 1.2.1), other compounds, or their metabolites, can interact with macromolecules and bind to them in a covalent, and therefore irreversible, manner. For example, the ability of many xenobiotics to be metabolically converted to reactive metabolites which can covalently bind to DNA has been known for a long time. In fact, DNA adduct formation by a reactive intermediate (the 'ultimate carcinogen') has been recognized to be an important step in carcinogenesis. However, reactive metabolites can also attack proteins, lipids, or other macromolecules. The toxicological significance of covalent protein binding is less clear than that of DNA binding, except for a small number of well-studied examples. Recently, the role of covalent binding of reactive metabolites to cellular target molecules, which act as stress signal enhancers and are involved in signal transduction, has been emerging as an important mechanism in gene regulation.

9.1. Electrophiles and nucleophilic targets

Certain xenobiotics or their metabolites are reactive because they exhibit an intramolecular center featuring low electron density (such molecules are called

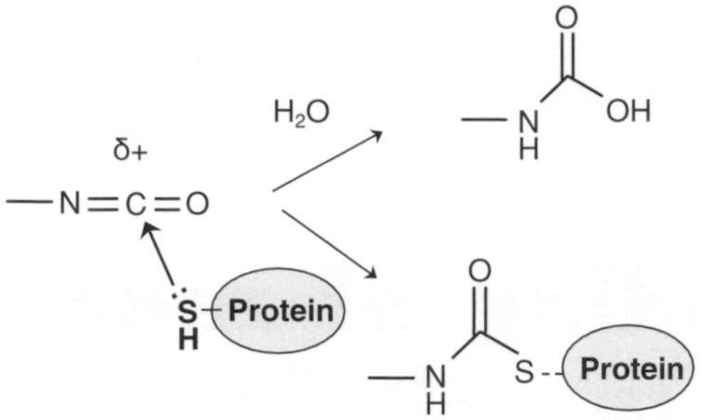

Figure 9.1. Methyl isocyanate is a strong electrophile that immediately reacts with detoxifying nucleophiles (water) or with nucleophilic sites of target proteins.

'electrophiles'). These electrophilic centers can preferentially be attacked by a center with high electron density (e.g. a free electron pair) of a another molecule (a nucleophile). The result is a covalent bond between the two reaction partners, with the xenobiotic now being present as an adduct to the target molecule.

The molecular size, charge density, and the degree of polarization of the electrophilic species will largely determine the type of nucleophilic reaction partner. For example, α,β-unsaturated carbonyls or quinoid compounds will preferentially react with sulfhydryl groups of amino acids or peptides, while aliphatic or aromatic carbon cations will preferentially react with oxygen of purine and pyrimidine bases. Thus, the type of target that will react with a specific electrophilic intermediate can in many cases be predicted.

Such reactive and electrophilic compounds, when they enter the body or when they are generated metabolically, are often inactivated by small molecular nucleophiles in body fluids or cells. The most frequent nucleophile and detoxifying molecule is water, but other compounds, e.g. sulfhydryl-containing peptides such as glutathione, can also effectively detoxicate the reactive compound. If the xenobiotic is extremely reactive, or if it escapes detoxication by scavengers, then such a compound may form adducts to critical cellular macromolecules, sometimes disrupting the structure and function of a cell or tissue as a consequence of this binding.

An example of extremely reactive electrophilic compounds, which readily form adducts to tissue macromolecules, is isocyanates (see Figure 9.1).

Methyl isocyanate is formed as an intermediary product during the industrial production of pesticides. The compound is volatile and extremely reactive. Therefore, methyl isocyanate features a high potential for inducing toxicity to the airways following accidental inhalation.

During an accident in a production plant in Bhopal, India in 1984, large amounts of methyl isocyanate were released into the air. More than 2,000 people died and many more were injured, as these people lived in close proximity to the plant. The major symptoms of toxicity were injury to the airways and lung edema.

In most cases, however, metabolic activation is required for a xenobiotic to become an electrophilic species. Thus, reactive intermediates, rather than the parent compound itself, are often responsible for forming adducts to cellular macromolecules.

Due to their abundance in a cell, proteins are major targets of an electrophilic attack by a xenobiotic (for example, hepatocytes consist of approximately 20 percent protein per weight). Not all protein binding is toxicologically relevant; however, in some cases, selective alkylation, arylation, or acylation of specific protein targets has been mechanistically linked to the xenobiotic's toxicity. Some drugs may similarly produce their intended therapeutic action by covalent binding to key targets (e.g. anticancer agents).

9.2. Covalent protein binding

The nucleophilic targets in proteins which most frequently undergo reactions with electrophiles are the sulfur-containing amino acid residues, i.e. cysteine and methionine, or the nitrogen of lysine and histidine residues. However, at the cellular level, it seems plausible that not all proteins are equally adducted by a reactive metabolite. Rather than being random reactions, certain proteins are indeed selectively alkylated or arylated, while others are spared. What factors determine, mechanistically, which proteins are targeted by a reactive metabolite?

1 The reactivity of a metabolite determines the target selection. The greater the half-life of a reactive metabolite, the longer the potential time and range for possible interactions with a more distant target. Alternatively, the shorter the half-life, the more avidly will a reactive metabolite react with a target in its vicinity. For example, some reactive intermediates are so electrophilic that they immediately react with a nucleophilic site in close vicinity to the place where the metabolite was generated, and this is often the bioactivating enzyme (mostly CYPs). Indeed, there are examples where specific CYP isoforms are covalently modified by a reactive metabolite. This does not necessarily happen right at the active center of the protein, because the catalytic center has a low abundance of nucleophilic sites, but often at other sites of the hemoprotein, e.g. at the heme nitrogen. In contrast, if the metabolite is more stable, it can diffuse away from the site of generation and penetrate into other organelles, or even cross biomembranes.

2 High concentrations of a reactive metabolite may favor covalent interactions. This does not always happen at the site of generation. In contrast, certain metabolites diffuse away and are up-concentrated at more distant sites. For example, acyl glucuronides, which are protein-reactive ester glucuronide conjugates (see section 9.2.2.3), can attain high concentrations (up to 100-fold increased as compared to intracellular concentrations) in the biliary canaliculi, following active secretion from hepatocytes against a concentration gradient. If other microenvironmental conditions favor their reactivity even more (here, a slightly more alkaline pH in bile), then these electrophilic intermediates will avidly react with canalicular proteins.

3 It is not only the concentration of the reactive metabolite, but also the local abundance and differential subcellular distribution of anti-electrophilic defense mechanisms (e.g. nucleophilic scavengers which inactivate reactive metabolites), that greatly influences the net outcome of covalent binding.

The selectivity of protein binding, as well as the downstream toxicological consquences of adduct formation, will be best illustrated by the most extensively investigated compound and paradigm, acetaminophen.

9.2.1. *Selectivity of covalent adduct formation*

Acetaminophen (APAP, N-acetyl-p-aminophenol; in Europe called 'paracetamol') is an analgesic and antipyretic drug which, in contrast to aspirin, does not cause gastrointestinal irritation and microbleeding and, therefore, has been widely used since the 1950s. Therapeutic use of APAP is safe; however, ingestion of high doses is associated with acute liver injury (in multidrug therapy or accidental and intentional overdose). For example, in the UK >1,500 cases of APAP-related liver necrosis are reported each year, >50 with a fatal outcome.

The molecular mechanisms underlying APAP-induced liver injury are well known – at least those which are determined by toxicokinetic factors, including exposure, bioactivation, and detoxication pathways. APAP toxicity is a clear function of the dose; the threshold for acute toxicity (in the adult human) is >5–15 g. The pathogenesis of liver necrosis induced by APAP has been studied in animal models, in particular the mouse, which is a

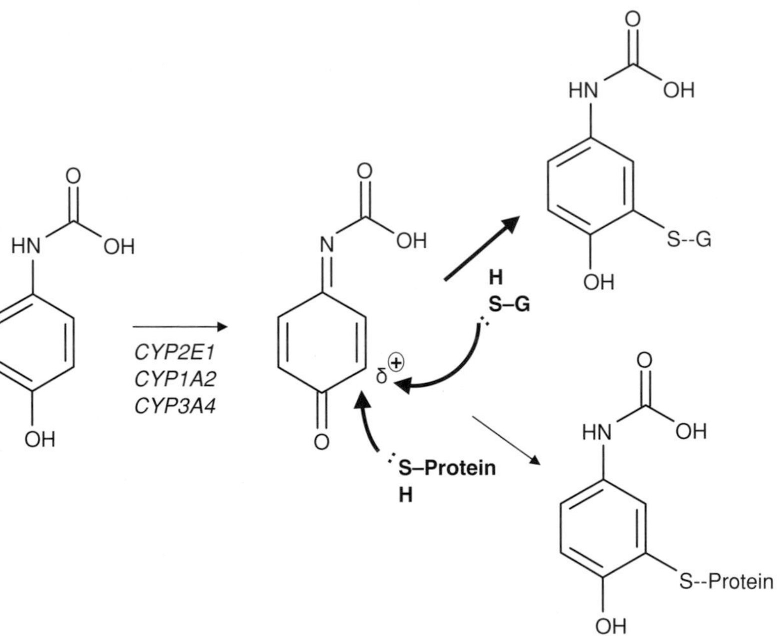

Figure 9.2. The oxidative metabolite of APAP, NAPQI, is an electrophilic quinoneimine which arylates peptides (e.g. glutathione, GSH) or proteins through interactions with nucleophilic thiol groups.

sensitive species and produces a similar phenotypic pattern of liver injury to that observed in humans. The toxicity is clearly associated with the production of a reactive intermediate (normally a minor pathway of biotransformation). This metabolite is produced by CYP-catalyzed oxidation of APAP to N-acetyl-p-benzoquinoneimine (NAPQI) (see section 4.2.1.2). Quinoneimines typically are electrophilic species which react with cellular nucleophiles and arylate hepatocellular proteins (see Figure 9.2).

Mechanisms of acetaminophen-induced hepatocellular injury: Acetaminophen toxicity is based on multiple cellular mechanisms. Bioactivation and production of a reactive quinoneimine is, however, an initiating event and crucial step proximal to the cascade of subsequent events. The protein-reactive metabolite, NAPQI, arylates a number of proteins and transactivates genes involved in an early stress response. NAPQI also induces massive oxidative stress, which is even enhanced because glutathione is being consumed. This leads to changes in the calcium homeostasis and induces damage to DNA. Finally, NAPQI also damages mitochondria by forming covalent adducts to mitochondrial proteins and posing an oxidative stress in mitochondria. This leads to a rapid fall in cellular ATP level. Thus, although apoptotic stimuli will be present at several levels including release of pro-apoptotic factors from mitochondria and signals from the cytosol, the liver parenchyma will primarily be subject to necrotic cell death, because the energy crisis in mitochondria will largely block the ATP-requiring pathways of apoptosis (see Figure 9.3).

The first and pioneering steps towards identifying the relevant target proteins arylated by APAP, using a specific anti-APAP antibody in liver homogenates of APAP-treated mice, revealed that a distinct number of intracellular proteins located in different subcellular compartments exhibit APAP adducts. In the mouse model, one target protein seems particularly intriguing. It is a cytosolic 58-kD protein, termed 'APAP-binding protein'. Although well characterized and sequenced, the protein's physiological function is not known. However, because it is also targeted by other xenobiotics (i.e. their reactive metabolites), it has been suggested that the APAP-binding protein may serve as a nucleophilic 'sensor' for electrophilic and potentially hazardous intermediates. Indeed, recent findings demonstrate that this protein, after arylation by NAPQI, is activated and then translocated into the cell nucleus, where it associates with chromatin. This is important as it raises the possibility that the APAP-binding protein might serve as a transcription factor, perhaps similarly to other electrophile-binding protein complexes which bind to specific response elements (e.g. EpRE) in the promoter region of stress genes and induce transcription of gene products involved in either cell rescue or cell demise (see section 5.4).

With the advent of more sensitive mass spectrometry methods of protein identification directly on two-dimensional gels, a host of additional target proteins have been identified in various organelles including mitochondria. Not all of them are equally abundant and equally critical for the survival of the cell (see Table 9.1).

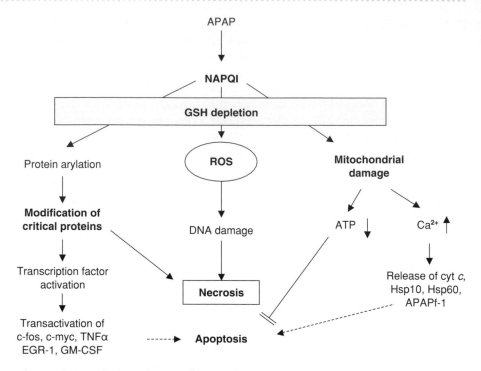

Figure 9.3. Multiple pathways of liver cell injury induced by acetaminophen. The reactive metabolite NAPQI causes protein arylation, mitochondrial damage, and oxidative stress. As apoptosis will be suppressed by both low levels of ATP and high levels of prooxidants, necrosis will be predominant.
Source: Modified from Ruepp, S.U., Tonge, R.P., Shaw, J., Wallis, N. and Pognan, F. (2002) Genomics and proteomics analysis of acetaminophen toxicity in mouse liver, *Toxicol. Sci.* 65: 135–150.

Table 9.1 Major hepatic target proteins arylated by acetaminophen

Hepatocellular organelle	Protein
Endoplasmic reticulum	Glutamine synthetase
	Glutathione-S-transferase
	Calreticulin
	Thiol–protein–disulfide oxidoreductase
Mitochondria	Glutamate dehydrogenase
	Carbamyl phosphate synthetase
	Aldehyde dehydrogenase
Cytosol	Acetaminophen and/or selenium-binding protein
	Glutathione-S-transfease
	Glyceraldehyde-3-phosphate dehydrogenase
	10-formyl-tetrahydroformate dehydrogenase

Is there a plausible causal link between covalent adduct formation and the downstream toxic effects? And which of these target macromolecules are critical and mechanistically relevant in the pathogenesis of liver injury?

9.2.2. Downstream toxicological consequences of covalent protein binding

Whether or not covalent modification of target proteins may be causally related to toxicity has been a matter of debate for many decades, and many arguments in favor and against have been discussed. The difficulty of defining a clear mechanistic role of chemically-altered proteins often lies in the fact that protein adduct formation (a result of bioactivation) cannot be dissociated from metabolic activation itself (if one blocks one process, then everything is blocked).

Interestingly, immunochemical localization of the covalent acetaminophen–protein adducts with a specific antibody (that was developed against activated APAP bound to a carrier-protein) revealed that the adducted proteins are located in the same sublobular areas where liver necrosis later develops. Although this alone does not allow one to conclude that there is a causal relationship between protein adduct formation and tissue injury, this technique can be used as a biomarker for exposure and reactive metabolite formation.

Meanwhile it has become clear that the reactive metabolite of APAP, in addition to causing protein arylation, also produces oxidative stress resulting in ROS formation and protein thiol oxidation. It also recruits immune cells, mediates cytokine release, and evokes a general cellular stress response. This multitude of cellular responses makes it particularly difficult to investigate the role of an isolated molecular mechanism.

Nowadays, in view of the rapidly growing understanding of the complexity of multiple processes involved in the pathogenesis of a toxic compound, the question of the mechanism underlying the toxicity of a reactive metabolite is perhaps less focused on covalent binding alone. In many cases, a reactive metabolite exerts other stress signals that accompany the interaction with target proteins, and it has become clear that it is seldom a single mechanism (e.g. covalent binding to a specific protein or to multiple proteins) that causes all the downstream toxic effects. Nevertheless, covalent modification of targets remains crucial (see Figure 9.4).

There are specific examples for which a clear causal relationship between covalent binding to a critical target protein and toxicity has been demonstrated.

9.2.2.1. Covalent modification and inactivation of protein phosphatases

An example of a protein that is of paramount importance for cell survival, and the covalent modification of which will invariably lead to cell demise, is the group of protein phosphatases. These enzymes are selectively targeted by toxins derived from cyanobacteria.

Bioactivation to reactive metabolite
Other cellular stress
+
Protein-selective covalent binding
Disruption of critical protein function/structure
Signal ('Stress')
Depletion of antioxidant/-electrophilic defense systems
Modification of protein to neoantigen
Accelerated protein degradation
Toxicity

Figure 9.4. Possible downstream molecular consequences of covalent modification of a protein by an electrophilic intermediate. This can result in adaptive compensation or organ toxicity.

Microcystins are a group of related cyclic heptapeptides produced by cyano-bacteria ('blue-green algae'), e.g. *Microcystis aeruginosa.* If there is an algal bloom in a lake or in a small pond, contamination with these toxins can become an environmental problem and affect both game and farm animals.

D-Glu
Mdha
Adda
D-Ala
L-Leu
Masp
L-Arg

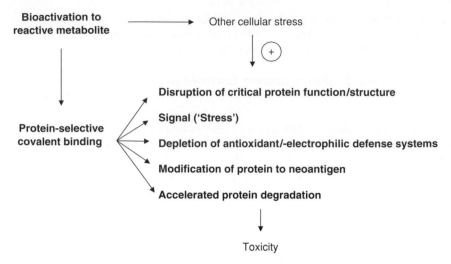

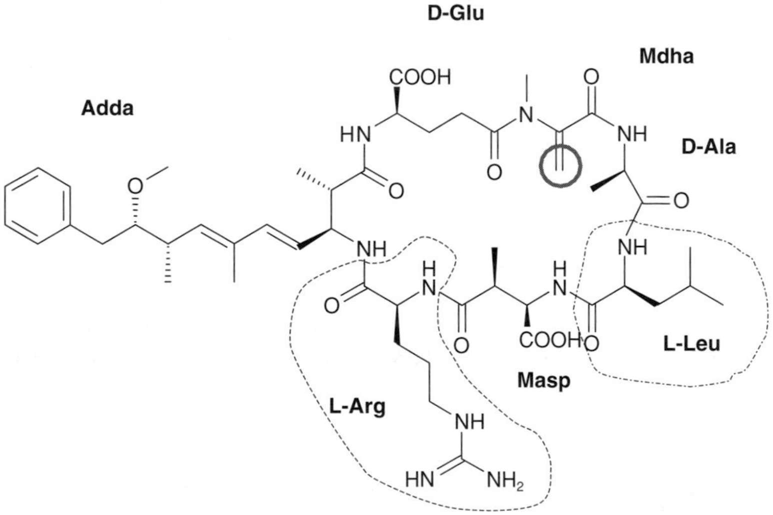

Figure 9.5. Chemical structure of microcystin-LR. The two variable amino acids are highlighted. The circle indicates the critical electrophilic carbon atom involved in covalent binding.

More than 20 different molecular species of microcystins have been identified. The molecule possesses two variable L-amino acids (leucine, arginine),
three D-amino acids, and two unusual amino acids (methyldehydro-alanine
(Mdha) and amino-methoxy-trimethyl-phenyl-decadienoic acid (Adda)).
Importantly, microcystins feature an electrophilic center; they do not need
to be bioactivated to become reactive species (Figure 9.5).

Microcystins exhibit a pronounced organotropic toxicity. In several species
it is the liver that is affected. Liver injury develops rapidly (i.e. within a few
hours) and is characterized by endothelial damage, apoptosis, intrahepatic
hemorrhage, and necrosis of the liver parenchyma.

Mechanisms of microcystin-induced liver injury: Two important mechanisms
have been detected that can explain both the organ-selective toxicity of microcystins and the rapid induction of parenchymal cell collapse and hemorrhage.

1 At the toxicokinetic level, microcystins are selectively taken up into hepatocytes
   by one of the multispecific organic anion transporters in the liver. Thus, they
   can reach high concentrations in the liver, where they subsequently damage the
   parenchymal cells (see section 3.1).
2 This mechanism, at the toxicodynamic level, is based on a highly selective molecular interaction between microcystin and molecular targets. The targeted proteins to which microcystins bind are protein phosphatases (PP), including PP-1,
   PP-2A, and PP-2B. Initially, hydrophobic and electrostatic interactions foster intermolecular interactions between the two molecules. Subsequently, the ethylene
   carbon of Mdha, an unusual amino acid residue of the microcystin molecule, is
   attacked by a cysteine residue of protein phosphatase, resulting in covalent adduct
   formation. Covalent binding readily inactivates the enzyme's function and leads
   to toxicity (see Figure 9.6).

Protein phosphatases (PP) are cytosolic enzymes that are critically involved
in cell homeostasis because they catalyze the dephosphorylation of proteins.
Reversible protein phosphorylation and dephosphorylation is a pivotal mechanism by which post-translational regulation of protein function is controlled.
These control mechanisms play an important role in cell differentiation, proliferation, cell metabolism, and turnover of structural proteins. On one side,
protein kinases transfer phosphate moieties from ATP to serine, threonine
or tyrosine residues. On the other side, protein phosphatases then hydrolyze
the phosphate bond and reverse the activation process.

Serine–threonine phosphatases are divided into the two classes, PP-1 and
PP-2. These share a catalytic site that exhibits a high degree of homology,
and both are targeted by microcystin.

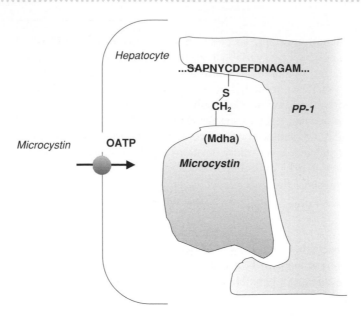

Figure 9.6. Microcystin is taken up into hepatocytes via a hepatocyte-specific organic anion transporter (OATP). Microcystin selectively interacts with and binds to protein phosphatase via a carbon–sulfur bond of a cysteine residue of PP-1.

Protein phosphatases have been implicated in regulating the mitogen-activated protein (MAP) kinase pathway, which in turn is involved in death-receptor-mediated apoptosis. How far the inactivation of PP2A by microcystin plays a role in the rapid induction of apoptosis that accompanies microcystin toxicity in the liver remains to be shown.

One pivotal function of protein phosphatases is to regulate the turnover of components of the cytoskeleton. In particular, protein kinases favor the disassembly of cytoskeletal components, while protein phosphatases favor the reassembly of the cytoskeleton. This might explain why microcystins rapidly disrupt the integrity of intermediate filaments, important components of the hepatocyte's cytoskeleton. Collapse of intermediate filament integrity is caused by a hyperphosphorylation state and rapid disassembly of vimentin, keratins, and nestin, which are components of the intermediate filaments. Similarly, the integrity of intercellular junctions is also highly dependent on PP function and is also rapidly lost after microcystin exposure (see Figure 9.7).

The effects of microcystins on these protein targets are highly selective. Therefore, it is perhaps not surprising that the toxic effects can occur at very low concentrations of microcystins. In fact, the IC_{50} of microcystin-LR required to inhibit PP-1 and PP-2A is 2×10^{-10} M! Due to their potent toxicity, microcystins can pose a hazard to the environment, and also for humans.

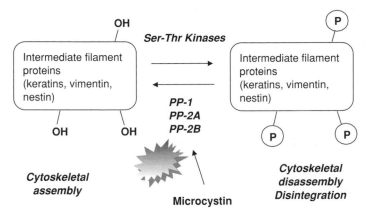

Figure 9.7. Phosphorylation of intermediate filament proteins favors dissassembly of the cytoskeleton, while dephosphorylation by protein phosphatases (PPs) favors assembly. Inactivation of PPs by covalent modification from microcystin results in a hyperphosphorylation state of these proteins, which causes rapid dissociation of the intermediate filament and collapse of the cytoskeleton.

'Algal blooms' are a problem worldwide. **Cyanobacteria** can cause a potential threat for cattle, water birds, and game, and intoxications in animals have indeed been reported. The toxins are not released from the cyanobacteria into the water but remain inside the cells. Thus, the toxic compound becomes active when whole cells are ingested. Therefore, chemical treatment of algal growth with $CuSO_4$ does not help, as the toxin is then released into the water and becomes toxic for the plankton, too. Besides microcystins, cyanobacteria also produce nodularins (produced by *Nodularia* species), which are cyclic pentapeptides and which are also hepatotoxic, as well as anatoxins, which are neurotoxic.

Microcystins can pose a potent human health hazard in drinking water. Contaminations of drinking water has, in isolated cases, caused similar pathology and symptoms of hepatotoxicity in humans to those seen in animals. For example, in 1996 contamination of drinking water with *Microcystis* toxins occurred in a clinic in Caruarù, Brazil. This was the first reported severe case, providing evidence that microcystins also inhibit PPs in human liver.

Another potential source of microcystin is the increasing marketing of algal products in health-food stores. These products are not always tested for microcystins and/or other toxic compounds, and highly toxic strains can potentially be present in these 'natural' foods.

9.2.2.2. Covalent modification of neurofilaments

Another typical example where selective covalent modification of proteins leads to toxicity is the neuropathy induced by *n*-hexane and related compounds.

> **n-Hexane** is an organic solvent widely used in the food industry (extraction of oils), in the industrial production of polymers, and in the oil industry (cracking). Hexane is also present in glues and paints and other household materials. Traditionally, the *acute* toxicity of n-hexane and other hydrocarbons has been considered minimal. In contrast, *chronic* exposure after a long transition phase (months) can result in neurotoxicity (sensoric–motoric or motoric polyneuropathies). Initially, the symptoms are non-specific and include weight loss and fatigue, but gradually they turn into more severe disturbances of the sensory function (numbness, distal paresthesia) in hands and feet, and also into muscle weakness in toes, fingers, arms, and legs.
>
> In the 1960s, the causal relationship between these symptoms and exposure to n-hexane became apparent. The neurotoxic effects were first observed in Japan, where home workers employed in the shoe industry (glueing of sandals) were exposed to relatively high concentrations of the volatile n-hexane for long periods. More recently, similar toxic symptoms have been observed in children who repeatedly and deliberately inhale high concentrations of this solvent (glue sniffers).

Mechanisms of n-hexane neuropathy: The clue to hexane's neurotoxic effects lies in the biotransformation to a protein-reactive metabolite. Specifically, n-hexane is metabolized in the liver by sequential (ω-1)-oxidation to the metabolite, 2,5-hexanedione (see Figure 9.8).

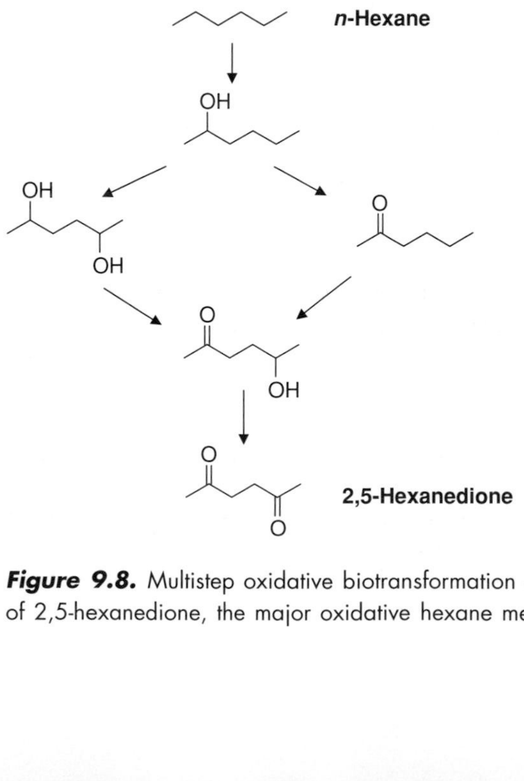

Figure 9.8. Multistep oxidative biotransformation of n-hexane results in the formation of 2,5-hexanedione, the major oxidative hexane metabolite in humans.

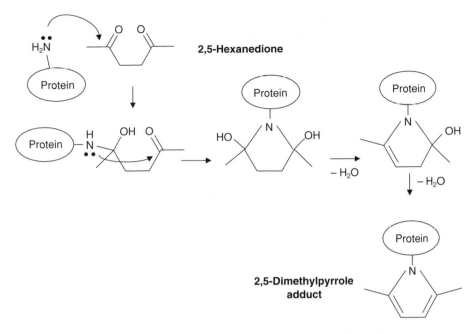

Figure 9.9. Sequential covalent binding of the electrophile 2,5-hexanedione to lysine residues of axonal proteins results in the formation of a 2,5-dimethylpyrrole adduct.

2,5-Hexanedione is the ultimate toxic metabolite that is responsible for inducing the neuropathy. The fact that 2,5-heptanedione is equally toxic, but 2,6-heptanedione and 2,1-heptanedione are not, suggests that there is a steric preference for the molecule in order to become toxic. In fact, all the compounds featuring similar toxicity are diketones with the two keto groups situated in the γ position. The reason can be found in the specific interaction of γ-diketones with target proteins; accordingly, this type of toxicity is also known as 'γ-diketone neuropathy'.

γ-Diketones interact with and form selective adducts to neuronal target proteins. Specifically, the carboxy carbons of 2,5-hexanedione represent electrophilic sites which are sequentially attacked by the nitrogen of a lysine residue, resulting in the formation of a hemiaminal and then a pyrrolidine. Finally, abstraction of water leads to the generation of a dimethylated pyrrole adduct (see Figure 9.9).

Many studies have provided evidence that the targeted proteins are compon-ents of intermediate filaments present in many cells, but particularly abundant in neurofilaments. Exposure to hexane or 2,5-hexanedione results in pyrrolation of ε-amino lysil residues of such neurofilamental proteins, which greatly affects their interaction with other cytoskeletal components. Ultimately, the neurofilament–microtubular network is disrupted as a consequence of interpolymer spacing. Such altered neurofilaments may accumulate at sites of axonal constrictions, such as the nodes of Ranvier. In addition, secondary autoxidation of the pyrrole rings can cause neurofilament–neurofilament crosslinks.

The selectivity of γ-diketones for this molecular target can also been demonstrated *in vitro*; selective binding of 2,5-hexanedione occurs to isolated rat neurofilament M and H proteins.

Neurofilaments are neuron-specific intermediate filaments and components of the peripheral axon (intermediate filaments, together with microtubules and actin, normally form the cytoskeleton in animal cells). Neurofilaments are composed of filamentous (not globular) substructures of three different types, and they are characterized by a high degree of phosphorylation.

In a nerve cell, all newly synthesized proteins, including the neurofilaments, arise in the body of the neuron. The neurofilaments are then transported distally along the axon by an ATP-consuming mechanism and at a low speed of approximately 0.2–1.0 mm/day. Not all neurofilaments migrate; some remain stationary. Proteolysis and protein turnover occur at the distal end of the neuron, near the synapses.

As a result of neurofilament pyrrolation, the axon gradually degenerates. The morphological hallmarks are greatly attenuated myelin sheaths, distally degenerated axon residues, and a club-shaped swelling in the preterminal region of the shortened axon (looking like 'giant axons' in cross-sections). These axonal swellings are filled with neurofilaments (see Figure 9.10).

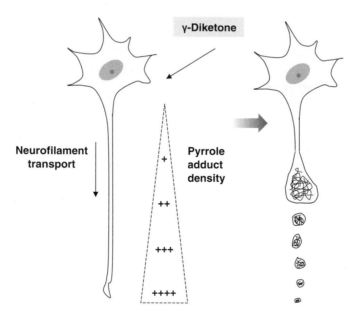

Figure 9.10. The most distally located neurofilaments exhibit the highest pyrrole adduct density, as a consequence of the slow migration of neurofilaments along the axon. This is also the site where the degeneration of the axon is initiated and from where the damage transgresses to more proximal sites.

Naturally the question arises as to the mechanistic basis of the neurotropic effects. Why is γ-diketone-induced toxicity most severe in the axon, although covalent binding and pyrrolation occur to many other proteins in the body? One important factor may be the longevity (half-life) of the axonal proteins; neurofilaments are extremely stable and have an extremely long lifetime, facilitating continued pyrrole adduct formation and cross-linking. Indeed, the highest adduct densities are found distally, where the oldest neurofilament proteins are present, while in the more proximal regions of the axon, where the newly synthesized proteins are located, fewer pyrrole adducts are present. In addition, the molecular cross-linking is likely to occur more avidly when the proteins are in close proximity, as is the case for neurofilaments.

9.2.2.3. Covalent modification of proteins in the biliary tree and small intestine

Certain reactive metabolites of drugs and other xenobiotics can form selective adducts to proteins of the biliary tree and small intestine. The reason for this tissue selectivity again can be found in toxicokinetics. Such metabolites include conjugated intermediates which are exported from the liver into bile against a steep concentration gradient and which, therefore, are abundant in the biliary tree.

Typical examples are acyl glucuronides (see section 4.2.2), which are protein-reactive intermediates generated from carboxylic acid-containing compounds. However, a causal relationship between protein acylation by these glucuronides and downstream toxic effects has not yet been unequivocally proven. It is also possible that acyl glucuronide–protein adducts are merely a molecular marker of the extent of covalent protein binding.

An example that illustrates the role of protein-reactive acyl glucuronides in the biliary tree is diclofenac.

Diclofenac is one of the most widely used nonsteroidal anti-inflammatory drugs (NSAIDs) for treatment of osteoarthritis, rheumatoid arthritis, ankylosing spondylitis, and acute pain. Although generally a safe drug, diclofenac can in rare cases produce severe hepatic injury, which is of an idiosyncratic nature (see section 10.3.3). Another adverse effect that diclofenac shares with many other carboxylic acid-possessing NSAIDs is gastrointestinal toxicity. While some of this toxicity (gastric irritation and bleeding) has clearly been related to the NSAID's pharmacological action (i.e. inhibition of cytoprotective prostaglandin production in the gastric mucosa), the pathogenesis of small intestinal irritation, erosions, and ulcer formation is less clear. Similarly, the mechanisms of hepatic injury are not known.

Diclofenac is metabolized in the liver by both oxidative metabolism (CYP2C9- and CYP3A4-catalyzed ring hydroxylation) and conjugation to glucuronic acid (catalyzed by UGT2B7 in humans and by UGT2B1, the rat homolog). The oxidized metabolites are mainly excreted renally, while the acyl glucuronide, in contrast, takes another route of elimination; a large portion of the glucuronide is excreted via the bile (in rats or dogs; in humans the fraction of biliary excretion of diclofenac is smaller). Being a large anion, the diclofenac acyl glucuronide is exported via the canalicular anion transporter Mrp2 across the hepatocellular apical membrane into the biliary canaliculus. The glucuronides leave the liver and reach the intestine, where a fraction is cleaved by bacterial β-glucuronidase, releasing the free aglycone, which is readily is reabsorbed. Thus, a substantial percentage of diclofenac (like other NSAIDs) is subject to enterohepatic circulation. Similarly to endogenous compounds (e.g. bile acids) which equally undergo enterohepatic circulation, reconjugation, and reexcretion, diclofenac goes through several cycles before all is excreted either renally or by the biliary route (see Figure 9.11).

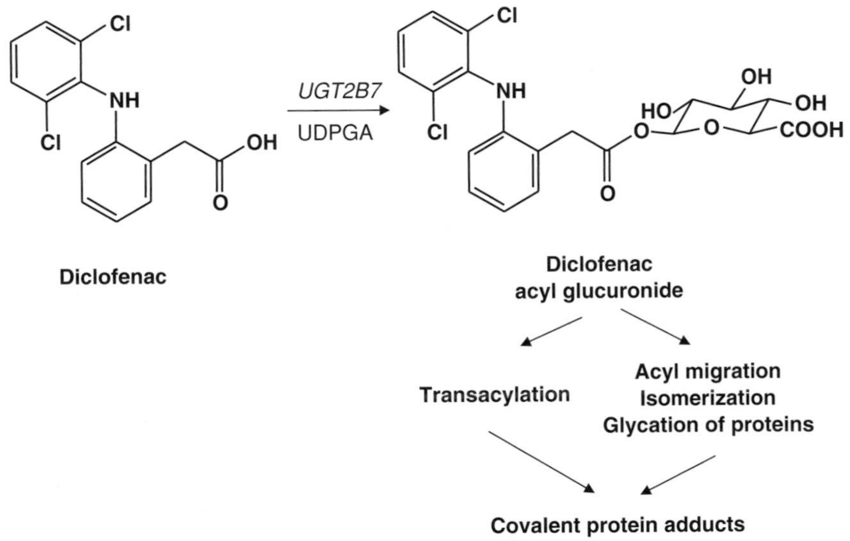

Figure 9.11. Diclofenac is conjugated to glucuronic acid to form a reactive acyl glucuronide.

Mechanisms of diclofenac acyl glucuronide acylation of hepatobiliary proteins: It is this repeated enterohepatic circulation that may provide a clue to the toxicity of diclofenac and similar drugs. First, the biliary tree and, hence, the small intestine are exposed to diclofenac for a prolonged time. Furthermore, and importantly, diclofenac metabolites in the biliary tree attain high local concentrations, as the acyl glucuronide is being actively up-concentrated for excretion. Calculations to determine the extent of up-concentration in bile for other acyl glucuronides have revealed that their canalicular concentrations can be up to 100-fold higher than intrahepatocellular concentrations, and up to 5,000-fold higher than those found in the peripheral blood! This is achieved by the function of a potent glucuronide export pump located in the canalicular membrane of hepatocytes (see section 3.3.1).

Mrp2 (multidrug resistance-associated protein-2), also termed 'conjugate export pump', is the canalicular isoform of a family of ATP-dependent transmembrane carriers belonging to the ABC (ATP-binding cassette) family. It features a broad substrate specificity and mediates the vectorial hepatobiliary transport of glutathione, glutathione conjugates, leukotriene 4, and, importantly, glucuronide conjugates of many endogenous and xenobiotic substrates, including that of diclofenac. The expression of Mrp2 is tightly regulated; not only can its abundance vary but it can also be relocated to other domains of the hepatocellular membrane (e.g. the basolateral side) if certain pathophysiological conditions require this. For example, during cholestasis, when bile flow is decreased or stopped (see section 3.3.1), relocation of the transporter to the basolateral membrane, together with up-regulation of other basolateral conjugate pumps, ensures that cholephilic compounds are excreted from the hepatocyte and thus excessively high (toxic) concentrations can be avoided.

Acyl glucuronides are protein-reactive (see section 4.2.2.2), and a number of protein adducts of diclofenac (metabolites) have recently been identified. Some adducts are present on circulating plasma proteins; others are confined to specific tissues. In the liver, large amounts of protein adducts are present at the canalicular membrane of hepatocytes. One important target has been identified as the canalicular ectoenzyme, DPP IV. Following exposure of rats to diclofenac, not only were adducts found on DPPIV, but the peptidase function of the enzyme was also decreased.

Dipeptidyl peptidase (DPP) IV is a multifunctional transmembrane glycoprotein and exopeptidase, featuring a post-proline peptidase activity. It is expressed by almost all mammalian cells, and it is identical to the adenosine deaminase binding protein on lymphocytes (CD26). DPP IV is also abundantly expressed in the canalicular domain of hepatocytes. Its exact role in the liver and the nature of the physiological substrates is still unclear. Typical for DPP IV is that it expresses a short cytoplasmic domain, a hydrophobic transmembrane domain, and that the bulk of the enzyme is extracellular. The extracellular part consists of three domains, the middle part of which harbors 10–12 highly conserved cysteine residues (this is also responsible for DPP IV binding to collagen I). Thus, this domain which exhibits many nucleophilic sites could become important in terms of DPP IV being a target for electrophiles.

Why do these reactive acyl glucuronides acylate preferentially DPP IV (and probably other canalicular proteins)? Several reasons may account for this.

1 DPP IV and other canalicular proteins are in close proximity to Mrp2, which mediates the vectorial transport of these conjugates.
2 DPP IV features many sulfhydryl groups and exposes these nucleophilic sites to the electrophilic metabolite.

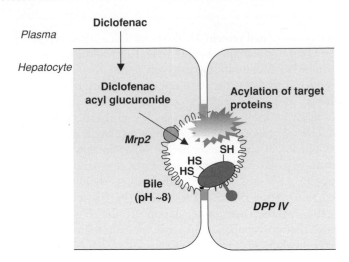

Figure 9.12. Mrp2-driven up-concentration of the reactive diclofenac acyl glucuronide in bile canaliculi favors covalent binding to the canalicular protein target, DPP IV.

3 The pH in bile is slightly more alkaline (~8) than in the cell. Acyl glucuronides are known to be more readily hydrolyzed (and thus react with nucleophiles) in alkaline pH.
4 Importantly, the reactive glucuronides are highly up-concentrated in the canaliculus (see above).

This example illustrates that many factors together may determine the targets for covalent interactions and adduct formation. Yet it is not known whether the inactivation of DPP IV is causally associated with cholestasis or even related to the rare idiosyncratic cases of drug hepatitis that are seen with many NSAIDs (see Figure 9.12).

Interestingly, diclofenac protein adducts also occur further downstream, i.e. in the small intestine. Again, it is not yet known whether these protein adducts to intestinal mucosal proteins are causally linked to the potential of diclofenac for small intestinal ulcer formation. Two points are interesting, however:

1 As in bile, the pH in the small intestine is more alkaline than in other places, which would favor covalent binding
2 The areas where adducts are present are congruent with those in which the ulcers appear (and adduct formation precedes ulceration).

9.3. Covalent DNA binding

Some electrophilic metabolites can also avidly interact with and covalently bind to nucleic acids including DNA. Because in a cell there is quantitatively much more protein, lipid or RNA present than there is DNA (in hepatocytes, DNA accounts only for approximately 0.2 percent per weight), only a small fraction of a bioactivated xenobiotic will covalently bind to DNA. Nevertheless, DNA adduct formation has been considered more dramatic and has received much more attention than protein

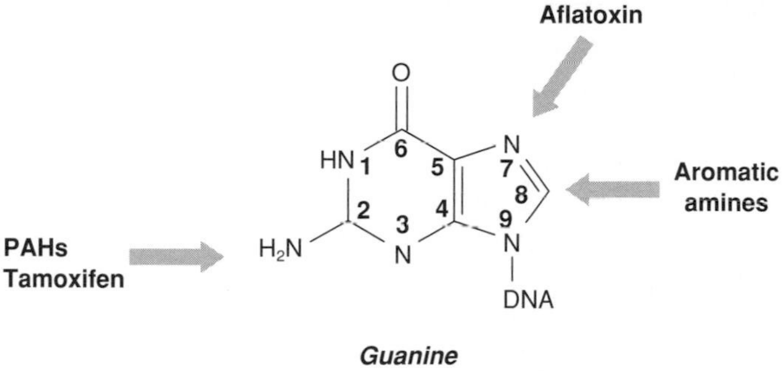

Figure 9.13. Electrophilic metabolites of xenobiotics differentially interact with and covalently bind to selective sites of DNA bases.

binding because such adducts can alter the DNA structure and, if it escapes repair, can result in erroneous DNA replication and in the induction of mutations. Ultimately, DNA alkylation has been implicated in carcinogenesis. In fact, for many genotoxic carcinogens, the amount of DNA adducts correlates with the incidence of tumor formation. However, it is not the overall extent of adduct formation but rather the specific site in a particular gene that is mechanistically important in carcinogenicity.

All four bases, as well as phosphate oxygen, can react with electrophilic metabolites. However, it is the guanine residue which is the predominant base to be attacked by an electrophilic species and potential carcinogen. The nucleophilic targets in the DNA are predominantly electron-dense sites, such as nitrogen and oxygen atoms in nucleic acids. The site and extent of binding is dependent on, among other factors (including sequence selectivity), the size and the reactivity of the electrophilic species and electrostatic and steric factors. For example, activated polycyclic aromatic hydrocarbons (PAHs) predominantly bind to the N-2 position of guanine, while the reactive metabolite of the mycotoxin aflatoxin preferentially the N-7 position. Aromatic amines, on the other hand, readily bind to the C-8 position of guanine after rearrangement; the carbon itself is not very nucleophilic (see Figure 9.13).

The consequences of nucleotide adduct formation can be dramatic; many adducted sites (e.g. guanine O-6 and N-2) are normally involved in forming hydrogen bridges with the partner base. These bonds are no longer possible, which will result in erroneous base pairing when the DNA undergoes replication. Such a mismatch can end up in base substitutions (point mutation), as shown below for benzo[a]pyrene. Fortunately, a number of control mechanisms continuously check the DNA for any type of damage, and in most cases these mistakes are repaired, as long as the second strand and DNA polymerase III remain intact. In addition, not all DNA adducts are stable; for example, the covalent bonds between N-alkylated purines and the reactive metabolite are readily cleaved by hydrolysis.

9.3.1. Toxicological consequences of DNA alkylation

It has long been known that covalent modification of DNA can lead to the formation of tumors. Some of the pioneering experiments were done with polycyclic aromatic hydrocarbons including benzo[a]pyrene.

Benzo[a]pyrene (BaP) (see also section 5.4) is a ubiquitous environmental pollutant and a potent mutagen and carcinogen. It is one of the most important carcinogens in cigarette smoke. In particular, BaP has been implicated in causing mutations in the tumor supressor gene p53 (see section 8.2); such mutations have been detected in lung tumors of smokers.

BaP is metabolized by CYP1A1 to a diol-epoxide, which has been considered the 'ultimate carcinogen' (i.e. the final electrophilic intermediate after a sequence of metabolic activation steps). The first step is oxidation to a 7,8-epoxide, which is followed by hydrolysis of the epoxide to its *trans*-7,8-diol catalyzed by epoxide hydrolase. This metabolite is then further oxidized to the 9,10-epoxide. This latter intermediate harbors an active center, i.e. the carbon atom at the C-10 position. The reason why it is at this site that adducts are preferentially formed lies in the fact that this so-called bay region of the molecule provides an area of steric hindrance for detoxifying enzymes, while oxidation can easily occur. Here, the epoxide can open to a carbonium ion and is thus very susceptible to nucleophilic attack (see Figure 9.14).

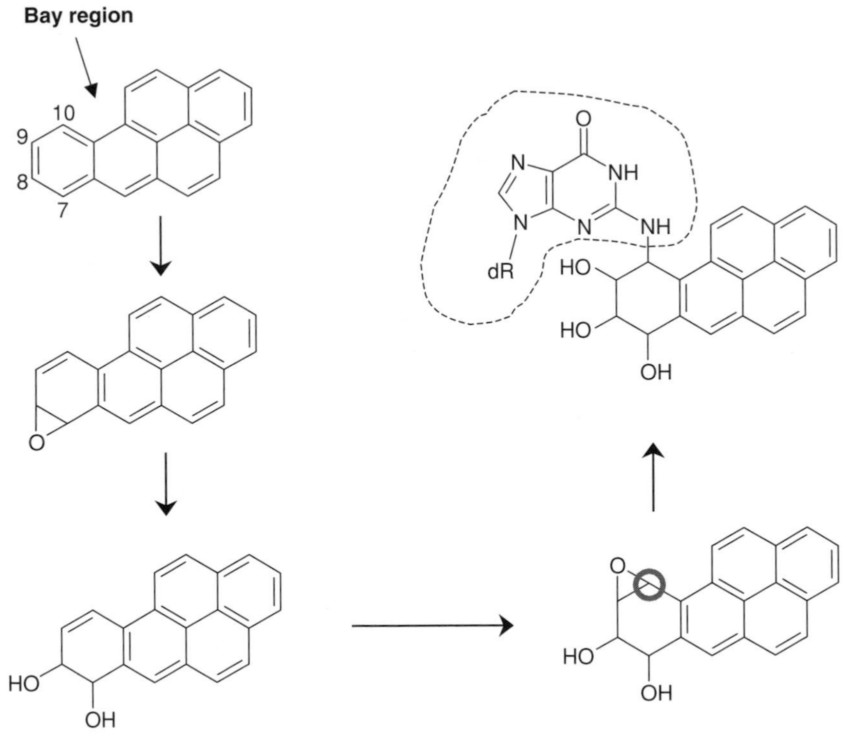

Figure 9.14. Bioactivation of benzo[a]pyrene to the ultimate reactive metabolite and carcinogen, 7,8-diol-9,10-epoxide, results in covalent adduct formation with deoxyguanosine. The circle marks the electrophilic center.

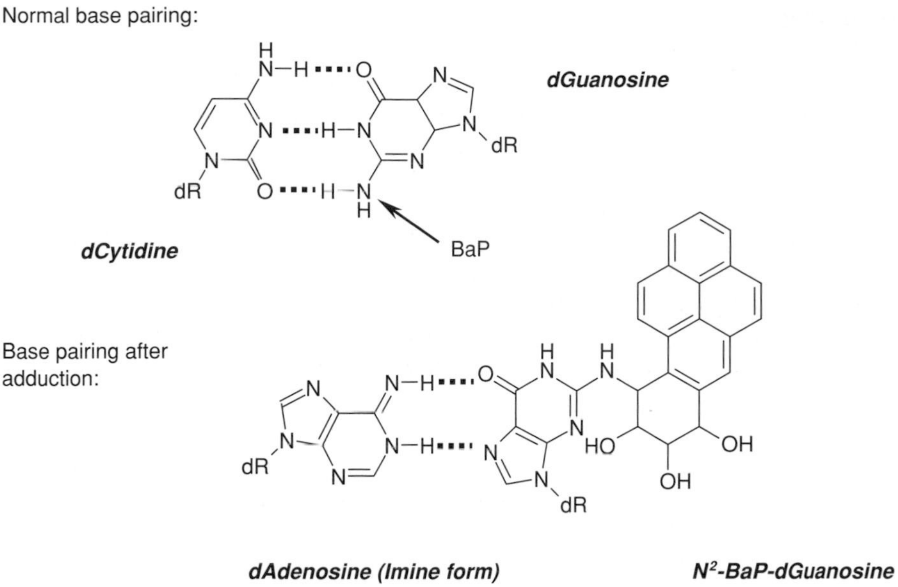

Normal base pairing:

dCytidine   BaP

dGuanosine

Base pairing after
adduction:

dAdenosine (Imine form)   N²-BaP-dGuanosine

Figure 9.15. The presence of a BaP adduct at the N-2 amine position of guanine precludes binding via three hydrogen bonds with cytosine. Instead, the adducted guanine will pair with adenine, and a base transversion will result.

Mechanisms of benzo[a]pyrene-induced DNA adduct formation and mutagenesis: The DNA-reactive metabolites of PAHs preferentially react with the exocyclic amino groups of DNA bases. Indeed, the major benzo[a]pyrene adduct on DNA is BaP-N²-dG. Several stereospecific isomers have been identified. But what are the downstream toxicological consequences of these adducts?

The presence of BaP adducts can have dangerous repercussions when the cell enters the cell cycle and undergoes DNA replication. As shown here, under normal conditions, guanine pairs with cytosine via three hydrogen bonds. However, one of these bonds involves the N-2 amine position, which is occupied after covalent binding because the BaP adduct sits right there. Consequently, the BaP-N²-guanine can only pair with adenine, building up two hydrogen bridges, but this is the wrong partner. In the next cell division cycle, the adenine (wrong base) will pair with thymine. The result is a base pair transversion; if this mismatch escapes repair, the change will become permanent and the result is a point mutation (see Figure 9.15).

Induction of a mutation alone need not necessarily result in a deleterious reaction for the organism. If the mutation occurs in a nontranscribed region or in a region of the genome that is inactive, then there may be little or no downstream biological effects. In contrast, if the mutation hits a proto-oncogene (abnormal activation or overexpression) or a tumor suppressor gene (inactivation), then this alteration can become potentially carcinogenic. For example, BaP induces G→T transversions in specific codons (the 12th) of the ras family of protooncogenes, which may convert the gene into an active oncogene.

Learning points

- Xenobiotics can be bioactivated to an electrophilic metabolite which irreversibly reacts with a nucleophilic partner and forms a covalent bond. These targeted nucleophiles are either small molecular scavengers in a cell (e.g. glutathione) or macromolecules such as proteins, DNA, and lipids.

- The selectivity of covalent binding is determined by the chemical nature of the electrophile, its subcellular localization and concentration, and the reactivity (nucleophilicity) of available targets.

- The consequences of covalent adduct formation to amino acid residues can be manifold and can include inactivation of enzymes (e.g. protein phosphatases), transporters, or structural proteins (e.g. neurofilaments), haptenation of a peptide, or induction of signaling pathways that are involved in the regulation of stress response genes. This is often mechanistically related to toxicity. For many other protein-reactive xenobiotics, however, the biological significance of covalent binding is not known; the adducts may serve as biomarkers to detect reactive metabolites.

- DNA bases can be alkylated by electrophilic metabolites (e.g. from PAHs). If they escape repair mechanisms, this can lead to a base mismatch during DNA replication and a possible mutation. If this occurs in critical genes, e.g. in a tumor suppressor gene, then this can disrupt the cell cycle control and ultimately result in increased tumor formation.

Further reading

Methyl isocyanate

Jeevaratnam, K. and Sriramachari, S. (1994) Comparative toxicity of methyl isocyanate and its hydrolytic derivatives in rats. 1. pulmonary histopathology in the acute phase, *Arch. Toxicol.* 69: 39–44.

Covalent protein binding

Boelsterli, U.A. (1993) Specific targets of covalent drug–protein interactions in hepatocytes and their toxicological significance in drug-induced liver injury, *Drug Metab. Rev.* 25: 395–451.

Nelson, S.D. (1994) Covalent binding to proteins, *Methods Toxicol.* 1B, 1: 340–348.

Pumford, N.R. and Halmes, N.C. (1997) Protein targets of xenobiotic reactive intermediates, *Annu. Rev. Pharmacol. Toxicol.* 37: 91–117.

Acetaminophen

Bartolone, J.B., Birge, R.B., Sparks, K., Cohen, S.D. and Khairallah, E.A. (1988) Immunochemical analysis of acetaminophen covalent binding to proteins, *Biochem. Pharmacol.* 37: 4763–4774.

Bessems, J.G.M. and Vermeulen, N.P.E. (2001) Paracetamol (acetaminophen)-induced toxicity: Molecular and biochemical mechanisms, analogues and protective approaches, *Crit. Rev. Toxicol.* 31: 55–138.

Birge, R.B., Bartolone, J.B., Hart, S.G.E., Nishanian, E.V., Tyson, C.A., Khairallah, E.A. and Cohen, S.D. (1990) Acetaminophen hepatotoxicity: Correspondence of selective protein arylation in human and mouse liver *in vitro*, in culture, and *in vivo*, *Toxicol. Appl. Pharmacol.* 105: 472–482.

Bulera, S.J., Birge, R.B., Cohen, S.D. and Khairallah, E.A. (1995) Identification of the mouse liver 44-kDa acetaminophen-binding protein as a subunit of glutamine synthetase, *Toxicol. Appl. Pharmacol.* 134: 313–320.

Fountoulakis, M., Berndt, P., Boelsterli, U.A., Crameri, F., Winter, M., Albertini, S. and Suter, L. (2000) Two-dimensional database of mouse liver proteins. Changes in hepatic protein levels following treatment with acetaminophen or with its non-toxic regioisomer 3-acetaminophenol, *Electrophoresis* 21: 2148–2161.

Halmes, N.C., Hinson, J.A., Martin, B.M. and Pumford, N.R. (1996) Glutamate dehydrogenase covalently binds to a reactive metabolite of acetaminophen, *Chem. Res. Toxicol.* 9: 541–546.

Hinson, J.A., Pumford, N.R. and Roberts, D.W. (1995) Mechanisms of acetaminophen toxicity: Immunochemical detection of drug–protein adducts, *Drug Metab. Rev.* 27: 73–92.

Hoivik, D.J., Manautou, J.E., Tveit, A., Mankowski, D.C., Khairallah, E.A. and Cohen, S.D. (1996) Evidence suggesting the 58-kDa acetaminophen binding protein is a preferential target for acetaminophen electrophile, *Fund. Appl. Toxicol.* 32: 79–86.

Pumford, N.R., Halmes, N.C., Martin, B.M., Cook, R.J., Wagner, C. and Hinson, J.A. (1997) Covalent binding of acetaminophen to n-10-formyl-tetrahydrofolate dehydrogenase in mice, *J. Pharmacol. Exp. Ther.* 280: 501–505.

Qiu, Y., Benet, L.Z. and Burlingame, A.L. (1998) Identification of the hepatic protein targets of reactive metabolites of acetaminophen *in vivo* in mice using two-dimensional gel electrophoresis and mass spectrometry, *J. Biol. Chem.* 273: 17940–17953.

Ruepp, S.U., Tonge, R.P., Shaw, J., Wallis, N. and Pognan, F. (2002) Genomics and proteomics analysis of acetaminophen toxicity in mouse liver, *Toxicol. Sci.* 65: 135–150.

Downstream consequences of covalent protein binding

Cohen, S.D., Hoivik, D.J. and Khairallah, E.A. (1998) Acetaminophen-induced hepatotoxicity, *Toxicology of the Liver*, Plaa, G.L. and Hewitt, W. (eds), 2nd edition, Raven Press, New York, NY, pp. 159–186.

Hart, S.G.E., Cartun, R.W., Wyand, D.S., Khairallah, E.A. and Cohen, S.D. (1995) Immunohistochemical localization of acetaminophen in target tissues of the CD-1 mouse: correspondence of covalent binding with toxicity, *Fund. Appl. Toxicol.* 24: 260–274.

Nelson, S.D. (1990) Molecular mechanisms of the hepatotoxicity caused by acetaminophen, *Sem. Liver Dis.* 10: 267–278.

Microcystin-induced liver injury

Mackintosh, R.W., Dalby, K.N., Campbell, D.G., Cohen, P.T.W., Cohen, P. and Mackintosh, C. (1995) The cyanobacterial toxin microcystin binds covalently to cysteine-273 on protein phosphatase 1, *FEBS Lett.* 371: 236–240.

Runnegar, M., Berndt, N., Kong, S.M., Lee, E.Y.C. and Zhang, L.F. (1995) *In vivo* and *in vitro* binding of microcystin to protein phosphatases 1 and 2A, *Biochem. Biophys. Res. Commun.* 216: 162–169.

Tencalla, F. and Dietrich, D. (1997) Biochemical characterization of microcystin toxicity in rainbow trout (*Oncorhynchus mykiss*), *Toxicon* 35: 583–595.

Toivola, D.M., Eriksson, J.E. and Brautigan, D.L. (1994) Identification of protein phosphatase 2A as the primary target for microcystin-1R in rat liver homogenates, *FEBS Lett.* 344: 175–180.

Toivola, D.M., Goldman, R.D., Garrod, D.R. and Eriksson, J.E. (1997) Protein phosphatases maintain the organization and structural interactions of hepatic keratin intermediate filaments, *J. Cell. Sci.* 110: 23–33.

Yoshida, T., Makita, Y., Tsutsumi, T., Nagata, S., Tashiro, F., Yoshida, F., Sekijima, M., Tamura, S.I., Harada, T., Maita, K. and Ueno, Y. (1998) Immunohistochemical localization of microcystin-LR in the liver of mice: A study on the pathogenesis of microcystin-LR-induced hepatotoxicity, *Toxicol. Pathol.* 26: 411–418.

n-Hexane neuropathy

DeCaprio, A.P., Kinney, E.A. and Fowke, J.H. (1997) Regioselective binding of 2,5-hexanedione to high-molecular-weight rat neurofilament proteins *in vitro*, *Toxicol. Appl. Pharmacol.* 145: 211–217.

Graham, D.G., Amarnath, V., Valentine, W.M., Pyle, S.J. and Anthony, D.C. (1995) Pathogenetic studies of hexane and carbon disulfide neurotoxicity, *Crit. Rev. Toxicol.* 25: 91–112.

Lehning, E.J., Jortner, B.S., Fox, J.H., Arezzo, J.C., Kitano, T.A. and LoPachin, R.M. (2000) γ-Diketone peripheral neuropathy. I. Quantitative morphometric analyses of axonal atrophy and swelling, *Toxicol. Appl. Pharmacol.* 165: 127–140.

Passarin, M.G., Monaco, S., Ferrari, S., Giannini, C., Rizzuto, N. and Moretto, G. (1996) Cytoskeletal changes in cultured human fibroblasts following exposure to 2,5-hexanedione, *Neuropathol. Appl. Neurobiol.* 22: 60–67.

Mrp2

Keppler, D. and König, J. (2000) Hepatic secretion of conjugated drugs and endogenous substances, *Sem. Liver Dis.* 20: 265–272.

Paulusma, C.C., Kothe, M.J.C., Bakker, C.T.M., Bosma, P.J., Van Bokhoven, I., Van Marle, J., Bolder, U., Tytgat, G.N.J. and Oude Elferink, R.P.J. (2000) Zonal down-regulation and redistribution of the multidrug resistance protein 2 during bile duct ligation in rat liver, *Hepatology* 31: 684–693.

Trauner, M., Arrese, M., Soroka, C.J., Ananthanarayanan, M., Koeppel, T.A., Schlosser, S.F., Suchy, F.J., Keppler, D. and Boyer, J.L. (1997) The rat canalicular conjugate export pump (Mrp2) is downregulated in intrahepatic and obstructive cholestasis, *Gastroenterology* 113: 255–264.

DPP IV

Dobers, J., Grams, S., Reutter, W. and Fan, H. (2000) Roles of cysteines in rat dipeptidyl peptidase IV/CD26 in processing and proteolytic acitvity, *Eur. J. Biochem.* 267: 5093–5100.

Acyl glucuronides

Atchison, C.R., West, A.B., Balakumaran, A., Hargus, S.J., Pohl, L.R., Daiker, D.H., Aronson, J.F., Hoffmann, W.E., Shipp, B.K. and Moslen, M.T. (2000) Drug enterocyte adducts: Possible causal factors for diclofenac enteropathy in rats, *Gastroenterology* 119: 1537–1547.

Bailey, M.J., Worrall, S., de Jersey, J. and Dickinson, R.G. (1998) Zomepirac acyl glucuronide covalently modifies tubulin *in vitro* and *in vivo* and inhibits its assembly in an *in vitro* system, *Chem.-Biol. Interact.* 115: 153–166.

Boelsterli, U.A. (1999) Reactive acyl glucuronides: Possible role in small intestinal toxicity induced by nonsteroidal anti-inflammatory drugs, *Toxic Subst. Mech.* 18: 83–100.

Hargus, S.J., Amouzedeh, H.R., Pumford, N.R., Myers, T.G., McCoy, S.C. and Pohl, L.R. (1994) Metabolic activation and immunochemical localization of liver protein adducts of the nonsteroidal anti-inflammatory drug diclofenac, *Chem. Res. Toxicol.* 7: 575–582.

Hayball, P.J. (1995) Formation and reactivity of acyl glucuronides: the influence of chirality, *Chirality* 7: 1–9.

Qiu, Y., Burlingame, A.L. and Benet, L.Z. (1998) Mechanisms for covalent binding of benoxaprofen glucuronide to human serum albumin. Studies by tandem mass spectrometry, *Drug Metab. Dispos.* 26: 246–256.

Seitz, S. and Boelsterli, U.A. (1998) Diclofenac acyl glucuronide, a major biliary metabolite, is directly involved in small intestinal injury in rats, *Gastroenterology* 115: 1476–1482.

Wang, M. and Dickinson, R.G. (1998) Disposition and covalent binding of diflunisal and diflunisal acyl glucuronide in the isolated perfused rat liver, *Drug Metab. Dispos.* 26: 98–104.

Wang, M., Gorrell, M.D., McCaughan, G.W. and Dickinson, R.G. (2001) Dipeptidyl peptidase IV is a target for covalent adduct formation with the acyl glucuronide metabolite of the anti-inflammatory drug zomepirac, *Life Sci.* 68: 785–797.

Benzo[a]pyrene-induced DNA adduct formation/mutagenesis

Jernstrom, B. and Graslund, A. (1994) Covalent binding of benzo[a]pyrene 7,8-dihydrodiol 9,10-epoxides to DNA – molecular structures, induced mutations and biological consequences, *Biophys. Chem.* 49: 185–199.

Kozack, R., Seo, K.Y., Jelinsky, S.A. and Loechler, E.L. (2000) Toward an understanding of the role of DNA adduct conformation in defining mutagenic mechanism based on studies of the major adduct (formed at N^2-dG) of the potent environmental carcinogen, benzo[a]pyrene, *Mut. Res. Fund. Mol. Mech. Mutagenesis* 450: 41–59.

Lutz, W.K. (1998) Dose–response relationships in chemical carcinogenesis: Superposition of different mechanisms of action, resulting in linear–nonlinear curves, practical thresholds, J-shapes, *Mut. Res. Fund. Mol. Mech. Mutagenesis* 405: 117–124.

Miller, K.P. and Ramos, K.S. (2001) Impact of cellular metabolism on the biological effects of benzo[a]pyrene and related hydrocarbons, *Drug Metab. Rev.* 33: 1–35.

Chapter 10

Immune mechanisms

Contents

10.1. Xenobiotic-induced activation of the innate immune system
10.2. Immunosuppression by xenobiotics
10.3. Immune-mediated toxicity

Immune-mediated toxicity is still a relatively new area in mechanistic toxicology. It is also one of the most complex fields in toxicology. Many aspects are poorly understood and a detailed understanding is only slowly emerging. As the immune system is vital to protect our body from foreign invaders, it harbors an intrinsic arsenal of potentially dangerous effector mechanisms which under certain conditions can become directed against our own cells or tissues. To prevent this, it is only logical that nature has endowed the immune system with many rigorous control mechanisms, redundancies to ensure proper function, inhibitors, and multi-pathway regulatory mechanisms.

In particular, three features have to be highlighted for a better understanding of immune-mediated mechanisms of toxicity.

1 The immune system, unlike other organ systems in the body, is not confined to one or two fixed organs. Instead, it is decentralized; there are a multitude of lymphatic organs distributed across the body. There are well-localized primary lymphatic organs (e.g. thymus, bone marrow) and secondary lymphatic organs (e.g. lymph nodes, spleen), but there are also circulating immune cells distributed across the whole body. Xenobiotics can exert effects on any of these lymphoid organs, and immune effector cells can be readily recruited to almost any site in the body.

2   In higher organisms (vertebrates) including humans, there is both a phylogenetically older immune system and a phylogenetically more evolved system, working in concert. The more primitive system, also called the innate immune system, which is the only functional immune system in invertebrates, consists of a number of immune cells featuring mainly phagocytic functions. These cells can also release proinflammatory and signaling mediators. Cells of the innate immune system include leukocytes, macrophages, natural killer (NK) cells, and γδ T cells. Importantly, they are not strictly antigen-specific; instead, they react upon a broad range of stimuli. On the other hand, the more modern immune system is antigen-specific, featuring an almost unlimited repertoire of specific responses directed against a given antigen. Importantly, this antigen response must be able to distinguish accurately between self and non-self. If this distinction is not rigorously maintained, the result can be potentially dangerous. For example, if the body does not recognize or insufficiently recognizes foreign proteins that invade the organism, an infection can ensue. On the other hand, if the immune system is unable to recognize self-proteins as self, it may attack its own tissues instead of exerting immune tolerance, and an autoimmune reaction may develop.

3   The effects of xenobiotics, which can modulate the function of the immune system at several levels, can have two opposing consequences: if xenobiotics push the normal function of the immune system out of balance, the result can either be an immunosuppression or an immune overstimulation. Both directions can bear danger and result in toxicity; immunosuppression can result in a diminished resistance against infections, while immunostimulation may result in hypersensitivity reactions, allergies, and autoimmune disease.

10.1. Xenobiotic-induced activation of the innate immune system

Leukocytes, macrophages, NK cells, and γδ T cells can greatly aggravate a signal stemming from a xenobiotic (or a reactive metabolite) and thus enhance tissue injury. These cells are present in many organs or tissues, but they can also be readily recruited to sites of action. Some organs are particularly rich in phagocytes. For example, in the liver there is a large population of macrophages (Kupffer cells) which can be activated by xenobiotics and which are mechanistically involved in enhancing the toxicity.

Kupffer cells are resident macrophages in the liver. They are the largest macrophage population in the whole body, representing approximately 80–90 percent of all fixed macrophages. Although small in size in comparison to the large hepatocytes, they represent approximately 15 percent of the total number of cells in the liver. They reside in the sinusoidal space, attached to the endothelial cells, and are thus directly exposed to the circulating blood. Their major function is to remove foreign material from the portal blood that streams into the liver. In fact, Kupffer cells have both F_c and C3 receptors, i.e. they are able to recognize and phagocytose both opsonized and non-opsonized particles (particles that are tagged with antibodies).

Another important function of these macrophages is to synthesize and release proinflammatory mediators, such as reactive oxygen species, reactive nitrogen species, and a number of cytokines. The production of these signaling molecules is often greatly increased during the initiation and progression of xenobiotic-induced liver injury. To amplify the signal further, the number of Kupffer cells in the liver is often increased during toxic liver injury, and extrahepatic macrophages are recruited and readily infiltrate the liver.

Activation of hepatic macrophages typically occurs if lipopolysaccharide (LPS, endotoxin produced from Gram-negative bacteria) is released from the intestine into the bloodstream, where it is bound to proteins and reaches the liver. In addition, there are many examples where toxic chemicals activate Kupffer cells. An example is carbon tetrachloride.

Carbon tetrachloride (see section 5.2.3) is bioactivated in the liver and induces centrilobular necrosis. A biomarker for this hepatic damage is the massive increase in hepatocyte-selective proteins (e.g. aminotransferase activities) in the serum. To demonstrate whether hepatic macrophages are indeed involved in the development of this injury, carbon tetrachloride toxicity can be examined in a liver where all the Kupffer cells have been selectively eliminated prior to administration of the toxin. In fact, Kupffer cells can be chemically destroyed by gadolinium chloride ($GdCl_3$). This treatment indeed protects (at least in part) from subsequent CCl_4-induced liver necrosis, emphasizing a mechanistic role of Kupffer cells in the toxic injury (see Table 10.1).

Mechanisms of Kupffer cell-mediated aggravation of liver injury: The roles of macrophages in enhancing the signals and aggravating liver injury are manifold. They include the presence of membrane-bound NADPH oxidase which can cause a burst in reactive oxygen production and release into the extracellular space (see section 5.1.4). In addition, nitric oxide is produced, proteases are released, and prostanoids and other bioactive lipids are generated. Finally, a number of cytokines

Table 10.1 Elimination of Kupffer cells by GdCl₃ protects from CCl₄-induced liver injury

Treatment	Liver injury	Presence of MΦ
Vehicle	–	+
CCl_4	++	+
$GdCl_3$ + CCl_4	(+)	–
$GdCl_3$	–	–

Note: Rats were given orally 4 g/kg CCl_4. After 24 h, serum aspartate aminotransferase (AST) activity was measured. Gadolinium chloride (10 mg/kg) was administered 24 h prior to CCl_4. Of course, the possibility that pretreatment with $GdCl_3$ might alter the CYP-mediated bioactivation of CCl_4 had to be considered; this was not the case.
Source: adapted from Edwards, M.J., Keller, B.J., Kauffman, F.C. and Thurman, R.G. (1993) The involvement of Kupffer cells in carbon tetrachloride toxicity, *Toxicol. Appl. Pharmacol.* 119: 275–279.

including TNFα and IL-1β are produced (see Chapter 11). These mediators act as signals and are involved in intercellular crosstalk; however, if released in excess quantities, they can also directly participate in tissue destruction.

All these mediators are produced by both resident macrophages and monocytes infiltrating from the circulation. In fact, infiltrating cells can further increase the number of phagocytes three-fold within the following 48 to 72 h. This has been observed not only after CCl₄ but also after other hepatotoxins including 1,2-dichlorobenzene and acetaminophen. Part of this cell recruitment is a result of chemokine secretion by hepatocytes and other cell types in the liver. Chemokines (e.g. monocyte chemoattractant protein, MCP-1) are compounds which build up a chemical gradient, attracting responding cells and causing them to migrate towards the site of production.

Recently, it has been shown that an additional immune cell type is coming into play. Dendritic cells (the most efficient antigen-presenting cells) circulate in the blood system and can be recruited to peripheral tissues by chemokines. For example, in the liver dendritic cells are attracted from chemokine release from Kupffer cells. These dendritic cells bind to the Kupffer cells via specific receptors on the dendritic cell membrane surface that recognize sugar residues on Kupffer cells. Importantly, dendritic cells can extravasate, i.e. leave the fenestrated endothelial wall of the hepatic sinusoid and come into direct contact with hepatocytes (see Figure 10.1).

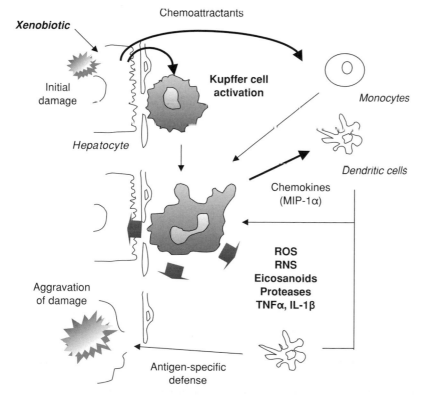

Figure 10.1. Activation of Kupffer cells in the liver and interactions with hepatocytes and phagocytes (crosstalk).

Some of the mediators released by Kupffer cells (TNFα, IL-1β, IL-8, and platelet activating factor (PAF)) are chemoattractants for another effector cell type, the neutrophils. Upon release of these mediators, β2 integrins on neutrophils are readily up-regulated. At the same time, the transcriptional activation of adhesion molecule proteins on endothelial cells and hepatocytes is also stimulated. This facilitates specific interactions between the adhesion molecules on neutrophils and their molecular partners on endothelial cells, allowing neutrophils to bind to the endothelial wall, extravasate, and infiltrate the liver. These neutrophils aggravate the damage by releasing tissue-damaging agents. PMNs thus represent a second wave of attack, following the initial wave of Kupffer cell activation, and it is often this second and more powerful attack that gives the chemically-damaged liver the final blow.

Neutrophils (PMNs, polymorphonuclear leukocytes) are circulating immune cells which play a major role in inflammatory processes and whose major function is to phagocytose and kill pathogenic organisms. However, in recent years it has become clear that neutrophils can also be mechanistically involved in the toxicity of xenobiotics. They are able to do this by releasing mediators (e.g. cytokines) and also directly-damaging agents (e.g. ROS, proteolytic enzymes). Neutrophils can also metabolize various chemicals through their myeloperoxidases. Although this is probably not important in the liver, it might become an efficient mechanism of bioactivation in other organs where otherwise little drug metabolism would occur. In order for such a toxic action to take place, PMNs must first receive a signal upon which they will accumulate in the particular tissue. Subsequently, they must receive a stimulus that activates them to release mediators and cytotoxic agents. This has been extensively investigated for the liver.

Normally, neutrophils circulate and are in random contact with endothelial cells but do not adhere to them. However, upon a stimulus (e.g. from Kupffer cells and/or hepatocytes), cellular adhesion molecules are up-regulated both on neutrophils and on the endothelial cells. The PMNs then slow down in their flow and roll along the surface of the endothelium. They finally become firmly adherent to the endothelial wall. PMNs are then activated and migrate through the endothelial wall (fenestrated in the liver), where they get in contact with parenchymal cells.

Mechanisms of hepatic tissue damage aggravation by neutrophils: Upon activation, neutrophils migrate across the endothelium and adhere to the parenchymal cells. Upon further stimulation by proinflammatory cytokines, neutrophils undergo oxidative burst and release large amounts of ROS. These alone are, however, not sufficient to induce full tissue damage; in addition, proteases (in particular elastase and cathepsin G) are released, which cause hepatocellular cell death and necrosis (see Figure 10.2).

In addition to macrophages, a large number of resident γδ T cells are present in the liver, which have also been implicated in playing a role in xenobiotic-induced non-specific immune reactions.

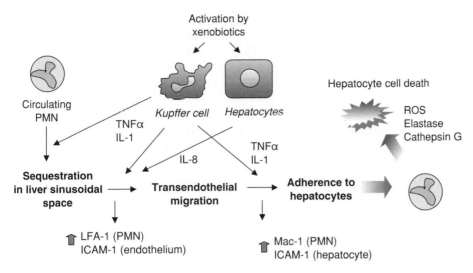

Figure 10.2. Neutrophil activation, transendothelial migration, and cytotoxic activity at the target tissue.

γδ **T cells** are specific lymphocytes featuring γδ receptors (as opposed to αβ T cell receptors). γδ T cell receptors recognize small molecules and intact proteins without prior processing and MHC-associated presentation of antigens by antigen-presenting cells (which would be required by αβ T cell receptors). However, cell–cell contact is required for proper function. This is possible in the liver as the endothelial cells are fenestrated, allowing T cells to leave the vasculature and to get into direct touch with the parenchymal cells. It is likely that non-MHC molecules on target cells present these small molecules to the γδ T cell receptor. Most of the γδ T cells have tissue-specific domains in their respective gene segments. Their distribution varies; for example, in peripheral blood ~5 percent of all T cells are γδ cells, while in the liver a large population of resident γδ T cells are present.

10.2. Immunosuppression by xenobiotics

A number of xenobiotics can suppress the maturation and development of immune cells and thus cause an immunosuppression (this involves both cells of the innate immune system and antigen-specific cells). For example, benzene (see section 5.1.1), which is bioactivated to reactive quinoid metabolites, is myelotoxic because these reactive metabolites can severely damage progenitor cells in the bone marrow. Because many cells in the bone marrow are damaged in a non-specific way, the result may be a pancytopenia (i.e. a loss of all cells). As this general hematopoietic cell destruction will also include the lymphocyte precursor cells (T and B cells), it is plausible that most of the specific immune system will be compromised.

Immunosuppression can also be caused by other mechanisms and can occur in other parts of the immune system. A widely cited example is the toxicologically important group of 'dioxins', including polychlorinated dibenzodioxins, dibenzofurans, and biphenyls. Among these xenobiotics, TCDD is the most powerful agent that has been implicated in causing dramatic immunosuppressant effects.

2,3,7,8-Tetrachloro-*p*-dibenzodioxin (TCDD) (see section 12.1) causes changes to the hematopoietic and mature immune system that can become apparent after a very small single dose (i.e. in the ng/kg body weight range). In animal experments, the number of peripheral lymphocytes is diminished after TCDD. In humans, a similar mechanism might become effective; evidence indicates that following exposure to polychlorinated biphenyls in rice oil, human populations in Taiwan and Japan exhibited distinct alterations in their T cell patterns, with a clear impact on health: these people developed increased sensitivity to respiratory infections, due to a suppression of the immune system.

The cause of dioxin-induced T cell depletion is found in the thymus, the major site where T cells differentiate. Indeed, after small doses of TCDD animals exhibit a decrease in thymus mass, leading to thymic atrophy.

The thymus is a primary lymphoid organ in which immature precursor cells develop into mature T cells that have attained the full ability to recognize non-self peptides in conjunction with self MHC molecules presented by antigen-presenting cells (APCs). During this maturation process, the immature T cell precursor cells, having migrated into the thymus from the bone marrow, differentiate into either CD4$^+$ or CD8$^+$ cells (CD4 and CD8 are both transmembrane glycoproteins belonging to the immunoglobulin superfamily. They are cell adhesion molecules with specificity for MHC molecules, facilitating signal transduction. CD4 binds to class II MHC and is a marker for helper cells; CD8 binds to class I MHC and is a marker for cytotoxic T cells).

In the thymus, three structures can be distinguished: the outer subcapsular zone, the cortex, and the medulla. The outer subcapsular zone is a relatively thin area that contains the most immature cells, which do not yet express CD4 or CD8. From here, the T cell precursors migrate deeper into the thymic tissue. In the second layer, the cortex, the T cell precursors begin to express both CD4 and CD8, and they rearrange their T cell receptor (TCR) α and β genes in such a way that each T cell will express a different type of rearranged heterodimer. Then the T cells migrate into the innermost part, the medulla, which contains the mature T cells. These cells either now express CD4$^+$CD8$^-$ and will later recognize MHC II (helper cells), or now express CD4$^-$CD8$^+$ and will later recognize MHC I (cytotoxic T cells). They will leave the thymus, enter the bloodstream and seed the secondary lymphoid tissues, where they will become activated by foreign peptide–MHC complexes.

A pivotal role in this differentiation process is played by specialized epithelial cells in the cortex. These epithelial cells not only provide trophic factors that are vital for T cell differentiation, but also express high levels of MHC I and MHC II molecules on their surface. Only those T cells that recognize MHC plus self peptide can survive (they are positively selected), while those T cells that do not recognize MHC plus self peptide will be eliminated by apoptosis. So all selected T cells originally recognize self peptide. Possibly self peptide/MHC recognition results in a higher activation threshold of those T cells. Therefore, a certain level of affinity is required to activate these T cells. In a further selection step, T cells recognizing self antigen with high affinity are being eliminated by apoptosis (negative selection). Therefore, T cells leaving the thymus have an activation threshold that is set too high for activation by self antigen. In other words, the major discriminator between positive and negative selection is the affinity for receptor binding. Furthermore, the organism has a number of additional peripheral control mechanisms for maintaining tolerance, and a number of additional factors, including inflammation, or the expression of costimulatory molecules, have to be present before this tolerance is broken.

Mechanisms of TCDD-induced thymic atrophy and T cell depletion: The mechanisms by which TCDD inhibits the differentiation of T cells involves thymic epithelial cells, but the exact molecular events are not known. There is compelling evidence, though, that the effects are mediated by the aryl hydrocarbon receptor (AHR; see section 12.1). First, it is striking that the AHR is abundantly expressed in the thymus. Second, and providing more direct evidence, is the fact that AHR-null mice were much more resistant toward the thymic toxicity inflicted by TCDD than wild-type mice. In fact, a high dose of TCDD (2,000 µg/kg body weight) did not decrease thymic weight nor decrease the cellularity of the thymic cortex in AHR −/− mice, while in heterozygous or AHR +/+ mice even with a ten-fold lower dose severe immunotoxicity was found. It is currently believed that TCDD damages thymic cortical epithelial cells, but also activates Ca^{2+}-dependent endonucleases which leads to apoptotic cell death in cortical thymocytes. The fact that the number of $CD4^+/CD8^+$ double positive thymocytes is not affected by TCDD, while the $CD4^+/CD8^-$ cell and $CD4^-/CD8^+$ single positive populations in the thymus and in the periphery are severely decreased in number, points to the possibility that TCDD affects a critical stage during the maturation and differentiation of T cells in the thymus (see Figure 10.3).

10.3. Immune-mediated toxicity

In contrast to xenobiotics such as TCDD, which suppress the function of the immune system, other xenobiotics can *enhance* the function of the immune system. Such an immunostimulatory effect can get out of control and result in harmful reactions. These forms of reactions are rare, but they are toxicologically relevant because the degree of the adverse effects can be severe.

Two basic forms of such xenobiotic-induced immunostimulatory effects are toxicologically relevant in humans. The first type comprises allergic reactions (also

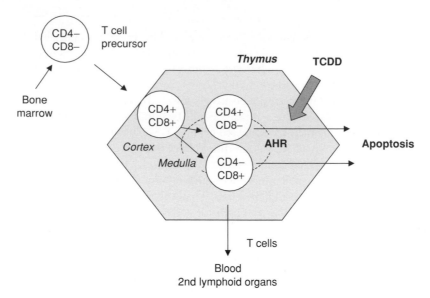

Figure 10.3. Activation of the AHR by TCDD and other dioxin-like xenobiotics prevents maturation of T cells into either CD4+ cells (T helper cells) or CD8+ cells (cytotoxic T cells) in the thymus.

called hypersensitivity reactions), which are most commonly known as chemically-induced respiratory tract allergies or contact allergies in the skin. In allergic reactions, the immune response is directed against drug-modified antigens, involving antibodies and/or T cells directed against drug and antigen.

The second type are called autoimmune reactions. Importantly, in autoimmunity antibodies/T cells are directed exclusively against true self antigens (and not against the drug or drug-modified antigens). Often the terms 'allergy' and 'autoimmunity' are used interchangeably, but in fact they are two distinct mechanisms.

In both cases, the immune reactions can be triggered by xenobiotics. This may be paradoxical at first thought, as most xenobiotics are small molecules, and typical immune reactions are only evoked against large peptides and other macromolecules featuring a cutoff molecular mass of >1,000 Da. However, the clue to this puzzle is that the 'small' xenobiotic that triggers an immune response is often a chemically reactive molecule (or it produces a chemically reactive metabolite) that can covalently bind to a target protein (haptenate the protein). The 'foreign' part of the protein (i.e. the covalently bound xenobiotic) is called a hapten. This hapten can theoretically induce an immune response via at least three different pathways:

1 The hapten is recognized by the immune system as part of a 'non-self' peptide fragment
2 Haptenation can induce a conformational change of the protein, thereby unfolding 'hidden' epitopes on the peptide, and thus promote an immune response against this new antigen
3 The hapten can modulate the immune system so that native 'self' peptides will be viewed as though they were non-self peptides and become subject to immune attack (autoimmune reaction) (see Figure 10.4).

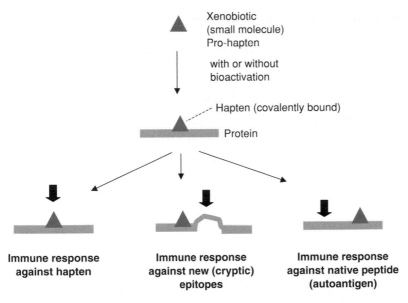

Immune response against hapten

Immune response against new (cryptic) epitopes

Immune response against native peptide (autoantigen)

Figure 10.4. Haptenation of a peptide by a reactive xenobiotic or a reactive metabolite can induce a specific immune response by different mechanisms. Source: adapted from Gut, J., Christen, U. and Huwyler, J. (1993) Mechanisms of halothane toxicity – novel insights, *Pharmacol. Ther.* 58: 133–155.

A typical example of a chemically-induced immunostimulatory reaction, which on one hand illustrates the toxicological significance but also shows the complexity of such multifactorial toxicity, is the 'Spanish Toxic Oil Syndrome'.

Toxic Oil Syndrome is the name of an epidemic intoxication that occurred in Spain in 1981, which affected more than 20,000 people and caused several hundred fatalities. At that time, a large number of patients were admitted to hospitals with respiratory symptoms and signs of autoimmune disease. These included interstitial pneumonitis, fever, rash, eosinophilia, joint pain, vasculitis, and the presence of antinuclear antibodies in the serum, as well as increased serum IgE levels. The etiology of this epidemic intoxication remained enigmatic for some time.

It later turned out that the cause of this immune-mediated disease was ingestion of rapeseed oil that had been illegally adulterated with oil labeled for industrial use, which had been denatured with 2 percent aniline. In an attempt to unravel the mechanism, several reaction products between aniline and fatty acids were identified, and these condensation products exhibited an excellent dose-dependent positive correlation with the risk of developing toxic oil syndrome. The exact etiology has still not been elucidated, but some candidate compounds have been identified, and their pathways of bioactivation and haptenation of proteins have been described.

Mechanisms of the induction of immune-mediated disease in Toxic Oil Syndrome: Aniline itself is not protein-reactive *per se*, but some of its oxidative metabolites, and some reaction products of aniline and fatty acids, clearly are pro-haptens or haptens. Specifically, two pathways can account for the generation of such reactive metabolites. First, aniline, an aromatic amine, can be oxidized to *N*-hydroxyaniline, which is further oxidized to nitrosobenzene. Aromatic *N*-hydroxy and nitroso compounds are notorious for undergoing redox cycling (see section 5.1.1) but also for being protein-reactive, forming adducts to sulfhydryl groups of target amino acid residues. Alternatively, aniline-coupled lipids, in particular fatty acid esters of 3-(*N*-phenylamino)-1,2-propanediol (PAP) can be metabolized to a protein-reactive species. The aromatic ring of the aniline moiety can be *para*-hydroxylated by CYP and further oxidatively metabolized by CYP or peroxidases to a quinoneimine. Quinoneimines are well-known electrophilic species that can arylate proteins (see section 9.2.1) (see Figure 10.5).

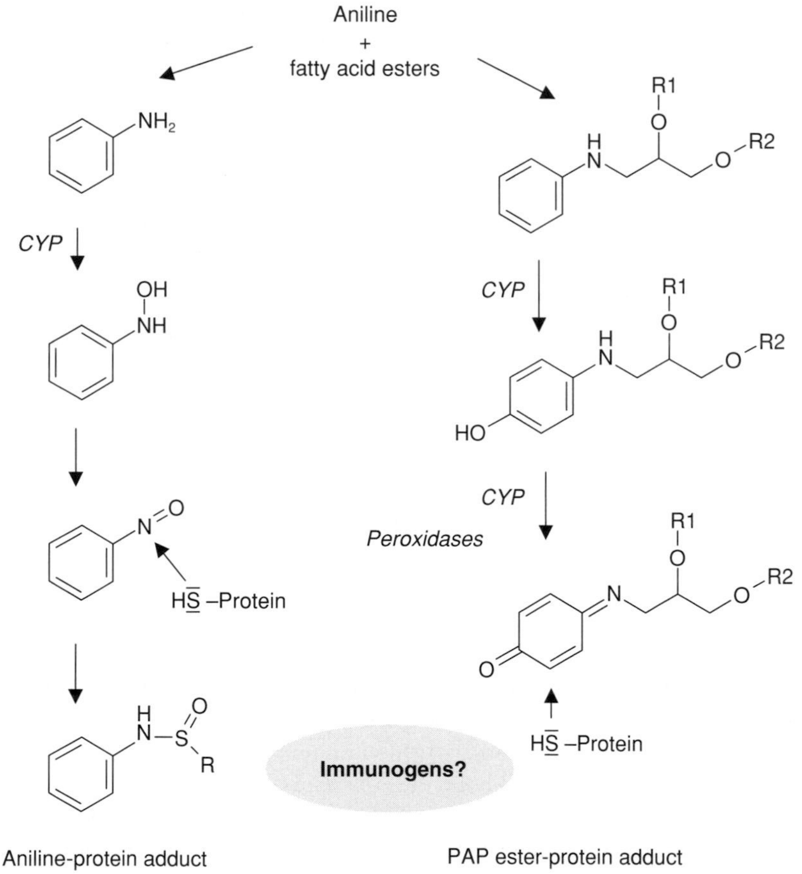

Figure 10.5. Pathways of bioactivation of putative pro-haptens to protein-reactive species implicated in Toxic Oil Syndrome. *Left,* aniline is oxidized via *N*-hydroxylation to the nitroso compound. *Right,* fatty acid esters of PAP (= 3-(*N*-phenylamino)-1,2-propanediol) are oxidized via *para*-hydroxylation to the phenol and further oxidized to a reactive quinone imine. *R1* and *R2,* oleyl-, linoleyl-, or linolenyl- residue.

It has been postulated that the metabolic generation of these reactive inter-mediates takes place in the bone marrow, immune system, or skin (and possibly in erythrocytes). This would explain why the immune reactions occur in these organs, and not in the liver.

The downstream molecular mechanism, where the immune system becomes involved, is even more speculative at this point. After haptenating unidentified protein targets (self proteins), the chemically-modified peptides likely represent neoantigens that can sensitize T cells. However, a sequence of additional biochemical and cellular events is necessary to elicit an immune response directed against self proteins and involving target tissues, and this is poorly understood. One factor, however, might be an important clue: the toxic agent possesses a lipid structure. Therefore, the lipid moiety of the fatty acyl anilide may act as an intrinsic enhancer (an adjuvant) of the immune reaction and may stimulate antigen-presenting cells (e.g. macrophages). In fact, the adjuvant effects of lipids, when covalently bound to the immunizing antigen, are well known.

10.3.1. Autoimmune reactions

Chemically-induced autoimmunity is a result of a modification of host tissues or immune cells by the chemical and not the chemical acting as an antigen/hapten. A typical example of a drug that has been implicated in such autoimmune reactions is procainamide.

Procainamide is an antiarrhythmic drug that has been associated with the development of autoimmune reactions. These are characterized by fever, involve-ment of the respiratory system, muscle and joint pain, arthritis, and other symptoms, summarized under the term systemic lupus erythematosus (SLE). Interestingly, the majority (~90 percent) of all patients develop anti-nuclear antibodies, i.e. circulating antibodies directed against chromatin components, which are clinically 'silent', and without outbreak of the disease. Actually, a large number of patients have antibodies against histones, but only symptomatic patients have antibodies against (H2A-H2B)-DNA, a specific component of chromatin. Apparently procainamide, or more likely one of its metabolites, induces an immune response by acting directly on T cells, possibly by inter-fering with T cell selection processes in the thymus resulting in the appearance of autoreactive T cells, which in turn recognize one or several autoantigens (chromatin). The autoimmune effector mechanisms would become active in only a small percentage of patients, though.

The mechanism of procainamide autoimmune toxicity has only recently become more clear. Two key events seem to play a crucial role: metabolic activation of procainamide to a protein-reactive intermediate, and abnormal maturation and differentiation of autoreactive T cells in the thymus.

Mechanisms of procainamide-induced lupus: Procainamide, like other aromatic amines, is metabolized through two major pathways. First, the amino group is acety-lated by NAT-catalyzed reactions (see section 4.2.4), and the *N*-acetylated product

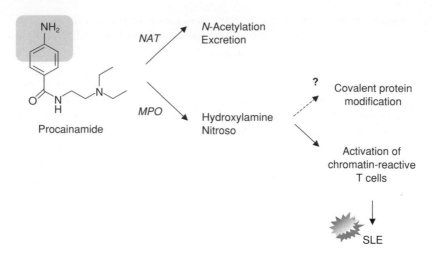

Figure 10.6. Bioactivation of procainamide can lead to an autoimmune response.

is readily excreted. Alternatively, procainamide is bioactivated by myeloperoxidase-catalyzed oxidation in white blood cells (neutrophils and monocytes) to the N-hydroxy and, subsequently, to the nitroso derivative (see above). As these metabolites are electrophilic protein-reactive species, they can covalently bind to protein targets. Because this second pathway is the crucial one that has been associated with the development of autoimmune reactions, while the first pathway is a detoxication reaction, one would predict that people featuring the polymorphic slow acetylator phenotype would exhibit an increased risk for developing procainamide-induced lupus; this is indeed the case (see Figure 10.6).

While this first (metabolic) portion is well established, the subsequent immunological mechanisms are still incompletely understood. Although it has been shown that metabolites can bind to proteins, this is unlikely to be important for inducing autoimmunity (in fact, no immune response against drug-altered antigens has been demonstrated in procanamide-treated patients). Why do all individuals not develop overt autoimmune disease? Obviously, there are rigorous control mechanisms that are only slowly being elucidated. Another puzzling question is, what is the significance of B cell-derived anti-chromatin antibodies?

Key to the understanding of procainamide-induced lupus is the thymus (see section 10.2). Normally, and essentially, the thymus is responsible in preventing autoimmunity by ensuring that the newly generated T cells do not react with self antigens. The maturing T cells undergo rigorous selection processes; T cell precursors with an avid reactivity for self proteins are killed by apoptosis, while cells with a low affinity for self peptides may survive. Although the surviving T cells recognize self peptides during positive selection, they are not autoreactive once they are in the periphery, indicating that during positive selection a higher threshold of activation is being set, possibly by inducing negative regulators of chemokine gene expression. A reactive metabolite of procainamide, the hydroxylamine, can 'break' this tolerance by preventing the establishment of unresponsiveness to self during the maturation process in the thymus. Indeed, recent data from a mouse model of procainamide-induced SLE-like disease has revealed that the normal immune repertoire does include nontolerant autoreactive B cells which are activated when the positive selection process in the thymus is disrupted.

10.3.2. Immunoallergy

Immunoallergic or hypersensitivity reactions generally imply that an immune response is triggered by a chemical and that the antibody or T cell-mediated attack is directed against the haptenated peptide. Although many of the immunological mechanisms involved in xenobiotic-induced autoimmune reactions are still obscure, one example is more completely understood and has given important insights into the immune activation pathways. This – and probably the single best understood xenobiotic – is the drug penicillin.

Penicillins are β-lactam antibiotics typically featuring a very low acute toxicity. High doses (≤1 g/kg body weight per day) given intravenously to patients are well tolerated. However, penicillins are among drugs that have been frequently associated with the appearance of immunoallergies. In fact, up to 1 percent of all recipients can develop some form of immune reaction directed against penicillin. Among these, hemolytic anemia is a frequent manifestation of the drug-induced toxic response.

For penicillin, too, haptenation of proteins is the first step in producing an immunoallergic reaction. However, penicillins are an exception in that

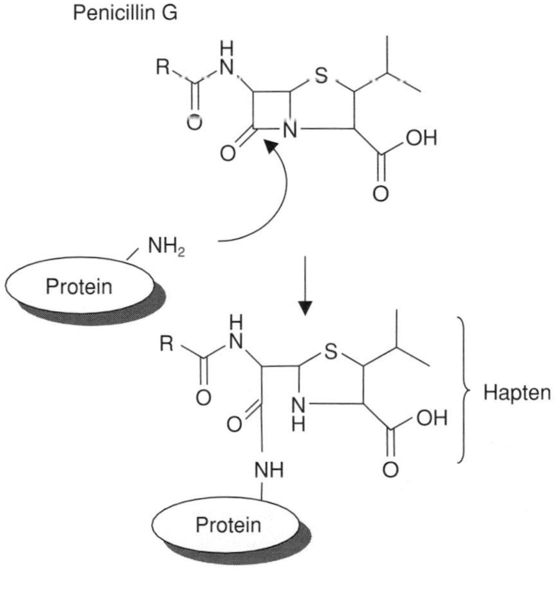

Penicillin G

Figure 10.7. Covalent interaction of penicillin G with nucleophilic sites of lysin residues of target proteins results in chemically-modified proteins (antigens).

---

they need not be activated to a reactive intermediate; they are chemically reactive by themselves (see Figure 10.7).

β-Lactam antibiotics of the newer generations are less allergenic than those belonging to the first generations. One reason, besides the reactivity of the compound, is the shorter half-life of the adducts. Unstable protein adducts are less likely to become antigens than adducts with a long half-life.

Mechanisms of penicillin-induced immune-mediated hemolytic anemia: The penicillin-modified peptide induces the production of specific IgG immunoglobulins (or IgM). These antibodies recognize and bind to the hapten on the surface of the erythrocyte membrane. The bound antibodies are recognized by natural killer cells or other phagocytes. These phagocytes, by virtue of their F_c receptor (a receptor which specifically recognizes the F_c portion of the immunoglobulin molecule), bind to the target cells and lyze it by the release of cytotoxic mediators from granules. Such an immune reaction (called Type II reaction according to the traditional classification of hypersensitivity reactions) is antibody-dependent and cell-mediated (see Figure 10.8).

Because for penicillin, metabolic bioactivation of the drug is not required to produce a reactive metabolite, the susceptibility of certain patients to developing these blood dyscrasias obviously cannot be reasoned on the basis of a differential expression of drug-metabolizing enzymes. What determines, then, whether or not a patient will develop immunoallergy? Interestingly, all patients treated with high doses of penicillin (i.e. $>10^7$ units per day) produce drug–erythrocyte adducts. However, only a small fraction of these patients produce anti-penicilloyl IgG. The reasons underlying this tolerance are still unresolved.

Other xenobiotics that have to be bioactivated by organ-selective metabolism can cause organ-specific autoimmune reactions. One of the best-known examples is immune-mediated hepatitis caused by a reactive metabolite of halothane.

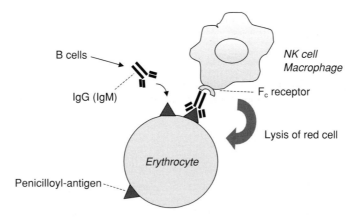

Figure 10.8. Antibody-dependent phagocyte-mediated lysis of red cells in penicillin-induced immunoallergy.

Halothane is an inhalation anesthetic which was introduced some 50 years ago. Preclinical safety trials had revealed minimal toxicity; clinical use of halothane, however, has been associated with two types of hepatic adverse drug reactions. The first one is a mild form of hepatotoxicity, occurring in approximately 20 percent of all recipients and characterized by mild and transient increases in serum aminotransferase activites. The second, much more serious but less frequent form is halothane hepatitis, characterized by post-operative liver necrosis and even hepatic failure.

This severe form of halothane-induced liver injury in humans resembles in many ways acute or chronic viral hepatitis. It is a rare event: the incidence is approximately 1:35,000 in patients who receive the first halothane anesthesia; however, the risk is ten-fold higher after repeated exposure, indicating that a sensitization has occurred. The mortality is high (approximately 35 percent in cases where hepatitis developed after the first exposure, and approximately 50 percent after repeated exposures!).

Meanwhile, newer anesthetics, featuring a lower potential of developing liver injury, have been introduced. Among these are the structural derivatives, isoflurane and desflurane. Interestingly, these congeners produce the same reactive metabolite as halothane. But what is the cause for the lower propensity of isoflurane or desflurane to cause hypersensitivity reactions in the liver? Similarly to the other examples, these new anesthetics have been associated with the generation of haptens. However, the most plausible reason is the rate of bioactivation; for isoflurane and desflurane, the extent of hepatic bioactivation to a reactive metabolite is more than 100-fold less than that for halothane.

Mechanisms of halothane-induced immune-mediated liver injury: As for many other drugs and xenobiotics which cause hypersensitivity reactions, it is usually the initial steps of the entire cascade leading to immune destruction of an organ that are best understood, while some of the downstream mechanisms involving positive and negative regulation of the effectors of the immune system are less clear.

Halothane is bioactivated in the liver by two distinct pathways, which are dependent on the availability of molecular oxygen. First, at low pO_2, CYP2E1 metabolizes halothane by bioreduction. This results in the cleavage of a bromide ion (a good leaving group) plus a trifluorochloroethyl radical. Analogously to the reactions caused by bioactivated carbon tetrachloride, this radical will react with a fatty acyl moiety and abstract a hydrogen (see section 5.2.3). This will cause direct toxicity due to lipid peroxidation.

Alternatively, in the presence of higher pO_2, this reductive pathway can be circumvented (and that is why during anesthesia with halothane, high oxygen pressure should be maintained). Under these circumstances, CYP2E1 oxidizes halothane by introducing a hydroxyl group. Again, a bromide is readily cleaved off, resulting in the formation of trifluoroacetylchloride (TFA). This metabolite is an electrophilic reactive species which can either hydrolyze water and become converted to trifluoroacetic acid, or else become attacked by a nucleophilic group (e.g.

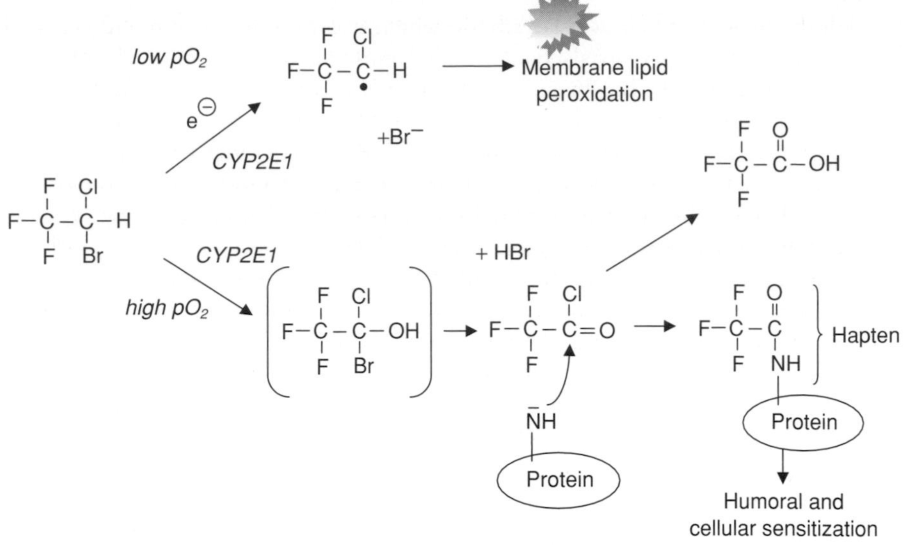

Figure 10.9. Oxidative biotransformation of halothane leads to the formation of covalent trifluoroacetyl adducts to lysine residues of hepatic proteins. In contrast, bioreductive metabolism produces the trifluorochloroethyl radical, which initiates lipid peroxidation.

a lysine residue) of a protein and thus form a protein adduct. In fact, haptenated proteins are likely to be the immunogens, ultimately leading to an immune response in the liver (see Figure 10.9).

A pivotal question is that of the identity of the trifluoroacetylated protein targets. Numerous adducted proteins have been isolated, sequenced, and identified. Among these is the CYP that bioactivates halothane, indicating that the reactive intermediate is very reactive and alkylates a target right at the site where it is generated. Other identified proteins include a protein disulfide isomerase, a 59 kD carboxylesterase, and calreticulin (and a large number of other targets). The targeted proteins are all located at the membrane of the endoplasmic reticulum, and it has been speculated that it is the location of these proteins, rather than their size, specific function, or other characteristics, that determines their role as a target. In addition, many of these TFA-adducted proteins are molecular chaperones, having a role in proper folding of other proteins.

Anti-TFA antibodies, produced in TFA-carrier protein-immunized animals, recognize all these adducted proteins, when the antiserum is incubated with electrophoretic-ally resolved proteins from liver exposed to halothane. This makes sense, as the antibody probably recognizes the hapten (plus some adjacent peptide sequences) covalently bound to proteins. However, interestingly, such antibodies also recognize some native proteins. For example, anti-TFA antibodies recognize specific mito-chondrial enzyme subunits (e.g. the E2 subunits of both pyruvate dehydrogenase and 2-oxoglutarate dehydrogenase). Specifically, the antibodies recognize the lipoic acid moiety, which is a component of these enzyme subunits. This becomes important in the context of a possible molecular mimicry mechanism that has been evoked to explain the low incidence of these autoimmune reactions (see below).

The downstream events that follow the TFA adduct formation to hepatic proteins are much less clear. Even if one assumes that there is a primary immune response, it is not clear what signals enhance this primary response, breaking the immune tolerance (which normally exists), and causes overt immune attack on the hepatic parenchyma. There are few experimental models to explore these mechanisms; nevertheless, evidence suggests that several mechanisms may be involved. One of these mechanisms is presentation of processed antigens by MHC I molecules on hepatocytes, which would be recognized by cytotoxic T cells, followed by cell lysis (see Figure 10.10).

It is important to recall that generally it is only a small proportion of a population receiving the potentially immune-stimulating xenobiotic that ultimately develops an immune reaction against that agent. What are the possible causes underlying this tolerance? Or, in other words, why is immunoallergic liver injury caused by xenobiotics (fortunately) such an infrequent event?

Two mechanisms will be discussed in this respect. First, it is well known that if individuals are exposed to the potentially immuno-enhancing xenobiotic via the oral route, the 'oral tolerance' phenomenon is observed.

Oral tolerance: This term implies that a potentially immunogenic xenobiotic taken by the oral route induces tolerance rather than an immune response. Why only very few recipients develop immune reactions against a hapten produced after oral exposure remains unclear. A current hypothesis involves 'suppressor cells' mediating this tolerance against subsequent immunization with the antigen by incomplete presentation of peptides. Such suppressor cells causing oral tolerance may include enterocytes and cells in the liver, both organs which are frequently exposed to protein-reactive metabolites but in which immune reactions to haptens are very rare. After ingestion of a pro-hapten (a drug that is not reactive *per se* but whose metabolites are protein-reactive), intestinal venous drainage through the liver is necessary for oral tolerance to develop. Indeed, experimental production of a portocaval shunt, circumventing the liver, abrogates oral tolerance to haptens.

A second mechanism that could account, in some cases, for the rare occurrence of immune reactions in the liver is molecular mimicry.

Molecular mimicry: Mimicry of antigens is a phenomenon that plays a possible role in xenobiotic-induced but also in other forms of immune-mediated disease of unknown etiology. It is based on the observation that all exposed patients develop drug–protein adducts, yet the immune tolerance is broken and overt disease develops only in a few of them. According to an intriguing hypothesis, the hapten (in the case of halothane, the TFA adduct) would structurally resemble very closely a native 'self' epitope of a normal protein, so that a natural tolerance would be established both against the self protein and the mimicking hapten. Indeed, in some patients who had *never received halothane*, at least two liver antigens were detected and recognized by anti-TFA antibodies. What is the nature of these natural antigens?

Sequence analysis of these isolated proteins revealed that the antigens are mitochondrial proteins. In fact, they are part of the E2 subunit of pyruvate dehydrogenase, which contains lipoic acid. Indeed, analysis of the three-dimensional molecular structure surprisingly revealed that TFA covalently bound to lysin mimics (at the molecular level) lipoic acid.

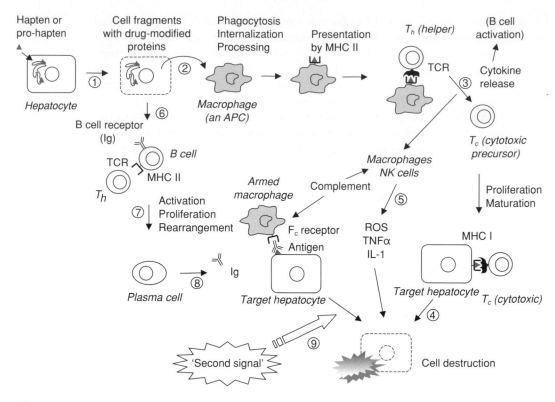

Figure 10.10. Putative mechanisms and pathways of immune-mediated hepatocyte injury by haptens or pro-haptens. *(1)* Covalent adducts to intracellular proteins will be accessible to immune cells following degradation of the hepatocyte (probably due to minor injury). Adducts may also be present on the plasma membrane. *(2)* Internalization of drug-altered proteins (immunogen) by antigen-presenting cell (ACP), followed by processing and presentation of the peptides in conjunction with major histocompatibility complex (MHC) class II molecules. The haptens (or conformational epitopes) of the peptides are recognized by the T cell receptor (TCR) of T helper (T_h) cells. *(3)* Cytokines are released, and B cells and cytotoxic T cell (T_c) precursors are activated, resulting in clonal expansion and maturation to functional T_c cells. *(4)* The drug-modified peptide fragment associated with MHC I molecules is recognized by T_c cells (and binding of accessory proteins is necessary), followed by lysis of the target cell via Fas receptor or perforin. *(5)* T_h cells release cytokines which results in activation of macrophages and NK cells. These cells can destroy target cells by secreting large amounts of ROS, complement factors (C3a), TNFα, IL-1, and other mediators. *(6)* Alternatively, haptenated proteins can be recognized by B cell receptors, followed by internalization, processing, and presentation of the peptide fragments by MHC II molecules. *(7)* B cells are activated and undergo clonal expansion and mature to plasma cells, secreting immunoglobulins (Ig). *(8)* Antibodies recognize and bind to epitopes on the plasma membrane of hepatocytes. Killer cells and macrophages can subsequently recognize and bind to the F_c portion of Ig via their F_c receptors, and/or complement activation can finally lead to the destruction of the hepatocytes. *(9)* Additional stimulators ('second signal') are, however, needed for T cell activation and killing of target cells.
Source: modified from Boelsterli, U.A., Zimmerman, H.J. and Kretz-Rommel, A. (1995) Idiosyncratic liver toxicity of nonsteroidal antiinflammatory drugs: molecular mechanisms and pathology, *Crit. Rev. Toxicol.* 25: 207–235.

According to this hypothesis, patients featuring genetic abnormalities of these enzyme subunits might not possess this tolerance mechanism and hence become prone to developing an immune response because the hapten would express a high degree of 'foreignity'. This hypothesis is currently being further explored.

As the trifluoroacetyl moiety of the halothane metabolite has been recognized to be an immunogen and antigen in drug-induced immune-mediated liver injury, it is important to investigate whether other xenobiotics that are metabolized to TFA also have the potential to induce autoimmune reactions in the liver. One such group of xenobiotics is the hydrated chlorofluorocarbons.

Hydrated chlorofluorocarbons (HCFCs) are a group of perhalogenated alkanes that have been been increasingly produced for use as refrigerants, in the foam plastic industry, and as propellants. They were developed to ultimately replace the hazardous chlorofluorocarbons (CFCs), which are widely banned because of their potential to deplete the ozone layer in the stratosphere.

It is striking that the molecular structure of these HCFCs closely resembles that of halothane. For example, in HCFC-123, only one chlorine atom distinguishes it from halothane (which features a bromine at the same position). Indeed, HCFC-123 is metabolized by the same CYP (CYP2E1) as halothane and produces the same reactive intermediate as halothane. Accordingly, HCFC-123 metabolism produces similar TFA adducts to liver proteins. The natural concern arises as to whether these industrial chemicals might have the same potential as halothane to induce immune-mediated liver injury in exposed individuals.

The answer was unexpected but clear. In 1997, industrial workers in Belgium who inadvertently were chronically exposed to a mixture of HCFC-123 and HCFC-124 developed liver toxicity. TFA adducts were found in liver tissue and, furthermore, auto-antibodies against human CYP2E1 (and p58) were found in the serum. Thus, some HCFCs can form the same adducts as halothane and also induce immune reactions. The extent of bioactivation, the overall exposure and toxicokinetics, as well as other factors, will determine the immunotoxic potential of these industrial chemicals, for which safer alternatives should be found.

10.3.3. Idiosyncratic reactions and the 'danger' hypothesis

Not everybody who is exposed to protein-reactive metabolites and who produces haptens develops an immune reaction directed against the hapten or an auto-antigen. In fact, for the majority of compounds that have been associated with immune-mediated toxicity the incidence of developing overt organ injury is very low (in the range of 1:10,000 to 1:100,000). Obviously, in addition to a wide range of control regulatory factors, there are host-related factors that will contribute to determining whether the xenobiotic will induce a full immune response (rare) or induce tolerance (in the majority of cases). These host factors are not known but may include both genetic and acquired (environmentally regulated) factors. Such a host (patient)-specific 'mixture' of characteristics is called an 'idiosyncrasy'.

Idiosyncratic reactions: Idiosyncratic toxicity delineates rare adverse reactions to drugs and other xenobiotics. The term implies that the reactions are based on a specific combination of factors that is characteristic for an individual and which predisposes this individual to succumb to the overt manifestation of toxicity. Because the potential to cause toxicity is inherent to many xenobiotics, one could define idiosyncratic reactions as the result of specific host factors which increase the penetrance and expressivity of the intrinsic toxic potential of a compound, while in the majority of other cases the patient does not develop signs of toxicity. Although such reactions are rare for an individual drug, they are common due to the large number of different drugs and other xenobiotics that can cause such reactions, and in view of the large patient number. Idiosyncratic drug reactions involve many different mechanisms, and immune-mediated toxicity is just one of them; abnormalities in biochemical pathways leading to metabolic idiosyncrasy have also been described.

Mechanisms of idiosyncratic immune-mediated toxicity: The mechanisms of induction of rare immunoallergy or autoimmunity for most drugs are not clear. Part of the enigma is that the reactions do not fit into one of the classical immunological categories of hypersensitivity reactions. Also, many observations are not compatible with the classical hapten theory. For example, anti-drug antibodies are not always found as a result of the immune response. Furthermore, in many cases, the onset of overt disease is delayed, and drug toxicity becomes clinically manifest after many months or even more than a year of continuous exposure when the autoimmune attack is suddenly triggered.

Certainly, other mechanisms than mere presentation to T cells of haptenated peptide fragments by antigen-presenting cells (APCs) must be involved. MHC-restricted recognition of the peptide by the T cell receptor is not sufficient to activate the T cell fully. Today it is known that additional costimulatory signals from the APC are needed before the T cells are activated. For example, such additional signals include the expression of the costimulatory molecular pairs, B7RP-1 (on APCs) and ICOS (inducible on T cells), or CD40 (on APCs) and CD154 (inducible on T cells). What causes the expression of these costimulatory signals to be induced?

One mechanism has been described by the 'danger hypothesis'. This theory is based on the assumption that normally exposure to an antigen causes tolerance, even if the degree of 'foreignness' of an antigen is high. Only if this tolerance is broken may immunity result. The trigger to this control mechanism is a 'danger' signal, with danger being defined as any sort of cellular or systemic stress. For example, slight tissue injury by subtoxic concentrations of a xenobiotic or reactive metabolite may provide the danger signal. However, extensive studies trying to identify up-regulation of costimulatory molecules by chemicals implicated in the induction of autoimmune diseases have been largely unsuccessful so far (see Figure 10.11).

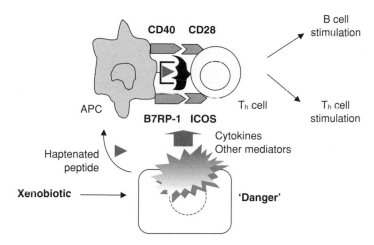

Figure 10.11. Expression of costimulatory factors is necessary for T cell activation. This could be initiated by, for example, cellular stress (danger signal).

Learning points

- Xenobiotics can either suppress the function of specific components of the immune system, thereby making the organism more sensitive to infections (can no longer recognize 'non-self'), or, alternatively, overstimulate the immune system, which will result in hypersensitivity including immunoallergic reactions, directed against specific drugs or other xenobiotics (attacks and damages 'self') or autoimmunity.
- Cells of the innate immune system (macrophages, PMNs, NK cells, γδ T cells) can be recruited and participate, in an antigen-independent way, in amplifying a toxic response to a xenobiotic.
- TCDD is a potent immunosuppressant by eliminating maturing T cells in the thymus. This is mediated via the AH receptor and kills immature T cells during their epithelial cell-regulated differentiation into either CD4$^+$ (helper) or CD8$^+$ (cytotoxic) single-positive T cells.
- Some xenobiotics can precipitate autoimmunity by directly interfering with the immune system, e.g. by disrupting the induction of T cell tolerance to self antigen (procainamide) or by directly stimulating cytokine release by T cells.
- Protein-reactive xenobiotics (e.g. penicillin) or their reactive metabolites (e.g. halothane and structural analogs) can act as haptens and form covalent adducts to proteins. If the adducts are stable enough, they can be taken up by professional antigen-presenting cells, processed, presented in conjunction with MHC II molecules, and trigger a primary immune response. However, many additional regulatory mechanisms have to be activated, and immune tolerance has to be broken, until secondary immune responses, culminating in antibody-mediated and/or cell-mediated effector mechanisms result in the destruction of self tissues (autoimmune reactions).

- Idiosyncratic immune-mediated reactions are rare manifestations of systemic or organ-selective toxicity occurring in very few exposed individuals only. The phenotypic manifestation of this immune toxicity is determined by individual susceptibility factors including genetic variability, environmental modulators, and underlying stress factors.

Further reading

Hepatic tissue damage aggravation by macrophages and neutrophils
Jaeschke, H. and Smith, C.W. (1997) Mechanisms of neutrophil-induced parenchymal cell injury, *J. Leukocyte Biol.* 61: 647–653.
Jaeschke, H., Smith, C.W., Clemens, M.G., Ganey, P.E. and Roth, R.A. (1996) Mechanisms of inflammatory liver injury: Adhesion molecules and cytotoxicity of neutrophils, *Toxicol. Appl. Pharmacol.* 139: 213–226.
Laskin, D.L. and Laskin, J.D. (2001) Role of macrophages and inflammatory mediators in chemically induced toxicity, *Toxicology* 160: 111–118.
Uwatoku, R., Suematsu, M., Ezaki, T., Saiki, T., Tsuiji, M., Irimura, T., Kawada, N., Suganuma, T., Naito, M., Ando, M. and Matsuno, K. (2001) Kupffer cell-mediated recruitment of rat dendritic cells to the liver: Roles of *N*-acetylgalactosamine-specific sugar, *Gastroenterology* 121: 1460–1472.

TCDD-induced thymic atrophy and T cell depletion
Fernandez-Salguero, P.M., Hilbert, D.M., Rudikoff, S., Ward, J.M. and Gonzalez, F.J. (1996) Aryl-hydrocarbon receptor-deficient mice are resistant to 2,3,7,8-tetrachlorodibenzo-*p*-dioxin-induced toxicity, *Toxicol. Appl. Pharmacol.* 140: 173–179.
Mondino, A., Khoruts, A. and Jenkins, M.K. (1996) The anatomy of T-cell activation and tolerance, *Proc. Natl Acad. Sci. USA*, 93: 2245–2252.

Toxic Oil Syndrome
Bujons, J., Ladona, M.G., Messeguer, A., Morato, A. and Ampurdanes, C. (2001) Metabolism of *(R)*- and *(S)*-3-(phenylamino)propane-1,2-diol in C57BL/6 and A/J-strain mice. Identification of new metabolites with potential toxicological significance to the Toxic Oil Syndrome, *Chem. Res. Toxicol.* 14: 1097–1106.
D'Cruz, D. (2000) Autoimmune diseases associated with drugs, chemicals and environmental factors, *Toxicol. Lett.* 112: 421–432.
Wulferink, M., Gonzalez, J., Goebel, C. and Gleichmann, E. (2001) T cells ignore aniline, a prohapten, but respond to its reactive metabolites generated by phagocytes: possible implications for the pathogenesis of Toxic Oil Syndrome, *Chem. Res. Toxicol.* 14: 389–397.

Autoimmune reactions
Kretz-Rommel, A. and Rubin, R.L. (2000) Disruption of positive selection of thymocytes causes autoimmunity, *Nature Med.* 6: 298–305.
Kretz-Rommel, A. and Rubin, R.L. (2001) Early cellular events in systemic autoimmunity driven by chromatin-reactive T cells, *Cell Immunol.* 208: 125–136.

Drug-induced immune-mediated liver injury
Boelsterli, U.A., Zimmerman, H.J. and Kretz-Rommel, A. (1995) Idiosyncratic liver toxicity of nonsteroidal antiinflammatory drugs: molecular mechanisms and pathology, *Crit. Rev. Toxicol.* 25: 207–235.

Bourdi, M., Amouzadeh, H.R., Rushmore, T.H., Martin, J.L. and Pohl, L.R. (2001) Halothane-induced liver injury in outbred Guinea pigs: Role of trifluoroacetylated protein adducts in animal susceptibility, *Chem. Res. Toxicol.* 14: 362–370.

Chen, M.L. and Gandolfi, A.J. (1997) Characterization of the humoral immune response and hepatotoxicity after multiple halothane exposures in guinea pigs, *Drug Metab. Rev.* 29: 103–122.

Furst, S.M. and Gandolfi, A.J. (1998) Immunologic mediation of chemical-induced hepatotoxicity, *Toxicology of the Liver*, Plaa, G.L. and Hewitt, W.R. (eds), Taylor & Francis, Washington, DC, pp. 259–295.

Gut, J., Christen, U., Frey, N., Koch, V. and Stoffler, D. (1995) Molecular mimicry in halothane hepatitis: Biochemical and structural characterization of lipoylated autoantigens, *Toxicology* 97: 199–224.

Kenna, J.G. and Jones, R.M. (1995) The organ toxicity of inhaled anesthetics, *Anesth. Analg.* 81: S51–S66.

Njoku, D., Laster, M.J., Gong, D.H., Eger, E.I., Reed, G.F. and Martin, J.L. (1997) Biotransformation of halothane, enflurane, isoflurane, and desflurane to trifluoro-acetylated liver proteins: association between protein acylation and hepatic injury, *Anesth. Analg.* 84: 173–178.

Park, B.K., Kitteringham, N.R., Powell, H. and Pirmohamed, M. (2000) Advances in molecular toxicology – towards understanding idiosyncratic drug toxicity, *Toxicology*, 153: 39–60.

Oral tolerance

Ju, C. and Pohl, L.R. (2001) Immunohistochemical detection of protein adducts of 2,4-dinitrochlorobenzene in antigen presenting cells and lymphocytes after oral administration to mice: Lack of a role of Kupffer cells in oral tolerance, *Chem. Res. Toxicol.* 14: 1209–1217.

Molecular mimicry

Albert, L.J. and Inman, R.D. (1999) Molecular mimicry and autoimmunity, *New Engl. J. Med.* 341: 2068–2074.

Christen, U., Quinn, J., Yeaman, S.J., Kenna, J.G., Clarke, J.B., Gandolfi, A.J. and Gut, J. (1994) Identification of the dihydrolipoamide acetyltransferase subunit of the human pyruvate dehydrogenase complex as an autoantigen in halothane hepatitis – molecular mimicry of trifluoroacetyl-lysine by lipoic acid, *Eur. J. Biochem.* 223: 1035–1047.

Gut, J., Christen, U., Frey, N., Koch, V. and Stoffler, D. (1995) Molecular mimicry in halothane hepatitis: Biochemical and structural characterization of lipoylated auto-antigens, *Toxicology* 97: 199–224.

Hydrated chlorofluorocarbons

Dekant, W. (1996) Toxicology of chlorofluorocarbon replacements, *Environ. Health Perspect.* 104: 75–83.

Hoet, P., Graf, M.L.M., Bourdi, M., Pohl, L.R., Duray, P.H., Chen, W.Q., Peter, R.M., Nelson, S.D., Verlinden, N. and Lison, D. (1997) Epidemic of liver disease caused by hydrochlorofluorocarbons used as ozone-sparing substitutes of chlorofluorocarbons, *Lancet* 350: 556–559.

Lind, R.C., Gandolfi, A.J. and Hall, P.D.L.M. (1995) Biotransformation and hepato-toxicity of HCFC-123 in the guinea pig: potentiation of hepatic injury by prior glutathione depletion, *Toxicol. Appl. Pharmacol.* 134: 175–181.

Idiosyncratic immune-mediated toxicity

Matzinger, P. (1994) Tolerance, danger and the extended family, *Annu. Rev. Immunol.* 12: 991–1045.

Pirmohamed, M. and Park, B.K. (2001) Genetic susceptibility to adverse drug reactions, *Trends Pharmacol. Sci.* 22: 298–305.

Schwartz, R.H. (2001) It takes more than two to tango, *Nature* 409: 31–32.

Uetrecht, J.P. (1999) New concepts in immunology relevant to idiosyncratic drug reactions: The 'Danger Hypothesis' and innate immune system, *Chem. Res. Toxicol.* 12: 387–395.

Chapter 11

Cytokine-mediated toxicity

Contents

Cytokines normally act as regulators of cell growth and differentiation, but they also play a pivotal role in the modulation and propagation of cell injury. For example, the groups of proinflammatory cytokines and chemokines are the controlling molecules of inflammatory events such as extravasation, cell migration, infiltration, and accumulation of leukocytes to the site of damage where tissue injury has occurred. Cytokines are also important in tissue repair by regulating cell proliferation and apoptosis (see Figure 11.1).

Proinflammatory cytokines are a group of signaling proteins with a characteristic set of features.

1 They are produced transiently, regulating important functions of cells, and they therefore have a short half-life.
2 Cytokines mainly act locally in an autocrine or paracrine fashion (i.e. sending the signal to the same cell or to the neighboring cells).
3 The released proteins act specifically with cytokine receptors expressed on the cell membrane.
4 Cytokines are not produced in specialized organs but are released from individual cells.

5 Most cytokines are not stored in cells. Instead, their expression is tightly regulated, and they are readily transcribed and synthesized after activation of the cell.
6 Cytokines have multiple biological functions, depending on the cell type on which they act and their concentration, as well as the presence of other cytokines. They can either potentiate or antagonize the function of other factors and fine-tune the effect of other cytokines. In addition, cytokines have overlapping functional activity, partially replacing and compensating each other if a particular member of the cytokine class is lacking. All these complex interactions make any predictions of a particular response to a given cytokine under a particular condition extremely difficult!

Upon binding of a cytokine to its membrane-spanning receptor, the receptor either undergoes a conformational change or oligomerizes, thereby activating the intracellular portion of the receptor. Two major signal transduction pathways are known to be involved in cytokine action. Upon binding of a cytokine to its receptor, some receptors can use their intrinsic tyrosine kinase activity to phosphorylate and activate the MAP kinase pathway. The other type of receptor does not possess tyrosine kinase activity, but equally activates kinase cascades, e.g. the STAT (signal transducers and activators of transcription) pathway. One characteristic of cytokines is that different ligands can bind to the same receptor and share common signaling pathways. In addition, individual ligands can bind to several receptors, which might explain in part their redundancy and pleiotropic response.

Cytokines can be grouped into proinflammatory cytokines (including tumor necrosis factors, interleukins, and interferons), growth factors (including epidermal growth factor and hepatocyte growth factor), and chemokines (including macrophage inflammatory proteins).

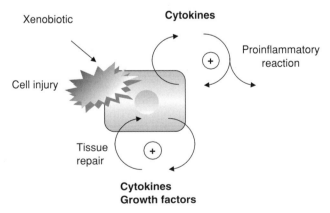

Figure 11.1. Roles of cytokines in promoting inflammatory reactions and cell and tissue repair.

11.1. Tumor necrosis factor-α and other proinflammatory cytokines

Tumor necrosis factor-α (TNFα) has been implicated in mediating the toxicity of many xenobiotics in a variety of organs. Its major roles are in crosstalking with other cells and other cytokines (see section 5.1.4), in modulating an inflammatory response, in promoting apoptosis (see section 7.2.2), but also in inducing tissue repair (see section 8.4). These obviously paradoxical roles and dual pathways are not fully understood.

Tumor necrosis factor (TNF) is a proinflammatory cytokine consisting of two closely related forms, TNFα and TNFβ (today called lymphotoxin-α). Both interact with the same receptors and share a variety of responses. TNF is produced mainly by macrophages/monocytes (but T and B cells also can produce TNF). TNF originates as a membrane-bound precursor-TNF, which is cleaved and secreted. The secreted TNF then aggregates into trimers and binds to and activates the TNF receptors.

TNF can be rapidly up-regulated upon a stimulus, but is also rapidly degraded; this seems plausible in view of its potent biological effects. For example, if macrophages are stimulated by bacterial endotoxin (LPS, lipopolysaccharide), mRNA production is increases up to 100-fold, and TNF protein secretion will shoot up to 10,000-fold! However, the $t_{1/2}$ of human TNF in macrophages is only ~12 min.

Two TNF receptors are known, TNF-R1 and TNF-R2. TNF-R1 is widely expressed on many cell types (while TNF-R2 is mainly expressed on leukocytes and endothelial cells). The intracellular portion of the TNF-R contains a 'death domain' (see section 7.2.2). TNF homotrimers bind to the extracellular portion of the receptor and cause aggregation of three receptors. The aggregated death domains then recruit a number of accessory proteins; first the TRADD (TNF-R-associated death domain), which in turn recruits FADD (Fas-associated death domain), TRAF2 (TNF-R-associated factor 2), and RIP (receptor interacting protein). This activates signaling cascades. Interestingly, one pathway induces caspase activation and results in apoptosis. At the same time, other pathways activate kinase pathways which activate NF-κB (see section 5.4.). NF-κB transactivates a number of cytoprotective genes (including heat shock proteins, antioxidants, and others), which antagonize the apoptotic signaling pathway. Thus, the same initial signal triggers both a cell death-inducing and a cell-protecting pathway. The outcome of this activation and the ultimate fate of the target cell depends on many other factors including the amount of TNF produced and the rapidity of onset and duration of TNF production (see Figure 11.2).

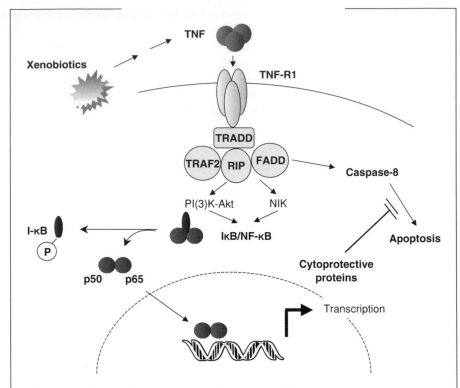

Figure 11.2. Signaling pathways of TNF-mediated activation of TNF receptor-1. The same signal potentially activates the pro-apoptotic and proinflammatory pathways, but also leads to the transcription of cell-rescuing proteins via activation of the transcription factor, NF-κB.

The possible role of TNF in mediating organ-selective tissue injury has been investigated in a number of animal models. For example, treatment of rodents with the hepatotoxic agents carbon tetrachloride or acetaminophen elicits increases in the hepatic expression of TNFα. The source of this cytokine is Kupffer cells. But what is the mechanistic role of this increased TNF production in the hepatotoxicity produced by these xenobiotics? To address this issue directly, experimental models have used TNF-null mice, TFNα and lymphotoxin-α double-deficient mice, or mice deficient in TNF receptor. When such genetically altered mice were treated with a hepatotoxic dose of acetaminophen, liver injury developed similar to that seen in normal mice. In contrast, injection of anti-TNF antibodies to mice afforded protection against acetaminophen hepatotoxicity.

These conflicting findings do not necessarily point to a lack of role of TNF in the development of hepatic injury. Instead, they indicate that the amount and local concentration of the cytokine may be crucial. Indeed, the minute amounts of TNF which are still present after injection of the antibody may be sufficient to trigger an anti-apoptotic response while sparing the cytotoxic effects inflicted by large amounts of TNF. At the same time, small levels of TNF are needed to stimulate post-injury

DNA replication and tissue remodeling (and this stimulus is absent in the genetically deficient mice).

Apart from modulating the effects of hepatotoxins, TNF has also been implicated in mediating the toxicity of a number of xenobiotics that exert adverse effects in the kidneys, skin, lung, and CNS.

Mechanisms of TNF-mediated potentiation of hepatic injury: TNF plays a multifunctional role in xenobiotic-induced liver injury. Three mechanistic pathways are crucial and interdependent.

1 After initial damage to hepatocytes, the resident macrophages at the site of damage become activated and secrete proinflammatory cytokines including TNFα. This signal recruits monocytes and neutrophils into the liver. These phagocytes in turn produce additional cytokines, ROS, RNS, and proteases, all of which will aggravate the tissue damage, which leads to the production of hepatic necrosis.
2 TNF can also mediate caspase activation and apoptosis if not counterbalanced by the simultaneously increased production of cell survival factors which protect from apoptosis. This latter, NF-κB-dependent process is dependent on transcriptional activation and de novo synthesis of proteins. If a xenobiotic (amanitin, actinomycin D, or acetaminophen at high concentrations) inhibits protein synthesis, then the apoptotic pathway may prevail, resulting in liver failure directly through TNF-mediated induction of apoptotic cell death.
3 TNF is also necessary for liver parenchymal regeneration following a toxic insult. In fact, TNF directly stimulates DNA replication in vivo through both interleukin (IL)-6 dependent and -independent mechanisms. This requires the induction of early immediate genes, including c-jun and c-fos, and activation of the transcription factors NF-κB, AP-1, and cEBP. Indeed, DNA-binding sites for these transcription factors have been found in the promoter region of the TNFα gene, indicating that induction of these genes by TNF is a self-amplifying process. The conditions that lead to an impairment of the stimulatory effects of TNF on cell proliferation and regeneration are, however, incompletely known.

11.2. Chemokines and inflammatory cell recruitment

Inflammatory chemokines are soluble small cytokines which chemoattract immunocompetent and inflammatory cells (e.g. macrophages, dendritic cells, T cells, PMNs) to the site of damage. Examples are the human IL-8 and the murine homologs, MIP (macrophage inflammatory protein)-1 and MIP-2. Chemokines are produced by various cell types and have been implicated in enhancing xenobiotic-induced inflammation.

For example, the hepatotoxicity induced by 1,2-dichlorobenzene in rats (see section 5.1.2) is greatly aggravated by activated macrophages and infiltrating PMNs. Following bioactivation of the compound in hepatocytes, these latter produce and secrete a number of chemokines which are responsible for activation and recruitment of proinflammatory cells. One of these chemokines is CINC (cytokine-induced neutrophil chemoattractant factor), which activates Kupffer cells in the liver. Indeed, following 1,2-dichlorobenzene administration, rat liver Kupffer cells express increased levels of the CINC receptor. Thus, chemokines signal the activation of Kupffer

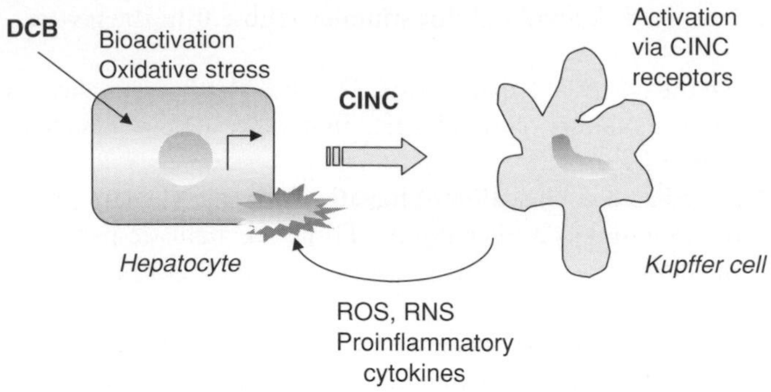

Figure 11.3. Activation of Kupffer cells by the chemokine CINC (cytokine-induced neutrophil chemoattractant factor). On exposure to 1,2-dichlorobenzene (DCB), hepatocytes respond with up-regulation of CINC and other chemokines, which in turn activates macrophages. The resulting hepatic necrosis associated with DCB is ultimately a consequence of Kupffer cell-mediated toxicity.

cells, which up-regulate an inflammatory response and ultimately are responsible for the progression of 1,2-dichlorobenzene-induced liver injury (see Figure 11.3).

Another example is the pulmonary inflammation caused by asbestos and other microfibers (see section 5.1.4) or by metals including vanadium.

Vanadium is used in the petrochemical, mining, and steel industries. Environmental or occupational exposure to vanadium dusts is characterized by respiratory problems including irritation of the upper and lower respiratory tract and impairment of pulmonary function. The mechanisms underlying vanadium toxicity are largely unknown, but pulmonary alveolar macrophages have been implicated as a biological target of inhaled vanadium. Aerosols of other metals (e.g. cadmium and cobalt) are also known to induce pulmonary inflammation. A hallmark is a dramatic increase in the number of macrophages, neutrophils, and lymphocytes in the lungs. Experimental evidence indicates that this toxic response is mediated by the production of chemokines.

Mechanisms of vanadium-induced pulmonary inflammation: Sodium metavanadate ($NaVO_3$) and vanadyl sulfate ($VOSO_4$) induce neutrophil influx into the lungs following rapid up-regulation of several chemokines. These include (in the rat) MIP-2 (the major neutrophil-recruiting chemokine) and MIP-1 (the major macrophage/monocyte-recruiting chemokine). Evidence suggests that vanadium-induced elevated MIP-2 mRNA levels in the lung are transcriptionally regulated through NF-κB. Indeed, the promoter region of the MIP-2 gene contains binding sites for NF-κB and AP-1.

The immune cells which have become activated by these chemokines rapidly infiltrate the pulmonary tissues and further aggravate the inflammatory response by releasing ROS, RNS, eicosanoids, proteases, and proinflammatory cytokines including TNF and IL-1β (see section 10.1).

Learning points

- Proinflammatory cytokines including TNFα are important mediators and enhancers of xenobiotic-induced toxicity. Their major functions include crosstalking with other cells, e.g. modulating inflammatory responses and promoting apoptosis.
- TNFα is also involved in cell proliferation and tissue repair. Transcriptional activation of a number of cell rescue genes is mediated via activation of the transcription factor NF-κB.
- Chemokines produced by macrophages after xenobiotic-induced tissue injury recruit proinflammatory cells (PMNs, macrophages and monocytes), which propagate and amplify the damage. This chemoattraction by cytokines occurs, for example, in metal-induced pulmonary injury.

Further reading

Proinflammatory cytokines
Foster, J.R. (2001) The functions of cytokines and their uses in toxicology, *Int. J. Exp. Pathol.*, 82: 171–192.

Tumor necrosis factor
Boess, F., Bopst, M., Althaus, R., Polsky, S., Cohen, S.D., Eugster, H.P. and Boelsterli, U.A. (1998) Acetaminophen hepatotoxicity in tumor necrosis factor/lymphotoxin-α gene knockout mice, *Hepatology* 27: 1021–1029.
Laskin, D.L. and Laskin, J.D. (2001) Role of macrophages and inflammatory mediators in chemically induced toxicity, *Toxicology* 160: 111–118.
Luster, M.I., Simeonova, P.P., Galluci, R. and Matheson, J. (1999) Tumor necrosis factor α and toxicology, *Crit. Rev. Toxicol.* 29: 491–511.
Papadakis, K.A. and Targan, S.R. (2000) Tumor necrosis factor: Biology and therapeutic inhibitors, *Gastroenterology* 119: 1148–1157.
Schümann, J. and Tiegs, G. (1999) Pathophysiological mechanisms of TNF during intoxication with natural or man-made toxins, *Toxicology* 138: 103–126.

TNF-mediated potentiation of hepatic injury
Leist, M., Gantner, F., Naumann, H., Bluethmann, H., Vogt, K., Brigeliusflohe, R., Nicotera, P., Volk, H.D. and Wendel, A. (1997) Tumor necrosis factor-induced apoptosis during the poisoning of mice with hepatotoxins, *Gastroenterology* 112: 923–934.

Chemokines and inflammatory cell recruitment
Baggiolini, M. (2001) Chemokines in pathology and medicine, *J. Int. Med.* 250: 91–104.
Chong, I.W., Shi, M.M., Love, J.A., Christiani, D.C. and Paulauskis, J.D. (2000) Regulation of chemokine mRNA expression in a rat model of vanadium-induced pulmonary inflammation, *Inflammation* 24: 505–517.
Younis, H.S., Parrish, A.R., Jang, J.J. and Sipes, I.G. (2002) 1,2-Dichlorobenzene mediates the production and release of factors in hepatocytes that enhance Kupffer cell activity, *Toxicol. Sci. Suppl.* 66: 42.

Chapter 12

Specific inactivation of enzymes and other proteins

Contents

Xenobiotics can very selectively target certain proteins (as opposed to damaging a protein at random). In the case of an enzyme, this is often due to highly selective primary interactions between the xenobiotic, being a potentially toxic 'pseudo-substrate', and the protein. Accordingly, this interaction will result in very specific and predictable toxic effects which will result from the compromised enzyme function. For example, if the enzyme is damaged or inhibited, its physiological substrate can no longer be converted (or is incompletely converted), and the substrate will eventually accumulate and cause a pathophysiological effect. One classical example is the interaction of organophosphate pesticides with acetylcholinesterase.

12.1. Disruption of acetylcholinesterase activity

Organophosphates (OPs) are a large class of chemically heterogeneous compounds used mainly as pesticides. They are important in the plant protection industry and are produced in enormous quantities worldwide and distributed in the environment. As OPs are usually non-persistent in the environment (featuring a $t_{1/2}$ of several hours to maximally several weeks), and because they do not accumulate in organisms and enter the food chain, they are not a major threat in ecotoxicology and environmental toxicology (although sometimes food products may be contaminated with small amounts of OPs). However, the flip-side of the story is the acute toxicity inherent to many OPs. In fact, some OPs are highly neurotoxic, a property which had been discovered by the 1930s and was later used for the development of insecticides. Unfortunately, these same characteristics and molecular mechanisms of OPs were applied for the derivatization and development of agents for chemical warfare (nerve gases).

Organophosphates are lipophilic compounds which are readily absorbed (including through the skin) and are rapidly distributed across the organism. Frequently, poisonings with OPs have a fatal outcome, and it is this acute toxicity of OPs which is the major cause of adverse reactions to agrochemicals. The potencies of this acute neurotoxicity however, vary greatly among different OPs. For example, for some nerve gas OPs the lethal dose for humans is in the low milligram range, while the lethal dose of the widely used insecticide, malathion, is as high as approximately 30 g.

The general structure of OPs involves a pentavalent P atom which is tetra-coordinated. For some compounds, there is an oxygen atom bound to the P by a double bond, and two ester substituents. For others (the phosphorothionates) P is bound to a sulfur atom via a double bond, and, in addition, one of the other oxygen atoms may be replaced by another sulfur. This structural diversity has important mechanistic implications, as these compounds (actually the phosphorus in the center) is electrophilic (see section 9.1). Its electrophilicity and reactivity are greatly determined by the substituents; for example, a P=O double bond renders the P highly electrophilic, and other substituents like halogens can even increase the reactivity (see Figure 12.1).

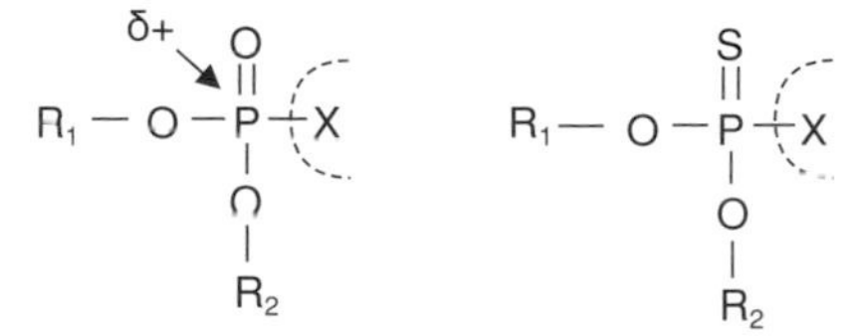

Figure 12.1. General chemical structure of organophosphate ester pesticides. The phosphorus represents an electrophilic center. X = good leaving group.

In biological sytems and at the toxicodynamic level, the primary molecular mechanism of OP action is its inhibition of acetylcholinesterase function by electrophilic attack of the enzyme. The manifestation of OP toxicity, however, is mediated by the downstream biological effects, secondary to the enzyme inhibition. Specifically, these effects are caused by the persistence and accumulation of acetylcholine, which plays a crucial role in the nervous system.

Acetylcholine esterase (AcChE) is a serine esterase whose function is to hydrolyze the neurotransmitter acetylcholine (ACh). Before focusing on this enzyme, let us briefly recall its substrate and the role it plays in the cholinergic nervous system, as this will be crucial for understanding the mechanism of OPs and the ensuing toxicity.

Acetylcholine (ACh) is an important neurotransmitter, abundant in the CNS and in the peripheral nervous system in various organs. It acts on cholinergic synapses, present in the parasympathetic nervous system, the first ganglion of the sympathetic nervous system, and at the motoric endplates. Acetylcholine is synthesized in the presynaptic neurons from choline and acetyl-CoA ('activated acetate') and is subsequently stored in vesicles. Upon a stimulus, the vesicle fuses with the terminal membrane and releases the ACh into the synaptic cleft, where it acts as a neurotransmitter across the synapse. At the surface of the postsynaptic neuron, ACh specifically interacts with ACh receptors. There are two types of ACh receptors which are anatomically and functionally different: the muscarinic receptors, involved in the function of the intestine, glands, heart, etc., and the nicotinic receptors, which are involved in the function of the skeletal muscle. Both receptors are present in the brain, and they are involved in controlling respiration and the cardiovascular system.

It is crucial that the activation of these receptors be terminated when the neuronal stimulus has ceased. This is achieved by the presence of AcChE, which is present on both the presynaptic and postsynaptic membrane, as well as in a soluble form. Upon hydrolytic cleavage of the neurotransmitter by AcChE, the choline moiety is taken up into the presynaptic neuron, and ACh is reassembled (see Figure 12.2).

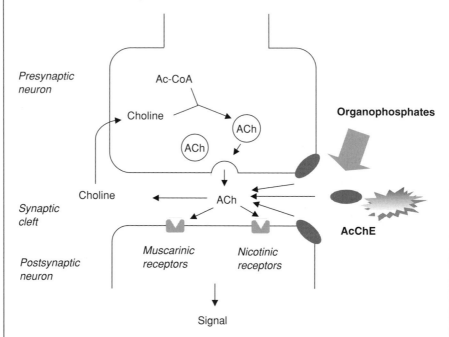

Figure 12.2. Because OPs inhibit the catalytic activity of AcChE, the neurotransmitter is not degraded but remains in the synaptic cleft and accumulates. Overstimulation of the ACh receptors at the postsynaptic membrane is the physiological basis for the ensuing toxicity.

Mechanisms of organophosphate toxicity: The molecular mechanism of OP inhibition of AcChE has been elucidated and many structural details are known. The key mechanism for understanding the inhibitory effect is the enzmye's serine hydroxyl group at the active center of the protein.

Normally, this serine hydroxyl group attacks the substrate, ACh, at the carboxyl carbon, and this will result in a covalent bond between the enzyme and the substrate. After release of the choline moiety, the enzyme remains transiently acetylated. After a short time, however (in the range of milliseconds), the acetylated enzyme is hydrolyzed, and the serine hydroxyl group (the active enzyme site) is regenerated.

In the presence of OPs, the active serine hydroxyl group of the enzyme is attacked by the highly electrophilic phosphorus in the center of the OP molecule, rather than by ACh. This is accompanied by the loss of the leaving group of the OP and the subsequent formation of a covalent bond between the enzyme and the OP. In contrast to the normal situation, this bond is very stable, and the modified enzyme is not readily hydrolyzed. In fact, the newly formed phosphate ester is very slowly degraded (days to weeks), and the enzyme remains in an inactivated form. Spontaneous hydrolysis is even further delayed after the so-called 'aging' of the inhibitor, i.e. release of an alkyl chain, which strengthens the phosphorus–enzyme bond (see Figure 12.3).

Irreversible inactivation of AcChE will lead to an increase in ACh. Indeed, the downstream biological consequences of OP toxicity largely reflect a high-dose ACh toxicity. In view of the importance of the cholinergic nervous system, many

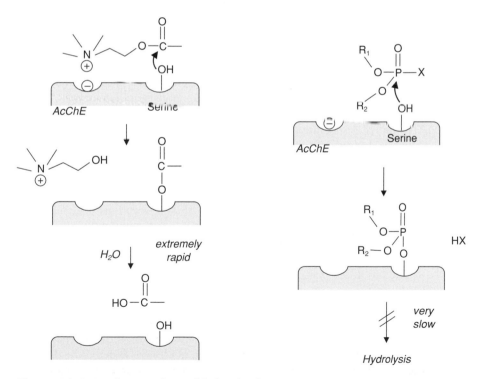

Figure 12.3. Mechanism of acetylcholine binding and organophosphate binding to the acetylcholinesterase.

Table 12.1 Downstream biological consequences of acetylcholinesterase inhibition and excess stimulation of acetylcholine receptors

Overstimulation at receptor	Downstream consequences
Muscarinic receptors (smooth muscles, heart, exocrine glands)	Bronchoconstriction, miosis, bradycardia, salivation, tears, increased peristaltic movements, diarrhea
Nicotinic receptors (skeletal muscles, autonomic ganglia)	Muscle weakness, tremor, hypertension, flaccid paralysis
Acetylcholine receptor (CNS)	Psychological disorders, disorientation, convulsions, respiratory depression, cardiovascular collapse

sequelae of these pathophysiological effects can be explained by the distribution and function of the ACh receptors in the body, following overstimulation. The major effects of OPs are summarized in Table 12.1.

The severity of OP-induced neurotoxicity is dependent on the relative amount of AcChE which becomes blocked. A 10–20 percent inhibition will result in mild symptoms, 50 percent inhibition in massive symptoms, and >90 percent inhibition is fatal. Time is crucial because the enzyme inhibition is irreversible; *de novo* synthesis of AcChE is required to restore the full capacity of the enzyme (normal turnover of AcChE is 50–100 days, depending on the isoform).

In addition to these effects on AcChE, OPs have additional targets in the nervous system. The compounds can alkylate or phosphorylate other macromolecules, including other esterases, and lead to a 'delayed-onset' neuropathy.

Because of the high potential toxicity for mammals including humans, some OP insecticides have been structurally modified to allow a more specific targeting of the insect nervous system. For example, some compounds require metabolic activation to inhibit AcChE effectively. The phosphorothionates (see above) need CYP-catalyzed oxidative desulfuration to become active (they are converted into the toxic oxygen analog). Indeed, insect CYPs readily bioactivate such compounds and turn them into highly toxic species. In contrast, mammalian tissues primarily detoxify phosphorothionates by another pathway; they hydrolyze them by carboxylesterases and other esterases (e.g. esterase A, which, in contrast to esterase B, is not inactivated by OPs). However, very large doses of phosphorothionates can also become toxic in mammals (see Figure 12.4).

Organophosphate pesticides provide a beautiful example to illustrate how the elucidation of the molecular mechanism underlying the toxicity of these compounds can be applied to develop antidotes which protect from the acute toxicity of OPs. Accordingly, two types of treatment have been designed: first, atropin, which is a muscarinic antagonist and will block these receptors, thus preventing overstimulation by excess ACh; and, second, oximes, which will accelerate the dephosphorylation of AcChE by the OP and thus regenerate the normal function of the enzyme. In addition, detailed knowledge of the mode of action of OPs has fostered the development of biomarker test systems to monitor possible exposure. Specifically, because OPs not only phosphorylate AcChE but also inactivate other esterases by this mechanism, measurement of nonspecific cholinesterase activity in the blood (erythrocytes) lends itself to use as a tool for biomonitoring exposure in humans.

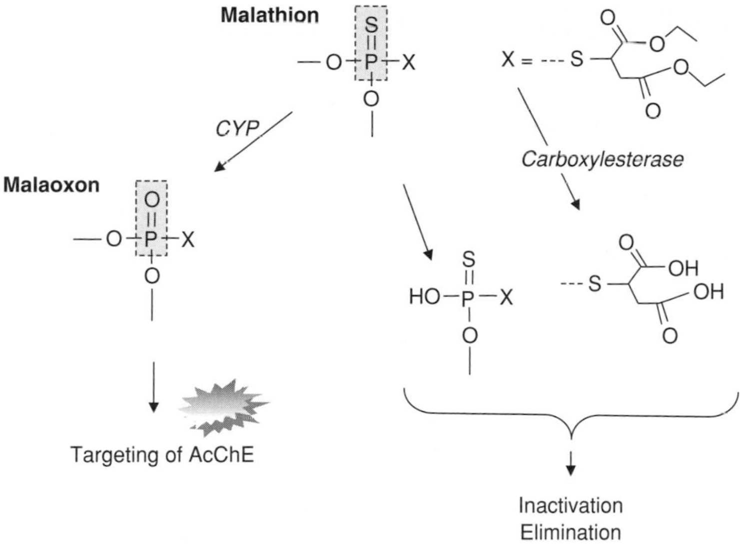

Figure 12.4. Phosphorothionates are bioactivated in insects by CYP to the oxygen analog (left pathway). Instead, in mammals, the predominant pathway is metabolic dealkylation or hydrolysis of carboxyl groups by carboxylesterases (right pathways).

12.2. Transthyretin binding and inactivation – disruption of thyroid function

Another mechanism underlying the toxicity of xenobiotics is based on specific interactions with the critical binding site on acceptor proteins which are normally involved in the transport of hormones and other regulators of body function and development. This specific targeting of proteins may cause pathophysiological effects that can be explained by a disruption of the kinetics of the particular hormone or regulator. A typical example is the binding of polychlorinated biphenyls to the thyroid hormone-binding protein.

Thyroid hormones (T_4 = tetraiodothyronin, thyroxine, and T_3 = triiodothyronine, which is formed from T_4 in liver, muscle and kidney) play important regulatory functions and determine metabolism, growth and differentiation in many tissues and organs. For example, the thyroid hormones are important regulators of testicular development in the early postnatal phase (indeed, the thyroid receptor is highly expressed on Sertoli cells in the testes).

To enable the normal transport of T_4 from the bloodstream to the brain (across the blood–brain barrier) and other target organs, T_4 is bound with high affinity to a specific transport protein, **transthyretin** (TTR, also called prealbumin). TTR exists in human plasma as a homotetramer and is present at concentrations of 200–300 µg/ml. TTR also indirectly binds and transports retinol (i.e. it binds the retinol-binding protein). Besides its major function in blood, TTR is also found in liver and other organs.

> Experimental evidence has indicated that exposure of animals to certain **PCBs** entails disruption of thyroxin homeostasis. This is manifested by enlarged thyroid and decreased blood T_4 levels. For example, PCBs decrease circulating T_4 levels in developing rats by ~90 percent! Blood retinol levels can be similarly decreased. In humans, it has been demonstrated that an inverse correlation exists between the PCB concentrations in mother's milk and plasma T_4 levels in their nursing infants. First it was speculated that these PCBs might bind to the thyroxin receptor and thus antagonize thyroxin effects. This was found to be true; however, the affinity of PCBs to the thyroxin receptor is much smaller (~10,000-fold) than that of thyroxine itself and is, therefore, unlikely to account fully for the hormone-disrupting effects of PCBs.

Mechanisms of PCB interactions with thyroid hormone activity: A likely explanation for the thyroid hormone-disrupting abilities of PCBs can be found in the fact that some PCBs avidly bind to transthyretin, and that they do so with equal or even higher affinity than T_4 itself (that is, with a K_i of 5–80 nM). This implies that certain PCBs (or their hydroxylated metabolites) are able to occupy the binding site of thyroxin at physiological concentration ranges. This will entail a sharp increase in the 'free' (non-TTR-bound) levels of thyroxin and, hence, an increased plasma clearance. Thus, the mechanism of thyroid function disruption by certain PCBs is based on a competitive interaction with T_4 for TTR binding sites.

This mechanism seems quite logical in view of the structural 'resemblance' of thyroxin and some laterally substituted PCBs. Interestingly, there is a clear structure–binding activity relationship among different PCBs. Most of the active PCBs are either 'T$_4$-like' (i.e. they have chlorine substitutions at the 3 *and* 5 (*meta-*) positions on one or both phenyl rings) or 'T$_3$-like' (i.e. they have chlorine substitutions at the 3 *or* 5 positions). Occupied *para*-positions are not essential for binding, but generally do not prevent binding. Increasing degrees of *ortho* substitution (i.e. all 2 and 6 positions chlorinated) cause the two phenyl rings in the PCB molecule to twist at an almost 90° angle, which causes lower rotational degrees of freedom and strongly precludes binding (see Figure 12.5).

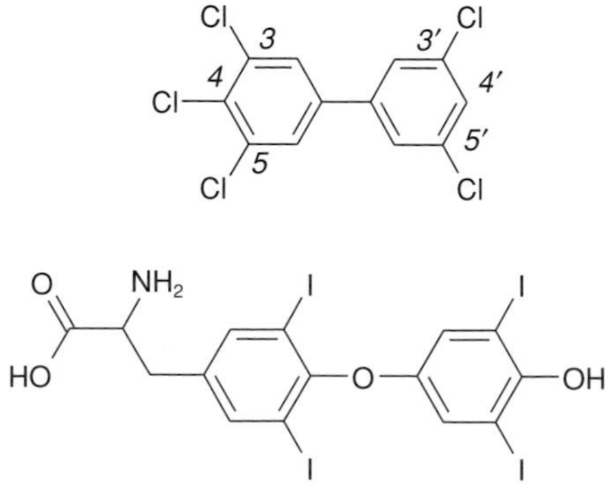

Figure 12.5. Structural similarity between thyroxin (T$_4$) and the *meta*-substituted PCB, 3,3',4,5,5'-PeCB, which features a high relative potency for binding to transthyretin.

Learning points

- Xenobiotics can specifically target and inactivate enzymes or inhibit binding proteins due to their structural similarities to a physiological substrate and high binding affinity for the protein.
- Organophosphates have a high affinity for a number of esterases and specifically phosphorylate and alkylate acetylcholine esterase. Irreversible inhibition of this enzyme prevents the degradation of the neurotransmitter, acetylcholine, resulting in overstimulation of the cholinergic nervous system.
- The neurotoxic potency of different organophosphates in humans can vary up to 1,000-fold. This is based on, among other factors, the prevalence of insect-specific bioactivation pathways versus mammalian-specific degradation reactions.
- Elucidation of the underlying molecular mechanism of OP toxicity has made possible the development of antidotes against acute poisoning, the availability of biomonitoring assays, and the specific design of OPs with minimal toxicity for humans.
- Certain *meta*-substituted PCBs bind to transthyretin, the thyroxin-binding protein, preventing binding of T_4 and T_3 and thus accelerating the plasma clearance of thyroid hormones. This results in hormone-disrupting effects.

Further reading

Organophosphate toxicity
Casida, J.E. and Toia, R.F. (1992) Organophosphorus pesticides: Their target diversity and bioactivation, *Tissue-specific Toxicity: Biochemical Mechanisms*, Dekant, W. and Neumann, H.G. (eds), Academic Press, London, pp. 33–70.
Ecobichon, D.J. (1997) Anticholinesterase insecticides, *Nervous Syst. Behav. Toxicol.* 11: 447–456.
Mileson, B.E., Chambers, J.E., Chen, W.L., Dettbarn, W., Ehrich, M., Eldefrawi, A.T., Gaylor, D.W., Hamernik, K., Hodgson, E., Karczmar, A.G., Padilla, S., Pope, C.N., Richardson, R.J., Saunders, D.R., Sheets, L.P., Sultatos, L.G. and Wallace, K.B. (1998) Common mechanisms of toxicity: A case study of organophosphorus pesticides, *Toxicol. Sci.* 41: 8–20.

PCBs and thyroid hormone activity
Chauhan, K.R., Kodavanti, P.R.S. and McKinney, J.D. (2000) Assessing the role of *ortho*-substitution on polychlorinated biphenyl binding to transthyretin, a thyroxine transport protein, *Toxicol. Appl. Pharmacol.* 162: 10–21.
Cheek, A.O., Kow, K., Chen, J. and McLachlan, J.A. (1999) Potential mechanisms of thyroid disruption in humans: Interaction of organochlorine compounds with thyroid receptor, transthyretin, and thyroid-binding globulin, *Environ. Health Perspect.* 107: 273–278.
Rickenbacher, U., McKinney, J.D., Oatley, S.J. and Blake, C.C.F. (1986) Structurally specific binding of halogenated biphenyls to thyroxine transport protein, *J. Med. Chem.* 29: 641–648.

Chapter 13

Nuclear receptor-mediated toxicity

Contents

13.1. The aryl hydrocarbon receptor (AHR)
13.2. Xenoestrogens and anti-androgens
13.3. Peroxisome proliferator-activated receptors (PPARs)

The toxicity of xenobiotics is often characterized by tissue specificity and compound selectivity. In many cases, this can be explained mechanistically by the tissue-specific expression of high-affinity intracellular receptors for many xenobiotics. These receptors may then mediate the toxicity through a number of signaling pathways or through direct interaction with specific response element on the DNA (there are other xenobiotic-binding proteins in cells; if they do not transmit a signal, they are not considered a receptor).

Further evidence that a receptor-mediated mechanism is involved in xenobiotic-induced effects is provided if

1 the effects are tissue-specific
2 the effects are predictable
3 increases in the transactivation of specific genes can be demonstrated
4 transcriptional responses occur rapidly
5 compounds bind reversibly to intracellular macromolecules
6 the effects are stereospecific.

Such receptors are often nuclear receptors.

A 'nuclear receptor' is a soluble receptor which binds a ligand, migrates into the cell nucleus and interacts with specific genomic response elements. Nuclear receptors are not always confined to the nucleus but are often abundant in the cytosol in an inactive form.

Toxicologically, two superfamilies of nuclear signaling molecules have gained enormous attention in the past years, in particular because our understanding of the molecular basis of their activation and downstream effects has been greatly increasing. These superfamilies comprise the steroid hormone receptors and the PAS receptors. The first family includes (each with different subtypes) the peroxisome proliferator-activated receptor (PPAR), the thyroid hormone receptor (TR), the estrogen receptor (ER), and the androgen receptor (AR), and others. The second family includes the aryl hydrocarbon receptor (AHR).

Steroid hormone receptors (also called zinc finger receptors) are a large family of receptors. They always form dimers (hetero- or homodimers). If they form heterodimers, the second partner is the retinoic X receptor (RXR, which binds 9-*cis*-retinoic acid). Receptors of this superfamily contain a ligand-binding domain, a DNA-binding domain (the 'zinc finger', i.e. a common motif which coordinates a Zn atom through cysteine and histidine and which fits into the major groove of DNA).

In some cases, steroid hormone receptors are kept in an inactive state in the cytoplasm by binding to a dimer of the 90 kDa heat shock protein (hsp90). This chaperone interaction holds the receptor in a conformation ready to bind ligand and prevents the receptor from binding to DNA. Upon binding of a ligand, the receptor undergoes a conformational change that dissociates the hsp90 moiety and facilitates recruitment of co-activators. The receptor then translocates into the nucleus, dimerizes, and binds to the response elements located in the promoter region of the specific genes.

PAS proteins comprise a growing family of signaling molecules that are identified by the presence of a region of sequence similarity named after the founding members PER, ARNT, and SIM. In the AH receptor, the PAS domain is also the region where agonists such as dioxin bind. PAS proteins commonly harbor basic helix-loop-helix domains, a DNA binding and dimerization motif found in many transcription factors. These proteins bind to DNA as heterodimers. They have been known to play an important role in embryogenesis and differentiation. The toxicologically most important PAS proteins are the AH receptor and its PAS partner ARNT, although members such as HIF1α and CLOCK play clear roles in environmental adaptation.

13.1. The aryl hydrocarbon receptor (AHR)

The aryl hydrocarbon receptor (AHR, also called 'dioxin receptor') is found in many cell types and is particularly high in epithelia. It is abundant in lung, thymus, and placenta, and exhibits intermediate expression in kidney, liver, heart, and spleen. Normally, the receptor resides in the cytoplasm as a complex with at least two other proteins. These other proteins include hsp90 and an immunophilin-like molecule that goes by a number of names (ARA9/AIP1/XAP2). These associated proteins act as chaperones, shielding the AHR from binding to DNA, imparting cytosolic localization and at the same time keeping the protein in a conformation that allows for ligand binding.

Upon binding to a ligand, the AHR sheds its chaperones and translocates into the nucleus. There it forms a heterodimer with another protein of the PAS family known as ARNT (AHR nuclear translocator). This heterodimer binds to xenobiotic responsive enhancers known as XRE (also called dioxine response elements or DREs) which are located proximal to the promoter region of specific genes that are activated by this signaling pathway. The target genes include CYP1A1, CYP1A2, and CYP1B1. In addition, some phase-II enzymes are also activated. Thus, the response of AHR activation is clearly pleiotropic.

AHR activity is further regulated by the presence of an AHR repressor (AHRR, another protein of the PAS family). The AHR repressor competes with AHR for associating with ARNT and also for binding to the XRE on the DNA. The AHRR–ARNT complex also acts as a repressor when bound to XREs. This repressor is induced by the AHR itself and thus forms a negative feedback loop for AHR regulation.

The natural ligands for the AHR are not known. However, the receptor, as well as ARNT, has been shown to be involved in normal developmental processes. For the AHR, this conclusion has been reached by the surprising findings that AHR-null mice exhibit (besides the expected unresponsiveness to CYP1A1 inducers) abnormalities in liver vascularization, and ARNT-null mice die before birth. The ARNT-null phenotype is unrelated to AHR signaling, but rather is related to ARNT's role as a partner of another PAS protein known as HIF1α.

Xenobiotic ligands include PAHs, but also many of the polychlorinated dibenzodioxins, polychlorinated dibenzofurans, and polychlorinated biphenyls.

13.1.1. AHR-mediated toxicity of polychlorinated dibenzodioxins, dibenzofurans, and biphenyls

The AHR binds many polychlorinated aromatic hydrocarbons with differing affinity.

Polychlorinated dibenzodioxins (PCDDs), polychlorinated dibenzofurans (PCDFs), and polychlorinated biphenyls (PCBs) are a large group of environmental chemicals of high toxicological relevance. Some of them are among the most toxic small molecules ever known. PCDDs and PCDFs are unwanted by-products that arise during chemical processes. For many years, PCBs were produced for industrial purposes. Now that their toxic potential has been recognized they are no longer produced commercially. These compounds are all lipophilic molecules that persist in the environment and also feature a long biological half-life. A good rule of thumb is that the higher the degree of chlorination, the less easily they are metabolically degraded; for example, TCDD has a biological $t_{1/2}$ in humans of 7–11 years!) (see Figure 13.1).

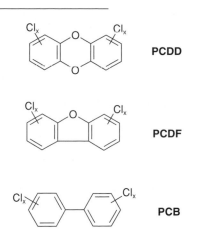

Figure 13.1. General chemical structures of polychlorinated dibenzodioxins (PCDDs), polychlorinated dibenzofurans (PCDFs), and polychlorinated biphenyls (PCBs).

Many congeners are possible due to the different degrees of chlorination. For example, 75 different forms of PCDDs or PCDFs and 209 forms of PCBs are possible. Their toxic potential varies greatly, but in qualitative terms the toxicity is similar. Because in the environment mixtures of many different compounds are found rather than pure chemicals, the composition of which are mostly unknown, a relative measure has been introduced to evaluate the toxicity of these compounds. This is given as toxicity equivalents (TEs) related to the most potent congener, TCDD, for which the TE has been arbitrarily set to 1.0.

The toxicological effects of PCDDs, PCDFs, and PCBs are pleiotropic (i.e. one trigger or one mechanism causes a multitude of transcriptional and phenotypic effects). Interestingly, the wide array of effects is mediated through one receptor, the AHR, and the differential potency can be explained by differential binding of a compound to the AHR.

Mechanism underlying the differential activity of polychlorinated dibenzodioxines, dibenzifurans, or biphenyls: The relative toxic potential of these compounds correlates excellently with and is dependent on their affinity to the AHR. Binding of a ligand to the AHR is then optimal when the two rings are co-planar, as in 2,3,7,8-tetrachlorodibenzodioxin (TCDD). Furthermore, in PCBs, the site of the chloro-substitution plays a pivotal role. For example, the 3,3′,4,4′,5,5′-hexachlorobiphenyl binds optimally, as all the chlorine atoms are in a non-*ortho*-substituted position. Chlorine atoms in an *ortho* position would cause steric hindrance, not enabling a co-planar orientation (see Figure 13.2).

The best-investigated species is undoubtedly TCDD, the most potent of all these congeners.

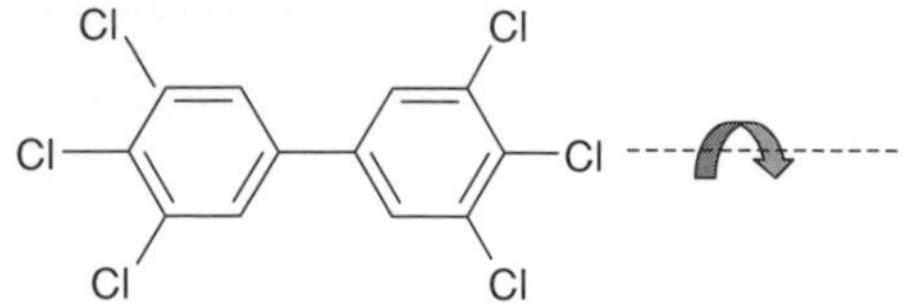

Figure 13.2. Co-planar orientation of 3,3',4,4',5,5'-hexachlorobiphenyl allows optimal binding with the AHR.

2,3,7,8-Tetrachloro-*p*-dibenzodioxin (TCDD, 'dioxin') is an environmental pollutant with a very high toxic potential featuring pleiotropic activity. TCDD is immunotoxic (thymocyte and B cell toxicity, see section 10.2.1) but also exerts endocrine toxicity, embryotoxicity and teratogenesis (laboratory animals; in primates at very high doses only). Furthermore, TCDD is a carcinogen (via non-genotoxic mechanisms) and has been classified as a Class 1 human carcinogen (implying that the molecular mechanism underlying its carcinogenic action also provides additional evidence for its carcinogenic potential). Finally, TCDD is also a very strong acutely toxic compound, with the effects becoming maximal after 2–4 weeks following a single exposure. The sensitivity is, however, species-specific; while guinea pigs are extremely sensitive (LD_{50} is approximately 500 ng/kg!), the hamster is at the other end of the scale (LD_{50} approximately 5 mg/kg), with a 10,000-fold difference in sensitivity in these two rodent species. The reasons are not known (both species express the AHR in the liver at similar levels). While TCDD in rodents produces the so-called 'wasting syndrome', during which the animals rapidly lose body mass and finally succumb (the mechanisms are not known), in humans the most conspicuous symptoms are the development of 'chloracne' (a persistent disturbance of epithelial cell differentiation in the skin).

   While the exact downstream mechanisms leading to these very diverse effects are mostly enigmatic, it has become clear that the initial underlying mechanism of all these effects is TCDD binding and activation of the AHR.

Mechanisms of AHR-mediated toxicity induced by TCDD: TCDD features an extremely high affinity for the AHR. The K_d (that is, that concentration with half-maximal receptor occupancy) in the most sensitive species can be as low as 10^{-11} M. Binding results in dissociation from hsp90 and other proteins. Now the AHR can translocate into the nucleus, where it heterodimerizes with ARNT and binds to the dioxin-response element (DRE) on the DNA. This results in transcriptional activation of a number of responsive genes including CYP1A1, glutathione transferase (GST), glucuronosyltransferase (UGT), and quinone oxidoreductase (NQO), i.e. a series of specific phase I as well as phase II xenobiotic-metabolizing enzymes (see Chapter 4 and Figure 13.3).

   A logical connection between induction of these enzymes and the development of the downstream effects with all the different forms of manifest toxicity associated with TCDD can, however, not be easily made. It is not probable that there is a single

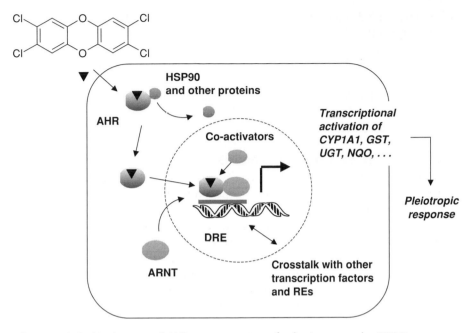

Figure 13.3. Mechanism of AHR transactivation of selective genes by TCDD.

'toxicity gene' the transactivation of which might not yet be discovered. Similarly, there is no known endogenous ligand that would give us a clue to a better mechanistic understanding of TCDD toxicity (although some plant flavonoids have been found to bind to AHR). What is known, however, is that the AHR has a pivotal role in the normal ontogenic development; for example, AHR-deficient mice exhibit abnormal vascular development and decreased liver size. But we cannot yet answer the questions referring to which genes are critical for AHR-mediated toxicity.

There is, however, compelling evidence showing that it is indeed the AHR receptor which is involved in mediating most TCDD-related downstream toxicological effects. This evidence includes the findings that:

- the responsiveness to TCDD positively correlates and segregates with the Ah^{b-1} allele
- the K_d for TCDD of non-sensitive mouse strains is 10–20 times higher than that in sensitive mouse strains
- AHR-null mice are resistant against the toxic effects of TCDD. For example, AHR −/− mice given 2 mg/kg did not exhibit toxicity, whereas in wild type AHR +/+ mice administered 200 µg/kg about half of all mice died!

Because TCDD toxicity has clearly been shown to be mediated by the AHR, the question arises as to whether there is a threshold dose for eliciting the downstream effects or whether the toxicity follows a linear dose–response curve. In other words, one might ask whether theoretically one molecule of the ligand (TCDD) would suffice to activate the AHR. Compelling evidence suggests that, similar to other dose–responses, TCDD toxicity via AHR activation follows a classical sigmoid curve. This would imply that a certain minimal amount of the ligand must be present for a cell to become transactivated.

It has also become clear, however, that it is the concerted interactions of several genes that mediate the complex array of toxic effects. Also, it is known that there is a crosstalk between the AHR and other receptors, e.g. the estrogen receptor (ER). Specifically, TCDD is known to regulate ERα activity negatively. The mechanisms are complex and not known in detail, and involve proteasome-dependent degradation of the ERα by AH receptor agonists.

13.2. Xenoestrogens and anti-androgens

Estrogen and androgen receptors have become increasingly important in toxicology because of their role in mediating xenobiotic-induced effects that mimic estrogenic or anti-estrogenic action. This is one of several mechanisms underlying the toxicity of the collectively called endocrine disrupters (some of them are 'xenoestrogens').

Xenoestrogens (or environmental estrogens) are a diverse and chemically unrelated group of xenobiotics that can elicit an agonistic (enhancing) response mediated by the estrogen receptor. Although for some environmental compounds the risk for humans and animals is still a matter of debate, some other compounds are strongly suspected to be related to increased incidences of hormonally-controlled cancers (e.g. mammary, testicular, and prostate cancer) and also in interfering with normal reproduction in wildlife. Examples include environmental pollutants (e.g. DDT, hydroxy-PCBs), and products used in the detergent and polycarbon industry (e.g. alkylphenols, bisphenol A).

Most xenoestrogens are weak agonists of the receptor (there are exceptions such as the synthetic estrogen diethylstilbestrol, DES, which was used to prevent abortions during pregnancy and which is a potent human carcinogen due to its estrogenic potency, equaling that of natural estrogen). Risk assessment is difficult as it is the relative estrogenic potency of a xenobiotic that has to be taken into account and this is sometimes very low in comparison with physiological estrogens. In other words, rather high concentrations of a given xenoestrogen would be required to elicit an adverse effect. On the other hand, the environmental stability and the bioaccumulating potential of many lipophilic compounds can make them more dangerous, in spite of the relatively low concentrations in the environment.

One mechanism by which these xenobiotics mediate their estrogenic or antiandrogenic effects is binding and activation of the estrogen receptor.

13.2.1. Estrogen receptor (ER)-mediated toxicity

The estrogen receptor (ER) includes at least two forms, ERα and ERβ. The latter has only recently been discovered, and its specific function has remained unclear. They are, however, distinct proteins and some differences exist in the transcriptional activity of these forms. The ER tissue expression also exhibits differences for ERα and ERβ. For example, ERα transcripts are found in the ovary, uterus, mammary gland, testes, pituitary, liver, kidney, heart, and skeletal muscle, while ERβ is predominantly found in ovary, prostate, lung, and bladder.

The ER is composed of six functional domains including a DNA-binding domain, a ligand-binding domain, and additional regions critical for gene expression. In the absence of ligand, the receptor is sequestered within the cell nucleus and maintained in an inactive state. Similarly to the other nuclear receptors, the protein is prevented from binding to DNA and kept in a conformation that facilitates ligand binding by heat shock proteins. Upon ligand binding, the ER receptor undergoes a conformational change and forms homodimers (but ERα preferentially dimerizes with ERβ). The ligand-receptor complex then binds to specific estrogen response elements (ERE) on DNA.

One characteristic of the ER is its 'promiscuity'; the receptor can bind a large variety of chemically unrelated ligands. Structural requirements include a ring structure and often a phenolic group in *para* position to a bulky hydrophobic structure, unhindered in the *ortho* position. One such group of xenobiotics is the alkylphenols.

Alkylphenol ethoxylates are ubiquitous products for industrial and household use as detergents and emulgators. They are distributed into the environment, where they are degraded by bacteria to **alkylphenols**. The lipophilic alkylphenols are relatively stable, building up in sediments and also bioaccumulating in organisms. They can therefore pose a potential hazard for aquatic organisms (see Figure 13.4).

The acute toxicity of alkylphenols is extremely small. However, alkylphenols have estrogenic activities, especially if they have a large hydrophobic chain.

In 1991 it was discovered by serendipity that an estrogen-dependent mammary tumor line proliferated even in the absence of added estrogens, and that this was due to contamination with **p-nonylphenol** which was present in the polystyrol culture dishes. Later it was found that p-nonylphenol could induce in male fish the synthesis of vitellogenin (a precursor of yolk protein), which normally is only produced in female fish. Thus, p-nonylphenol was able to imitate the pharmacological action of the natural estrogen, at least *in vitro* and in some fish and rodent assays. This effect is clearly mediated through the ER.

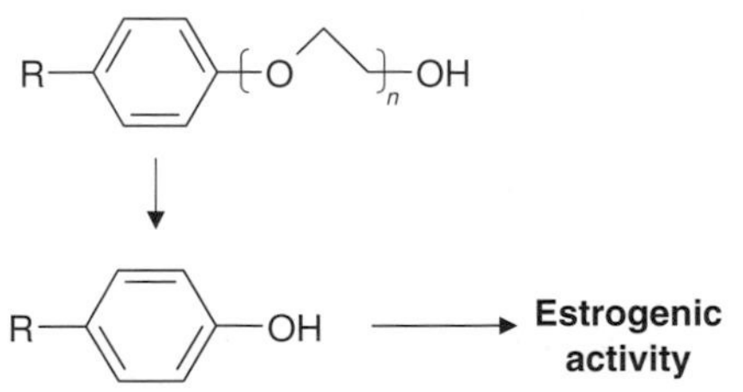

Figure 13.4. Degradation of alkylphenol ethoxylates to alkylphenols, featuring a phenolic group and a larger hydrophobic tail.

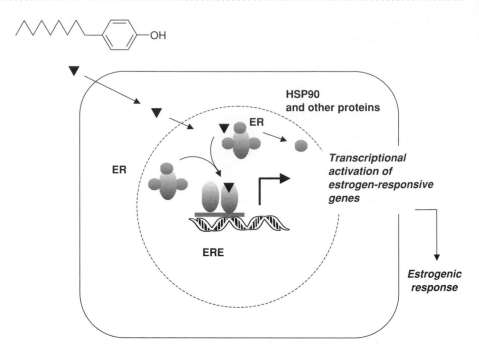

Figure 13.5. Mechanism of *p*-nonylphenol-induced activation of the estrogen receptor (ER). The lipophilic compound diffuses across biomembranes into the nucleus, where it binds to the ER. The ER forms homodimers and binds to estrogen-response elements (ERE) on DNA.

Mechanism of *p*-nonylphenol estrogenic activity: Nonylphenol binds to and activates the ER and transactivates a number of estrogen-responsive genes (see Figure 13.5). However, the relative affinity of *p*-nonylphenol is small (approximately 30,000-fold lower!) in comparison to estradiol. In addition, nonylphenol (and other alkylphenols) are rapidly and extensively metabolized by glucuronide conjugation in rats, and in contrast to the parent molecules the glucuronides do not exhibit any evidence of estrogen or anti-androgen activity. Could the *p*-alkylphenols pose a potential endocrine hazard to humans? In view of the low exposure to humans, the low estrogenic activity of these compounds, and the rapid clearance, a human health risk seems very small.

Another mechanism by which endocrine-disrupting xenobiotics may exert anti-androgenic effects is by interacting with the androgen receptor.

13.2.2. Androgen receptor (AR)-mediated toxicity

The androgen receptor (AR) is a ligand-activated steroid hormone receptor which plays a pivotal role in the development of male gonadal tissues. It has also been implicated in the development of some tumors, including prostate cancer. The AR is present in most tissues, but is most abundant in all male reproductive organs. Low levels of expression were demonstrated in liver, kidney, neuronal tissues, muscle, and female reproductive organs.

In its unliganded state, and in contrast to the ER, the AR is located primarily in the cytosol, and it is only after ligand binding that the receptor translocates into the nucleus. After ligand binding, the AR is phosphorylated and dimerizes, followed by binding to specific androgen response elements (ARE) on DNA.

Similarly to other steroid hormone receptors, the AR consists of several functional domains including a transactivation, a DNA-binding, a nuclear localization, a dimerization, and a ligand-binding domain.

The AR is regulated at the transcriptional as well as at the protein level. The expression is regulated mostly by androgens, but several other hormones and growth factors can also participate.

Physiological ligands for the AR are testosterone and dihydrotestosterone. However, a number of xenobiotics can also bind to the receptor, and these compounds have indeed been shown to elicit their endocrine-disrupting effect through interacting with the AR. Among these chemicals are vinclozolin, a dicarboximide fungicide, and, probably better known, a metabolite of the pesticide DDT.

1,1-Dichloro-2,2-bis(*p*-chlorophenyl)ethylene (*p,p′*-DDE or DDE), is a metabolite of DDT, which is widespread in the environment, although DDT is no longer produced in the Western world (see Figure 13.6).

Male rats exposed to DDE exhibit altered sexual differentiation and signs of feminization. In addition, if present at high concentrations, DDE can exert endocrine-disrupting effects in wildlife. This has been exemplified from an environmental toxicological case in Florida. Alligators in Lake Apopka, which was heavily contaminated with DDE, exhibited dramatically altered sex hormone levels and morphological alterations, as compared to alligators in a control lake. In particular, the basal plasma testosterone levels were greatly decreased in alligators from the contaminated lake. Furthermore,

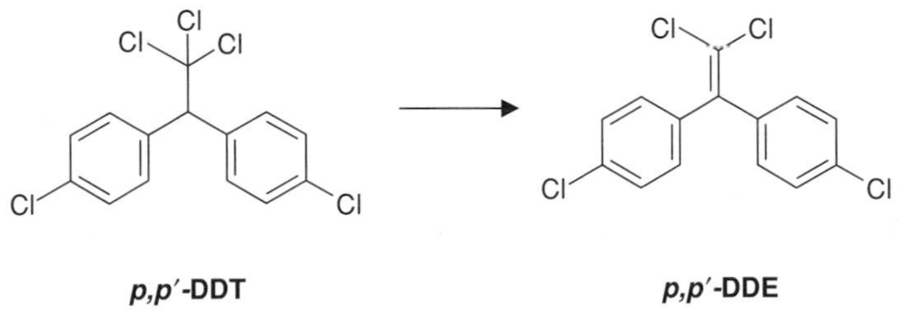

p,p′-DDT   *p,p′*-DDE

Figure 13.6. *p,p′*-DDE is a major metabolite of *p,p′*-DDT (1,1,1-trichloro-2,2-bis(*p*-chlorophenyl)ethane). Both the parent compound and its degradation product are lipophilic and persistent in the environment (DDE > DDT). Originally, the endocrine toxicity of DDT was attributed to DDT (the *o,p′*-isomer exhibits very weak binding activity to the estrogen receptor). However, more recently it has been demonstrated that the metabolite, DDE, is an anti-androgen interacting with the androgen receptor.

Table 13.1 Plasma concentrations of sex steroid hormones in alligators from Lake Apopka (contaminated with DDE) and Lake Woodruff (control lake)

Hormone	Lake Apopka alligators		Lake Woodruff alligators	
	Males	Females	Males	Females
Basal levels				
Estradiol (pg/ml)	36.2 ± 4.9	118.1 ± 19.7	40.3 ± 8.8	76.2 ± 10.3
Testosterone (pg/ml)	13.4 ± 3.9	13.1 ± 1.7	50.4 ± 9.0	18.5 ± 3.9
After LH				
Estradiol (pg/ml)	118.6 ± 32.5	170.7 ± 14.8	62.3 ± 12.7	82.0 ± 14.3
Testosterone (pg/ml)	15.8 ± 3.1	12.3 ± 2.9	44.5 ± 12.5	28.1 ± 8.1

Note: Plasma concentrations of estradiol-17β and testosterone were determined in 6-month old alligators prior to or after stimulation with luteinizing hormone (LH). LH is a powerful physiological stimulator of sex steroid hormone synthesis. Mean ± SEM.
Source: data (modified) are from Guillette, L.J., Gross, T.S., Masson, G.R., Matter, J.M., Percival, H.F. and Woodward, A.R. (1994) Developmental abnormalities of the gonad and abnormal sex hormone concentrations in juvenile alligators from contaminated and control lakes in Florida, *Environ. Health Perspect.* 102; 680–688.

after stimulation with the luteinizing hormone (LH), which greatly induces the production of sex steroid hormones, estrogen levels were increased not only in females (as would be expected) but also in males of the contaminated lake. This indicates that DDE had severely interfered with sexual differentiation and maturation (see Table 13.1).

These anti-androgenic effects have several causes, including induction of hepatic aromatase (a CYP which is involved in catalyzing the A ring aromatization of steroids and thus the production of estrogens). However, the most compelling mechanism involves interaction with the androgen receptor.

Mechanisms of *p,p'*-DDE-induced endocrine-disrupting effects: DDE is an anti-androgen, altering the expression of specific androgen (testosterone, dihydrotestosterone)-regulated genes. This is clearly an AR-mediated mechanism. However, the molecular mechanism differs from that elicited by xenobiotics activating the ER because the anti-androgen ligand/AR complex is not stable and does not lead to binding of the complex to the ARE. Instead, there is increased cytoplasmic degradation of the AR. In addition, DDE is able to displace androgen ligands from receptor binding. Thus, anti-androgenic activity of DDE results in an inhibition (transcriptional repression) of the AR-mediated gene transactivation and the related downstream biological effects (see Figure 13.7).

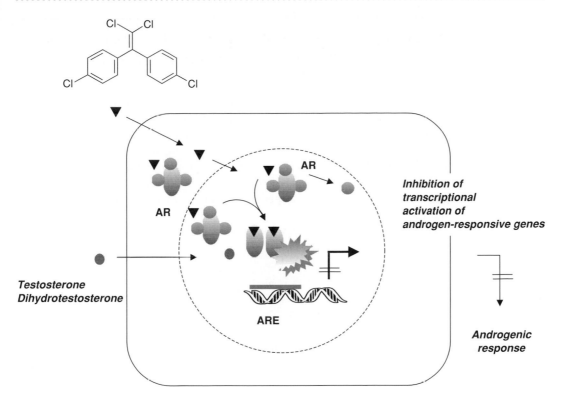

Figure 13.7. Mechanism of p,p'-DDE-induced inactivation of the androgen receptor (AR). The lipophilic compound diffuses into the cell, where it binds to the AR. This inactivates the receptor and prevents it from binding to the androgen response element (ARE) on DNA.

Again, if these mechanistic (toxicodynamic) considerations are taken as a basis for assessing the human risk, other (toxicokinetic) factors have also of course to be considered. For example, just because a xenobiotic binds to a steroid receptor *in vitro* (or *in vivo* after administration of very high doses), this does not necessarily mean that it is a relevant endocrine disruptor, nor that the possible effects are mediated through the ER or AR. Often the critical concentrations needed to elicit such a receptor-mediated response are not expected to be attained in humans. Nevertheless, the fact that there is clear endocrine toxicity in environmental organisms warrants great caution, and specifically in areas where DDT is still being used, DDE concentrations in human tissues or mother's milk have been found which may be higher than those eliciting anti-androgenic effects *in vitro*.

13.3. Peroxisome proliferator-activated receptors (PPARs)

The toxicological relevance of PPARs is relatively new; in fact, the first PPAR was detected in 1990. Since then the PPARs have become of paramount importance, and some of their effects have been implicated in the toxicity of drugs or industrial chemicals.

Peroxisome proliferator-activated receptors (PPARs) are ligand-dependent transcription factors belonging to the nuclear hormone receptor superfamily. They bind and are activated by fatty acids and some of the eicosanoid metabolites, although relatively high concentrations are required (i.e. concentrations higher than for some of the synthetic ligands). So far, there are three PPAR subtypes: PPARα, PPARδ (also called PPARβ), and PPARγ. The three types have different tissue distribution and different functions (see Table 13.2).

There are historical reasons for the name, but it might be slightly misleading: ligands for PPARα had been known to cause proliferation of peroxisomes in rodents; however, in humans, PPARs do not cause peroxisome proliferation (therefore, the receptor would perhaps better be termed 'fatty acid-activated receptor').

Peroxisomes are subcellular organelles which function as sites of fatty acyl-β-oxidation, cholesterol metabolism, glycerolipid biosynthesis, and other pathways of lipid metabolism. Peroxisomes, in contrast to mitochondria, can oxidize very-long-chain fatty acids (mitochondria have a cutoff at C_{22}-fatty acids). Again in contrast to mitochondria, peroxisome-mediated β-oxidation leads to an incomplete shortening of the fatty acyl carbon chain.

Table 13.2 Biological characteristics of PPAR subtypes

	PPARα	PPARδ	PPARγ
Tissue distribution	Liver, kidney, heart, muscle	Ubiquitous	Adipose tissue, intestine, immune cells
Regulatory function	Enzymes involved in β-oxidation of fatty acids, lipoprotein metabolism	Unclear (adipocyte differentiation?)	Genes involved in adipocyte differentiation, lipid and glucose metabolism
Major effect	Stimulates fatty acid β-oxidation		Stimulates storage of fat
Natural ligands	Arachidonic acid + analogs, leukotriene B_4	Fatty acids	Polyunsaturated fatty acids, prostaglandin J_2
Ligands (drugs)	Fibrates		Thiazolidinediones, NSAIDs

All PPARs form heterodimers with the retinoid X receptor and bind to specific PPAR response elements in the promoter region of their target genes.

13.3.1. PPARα-dependent toxicity

Two different aspects relevant to the toxicity of xenobiotics have been closely related to PPARα. The first one is the role of peroxisome proliferators in promoting liver tumors in rodents; the second one deals with their role as possible cytoprotecting agents against a number of hepatotoxins. Although not yet clearly understood, the basis for the two mechanisms might be similar.

Members of the peroxisome proliferators, although a chemically diverse group of compounds, have long been known to cause liver tumors in rodents. What is the mechanism underlying this effect, and how relevant is it for humans?

Peroxisome proliferators are a group of chemically diverse compounds, including hypolipidemic drugs of the fibrate type (e.g. clofibrate, ciprofibrate, gemfibrozil, and nafenopin) but also other, structurally unrelated compounds (e.g. plasticizers including di-(2-ethylhexyl) phthalate (see section 2.1.3), and some industrial solvents). What they have in common is that they cause liver tumors in mice and rats. Because all these compounds induce the proliferation of peroxisomes, it was speculated that this could be the common basis underlying the tumor-enhancing effects. However, it turned out that peroxisome proliferation, which is a rodent-specific effect, is just one of several pathways which is induced by these compounds. The basis for this and other effects, and what they all share, is that peroxisome proliferators all are ligands and activators of PPARα. Because PPARα is most abundant in liver, this is the target organ for most of their effects, including hepatomegaly due to hyperplasia and hypertrophy. They also induce the expression of a large number of genes involved in peroxisomal β-oxidation. Interestingly, these compounds do not elicit peroxisome responses in guinea pigs or nonhuman primates.

It has become clear that clofibrate-type drugs are not genotoxic carcinogens. Instead, they act as tumor promoters. That the PPARα is directly involved in mediating the tumorigenic response for all these chemicals has been convincingly demonstrated with PPARα-null mice, which did not produce liver tumors.

Mechanisms of PPARα ligand/activator-mediated hepatocarcinogenesis: Several mechanisms might be involved, and their interdependency has not yet been unraveled. All these effects are mediated by PPARα. For example, peroxisome proliferators stimulate replicative DNA synthesis and liver growth, a known tumor-promoting characteristic. In addition, the peroxisome proliferators inhibit hepatocyte apoptosis both *in vitro* and *in vivo*. Again, this is a key factor involved in tumor promotion, as apoptosis normally eliminates cells with potential preneoplastic changes.

The sequence of events is not yet clear. On the one hand, tumor necrosis factor-α has been implicated in mediating these effects, because TNFα both stimulates DNA replication and suppresses apoptosis in hepatocytes. On the other hand, activation of the mitogen-activated protein (MAP) kinase pathway (see section 5.4), including p38 MAP kinase, has been implicated in the cell growth. These MAP kinases, which form a self-amplifying cascade, are strongly activated by oxidative stress. But what is the connection between peroxisome proliferators and oxidative stress? The increase in peroxisomal fatty acyl β-oxidation, resulting from exposure

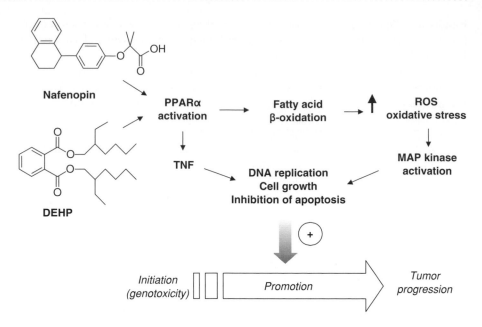

Figure 13.8. Mechanisms related to PPARα activation by nafenopine and other fibrates or by plasticizers, leading to net cell growth and tumor promotion in the liver. DEHP, diethylhexylphthalate.

to these compounds, involves also increases in the activity of fatty acyl CoA oxidase, a process by which large amounts of hydrogen peroxide are generated. This rise in H_2O_2 production is, however, not paralleled by an increase in catalase activity, which would detoxify hydrogen peroxide. Therefore, vigorous enzymatic production of hydrogen peroxide leads to increased oxidative stress. Indeed, sustained oxidative stress has been associated with nongenotoxic carcinogenesis in the liver (see Figure 13.8).

Because peroxisome proliferation and increases in peroxisomal β-oxidation are rodent-specific effects, it is unlikely that PPARα-ligand-mediated peroxisome proliferation and, hence, liver tumor promotion, is a relevant factor in humans.

The second toxicologically interesting role of PPARα is its participation in conveying cytoprotection against a variety of hepatotoxins. The best investigated example is the hepatoprotective effect provided by clofibrate against acetaminophen-induced liver injury.

Clofibrate is a widely used hypolipidemic drug that belongs to the class of fibrates, which are peroxisome proliferators in rodents. A number of studies have revealed that chronic pretreatment of mice with clofibrate, but also acute treatment with a single dose, protects from liver injury inflicted by a hepatotoxic dose of acetaminophen (APAP, see section 9.2.1). The possible mechanisms have been explored, but it seems that it is neither bioactivation of APAP to a reactive metabolite nor alterations in the hepatic cytoprotective GSH content that is affected by clofibrate. It turned out that clofibrate conveys protection against a large number of other, chemically different and mechanistically distinct, hepatotoxic compounds (e.g. carbon tetrachloride, bromobenzene, chloroform). Thus, because the mechanism of protection is unlikely to be related to mechanisms of liver injury, the possibility that the protection is mediated by PPARα has to be further explored.

Mechanism of clofibrate-mediated cytoprotection against hepatotoxicants: The mechanisms have not yet been fully elucidated. However, an important clue was given by the demonstration that PPARα-null mice had lost the ability to be resistant against APAP when given clofibrate, implicating a role of PPARα in this mechanism.

Because it is known that PPARα controls, among others, growth regulatory genes including *c-myc*, c-Ha-*ras*, *fos*, *jun*, and *egr-1*, which are involved in the progression of cell cycle (see section 8.4) and the transition from G_o to S, clofibrate, as a ligand for PPARα, could activate cell cycle progression. It is tempting to speculate that the hepatoprotective effect of clofibrate may be based on stimulating a mitogenic response. This would provide an advantage in restoring the injured parenchymal tissue and would help to restore the cell mass rapidly.

Indeed, stimulation of mitogenesis and cell replacement is an important mechanism that helps to compensate for the loss of cell mass during xenobiotic-induced liver injury (see section 8.1 and Figure 13.9).

13.3.2. PPARγ-mediated toxicity

In comparison to PPARα, PPARγ has often been called the 'opposing' receptor, because its activation mediates biological functions distinct from (and sometimes diametrically opposed to) those activated by PPARα ligands. For example, PPARγ has anti-tumor effects on a variety of cancers, rather than being a tumor-promoting factor. Similarly, PPARγ activation (being another 'lipid sensor' in the body) does not result in an induction of fatty acid oxidation, but rather causes an increase in storage lipids, which is another strategy of reducing an acute load of the organism with fatty acids.

The peroxisome proliferator-activated receptor-γ is encoded by a single gene which features a highly conserved structure in mice, rats, and humans. Three transcript forms, PPARγ1, γ2, and γ3, arise from alternative promoter usage and by alternative splicing, while at the protein level two isoforms, PPARγ1 and PPARγ2, have been identified. The differential function of these splice variants is not known, but their distinct tissue distribution (PPARγ1 is abundant in extra-adipose tissue, while PPARγ2 is abundant in adipose tissue) suggests that they may have different physiological roles.

Upon binding of a ligand, the receptor undergoes a conformational change. It is converted into an activated form that facilitates the recruitment of co-activators including the steroid receptor co-activator (SRC-1). Their function is not entirely

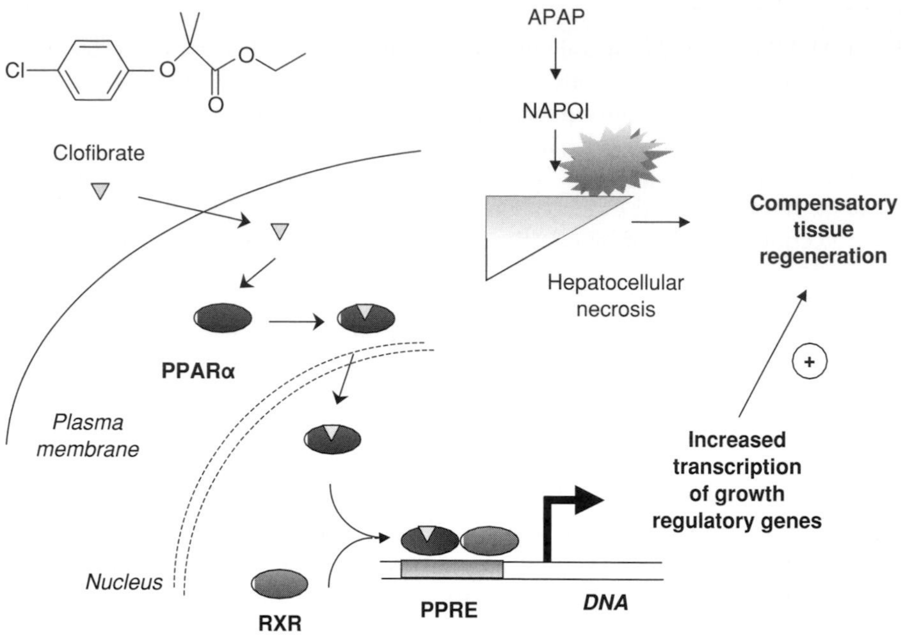

Figure 13.9. Hypothetical mechanism of hepatoprotection provided by the PPARα-activator clofibrate against acetaminophen and other liver toxicants. Transactivation of growth regulatory genes stimulates cell cycle progression and regeneration of injured hepatic tissue.

clear, but they could link the regulatory signal to the transcriptional machinery. This could explain why different (synthetic and natural) ligands exert differential responses upon binding and activation of the receptor.

PPARγ levels in fat tissue are 10–100 times higher than those in extra-adipose tissues; therefore, PPARγ has long been considered an 'adipose-selective' nuclear receptor. However, other tissues, including liver and skeletal muscle, also express PPARγ, although much less abundantly.

Importantly, epigenetic factors, including nutrition and obesity, can dramatically change the expression levels of PPARγ. For example, in a number of murine models of obesity and type 2 diabetes, the hepatic expression levels of PPARγ mRNA and receptor protein were highly increased. Activation of the receptor under these pathophysiological conditions can have totally different downstream biological consequences than under normal conditions. Because some currently used drugs (the thiazolidinediones) are used to treat these same pathophysiological conditions (type 2 diabetes), and because they are specific ligands and activators of PPARγ, the hepatic effects of these drugs should be closely monitored.

Although PPARγ has been gaining enormous attention as a target for anti-diabetic drugs and also as a possible target for anticancer drugs, e.g. in the colon, it is not often mentioned in a toxicological context. However, two aspects will be briefly discussed here where ligands and activators of PPARγ have been implicated. The first is receptor-mediated adipogenesis-promoting effects in the bone marrow.

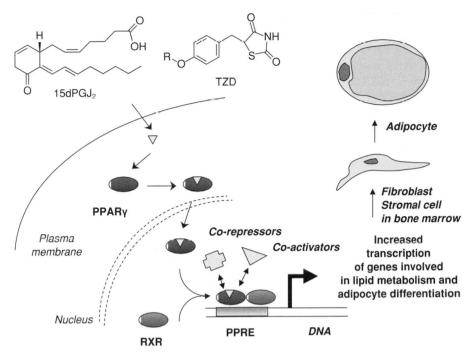

Figure 13.10. Transactivation of PPARγ-regulated genes leads to expression of genes involved in lipid metabolism and adipocyte differentiation. PPARγ ligands and activators include natural (prostaglandins) and synthetic (thiazolidinediones, TZD) compounds. 15dPGJ$_2$, 15-deoxy-$\Delta^{12,14}$ prostaglandin J$_2$.

The second example is the development of hepatic steatosis. The two effects have the same basis: activation of PPARγ by selective ligands, and modulation of these effects by regulation of the expression of the PPARγ genes (see Figure 13.10).

Thiazolidinediones (TZDs), also called glitazones, are a novel group of therapeutics used to treat insulin resistance and type 2 diabetes. They were the first chemical class of drugs found to specifically bind to and activate PPARγ. Especially when given in combination with other antidiabetic drugs, TZDs effectively reduce hyperinsulinemia, hyperlipidemia, and hyperglycemia.

The first TZD on the market was troglitazone, which was later withdrawn because of idiosyncratic hepatic toxicity. The mechanisms underlying troglitazone-induced liver injury are not known; they could involve reactive metabolites. Subsequently, new glitazones have been used, including rosiglitazone and pioglitazone. There have been hardly any reports of liver liability with these second-generation TZDs; it has to be mentioned, however, that it is not yet clear whether the common thiazolidinedione ring is involved in the formation of a reactive metabolite, and whether the greatly reduced therapeutic dose of the new TZDs (approximately 100-fold smaller than the dose used for troglitazone, due to much higher PPARγ affinity) is part of the reason that they are hepatic-safe.

Some TZDs, however, can induce fat accumulation in the bone marrow, which is a serious condition and which can lead to anemia. Indeed, both rosiglitazone and pioglitazone induced adipocyte differentiation in bone marrow stromal cells, and TZDs also cause bone marrow changes *in vivo*, although high doses are required for this effect to occur.

The second effect of TZDs is a fatty change in the liver which has been reported from experiments with mouse models of obesity and type 2 diabetes. Importantly, this effect has not been observed in normal wild type mice. Prolonged treatment with high doses of troglitazone, pioglitazone or rosiglitazone resulted in liver enlargement and microvesicular steatosis. Microvesicular steatosis is thought to be caused by an accumulation of fatty acids due to impaired degradation by β-oxidation, which is an important 'sink' for fatty acids in the liver. Microvesicular steatosis can be a very serious condition, because it can cause oxidative stress in the liver and progress to steatohepatitis or fibrosis. Whether there is any possible connection between these experimental results and the high incidence of fibrosis in patients who received troglitazone and who developed liver injury remains unclear.

Mechanisms of thiazolidinedione-mediated bone marrow adipogenesis and hepatic steatosis: Both the adipogenesis in the bone marrow and development of hepatic steatosis are most likely mediated through PPARγ activation. For example, in the bone marrow stromal cells, exposure to TZDs caused increased transcription of adipocyte-specific genes which are regulated by PPARγ.

In the liver, the striking microvesicular steatosis can be explained by recent findings in those obese mice which produce the hepatic toxicity. It turned out that these TZD-sensitive mice all exhibited highly up-regulated expression of PPARγ in the liver (where normally receptor expression is very low). Importantly, different murine models with distinct genetic alterations and different etiologies of insulin resistance and diabetes all had increased levels of hepatic PPARγ. Treatment of these obese mice, but not of their lean controls, caused increased transcription of genes involved in lipid metabolism (e.g. fatty acid-binding protein in the liver and fatty acid translocase), which is perhaps not unexpected.

The molecular mechanisms of PPARγ-mediated hepatic steatosis are not known, but the array of functional changes in these models allows a plausible model to be established.

1 There are increased fluxes of non-esterified fatty acids from the adipose tissue to the liver in obese animals, continuously exposing hepatocytes to high levels of fatty acids.

2 *De novo* synthesis of fatty acids from glucose is increased in liver cells as a consequence of PPARγ activation.

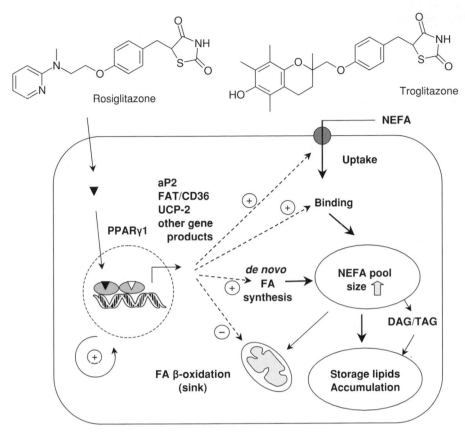

Figure 13.11. PPARγ-mediated pathways of altered fatty acid metabolism and disposition in hepatocytes of obese and diabetic mice exposed to glitazones. High expression levels of PPARγ are associated with the induction of PPARγ-responsive genes, resulting in enhanced uptake, binding, and *de novo* biosynthesis of fatty acids, as well as reduction of mitochondrial β-oxidation. This leads to a net increase in the hepatocyte's fatty acid pool and accumulation of storage lipids. PPARγ activation also enhances its own transcription. aP2, FAT/CD36, and UCP-2 are genes involved in fatty acid uptake, intracellular fatty acid binding, and mitochondrial uncoupling, respectively. NEFA, non-esterified fatty acids; DAG, diacylglycerol; TAG, triacylglycerol.

3 PPARγ-responsive genes that become up-regulated include fatty acid transporters and fatty acid-binding protein.
4 Degradation by β-oxidation of fatty acids is inhibited by TZDs (see Figure 13.11).

This example was also chosen because it demonstrates that a drug or xenobiotic may exert totally different downstream biological effects in healthy individuals (or wild type animals) versus individuals with pathophysiological changes. In particular, one should not forget that drugs are used in diseased patients, yet the preclincial safety assessment is made in healthy animals.

Learning points

- Activation of nuclear receptors by xenobiotics can mediate toxic responses through signaling pathways or direct interaction with specific DNA response elements.
- The aryl hydrocarbon receptor (AHR) mediates the pleiotropic toxicity of polychlorinated dibenzodioxins and dibenzofurans, and that of PCBs. While binding of TCDD to the AHR, receptor activation, and DNA binding to the XRE are well known, the downstream mechanisms leading from the induction of specific gene expression to the wide array of toxic effects are not known.
- Many endocrine-disrupting xenobiotics (xenoestrogens) in the environment are weak agonists for the estrogen receptor (ER). Although their estrogenic potency is low, many of these compounds can bioaccumulate.
- Binding and activation of the androgen receptor (AR) by a xenobiotic, e.g. a DDT metabolite, block the androgenic responses. The occupied receptor is rapidly degraded, and binding to the ARE on DNA is prevented, resulting in endocrine-disrupting effects.
- Peroxisome proliferator-activated receptors (PPARs) are ligand-activated transcription factors involved in lipid metabolism. Xenobiotics which activate PPARα can induce DNA replication and liver growth (they act as tumor promoters). Because clofibrate (a PPARα ligand and activator) promotes cell cycle progression, it could play a role in liver mass regeneration following toxic insult by chemicals.
- Activation of PPARγ by xenobiotics (e.g. thiazolidinediones) can cause adipocyte differentiation in the bone marrow and, in mice with up-regulated hepatic expression of PPARγ, severe hepatic steatosis by disruption of fatty acyl metabolism.

Further reading

AHR-mediated toxicity induced by TCDD

Fernandez-Salguero, P.M., Hilbert, D.M., Rudikoff, S., Ward, J.M. and Gonzalez, F.J. (1996) Aryl-hydrocarbon receptor-deficient mice are resistant to 2,3,7,8-tetrachlorodibenzo-*p*-dioxin-induced toxicity, *Toxicol. Appl. Pharmacol.* 140: 173–179.

Fernandez-Salguero, P.M., Pineau, T., Hilbert, D.M., McPhail, T., Lee, S.S.T., Kimura, S., Nebert, D.W., Rudikoff, S., Ward, J.M. and Gonzalez, F.J. (1995) Immune system impairment and hepatic fibrosis in mice lacking the dioxin-binding Ah receptor, *Science* 268: 722–726.

Kimbrough, R.D. (1995) Polychlorinated biphenyls (PCBs) and human health: an update, *Crit. Rev. Toxicol.* 25: 133–163.

Lucier, G.W., Portier, C.J. and Gallo, M.A. (1993) Receptor mechanisms and dose–response models for the effects of dioxins, *Environ. Health Perspect.* 101: 36–44.

Okey, A.B., Riddick, D.S. and Harper, P.A. (1994) The Ah receptor: Mediator of the toxicity of 2,3,7,8,-tetrachloro-*p*-dioxin (TCDD) and related compounds, *Toxicol. Lett.* 70: 1–22.

Safe, S. (2001) Molecular biology of the Ah receptor and its role in carcinogenesis, *Toxicol. Lett.* 120: 1–7.

Swanson, H.I. and Bradfield, C.A. (1993) The AH-receptor: Genetics, structure and function, *Pharmacogenetics* 3: 213–230.

Xenoestrogens and anti-androgens

Akingbemi, B.T. and Hardy, M.P. (2001) Oestrogenic and antiandrogenic chemicals in the environment: Effects on male reproductive health, *Ann. Med.* 33: 391–403.

Howdeshell, K.L., Hotchkiss, A.K., Thayer, K.A., Vandenbergh, J.G. and vom Saal, F.S. (1999) Exposure to bisphenol A advances puberty, *Nature* 401: 763–764.

Safe, S.H. (1995) Environmental and dietary estrogens and human health: Is there a problem?, *Environ. Health Perspect.* 103: 346–351.

Tyler, C.R., Jobling, S. and Sumpter, J.P. (1998) Endocrine disruption in wildlife: A critical review of the evidence, *Crit. Rev. Toxicol.* 28: 319–361.

ER-mediated toxicity

Witorsch, R.J. (2000) Endocrine disruption: A critical review of environmental estrogens from a mechanistic perspective, *Toxic Subst. Mech.* 19: 53–78.

Alkylphenol ethoxylates

Nimrod, A.C. and Benson, W.H. (1996) Environmental estrogenic effects of alkylphenol ethoxylates, *Crit. Rev. Toxicol.* 26: 335–364.

p-Nonylphenol estrogenic activity

Moffat, G.J., Burns, A., Van Miller, J., Joiner, R. and Ashby, J. (2001) Glucuronidation of nonylphenol and octylphenol eliminates their ability to activate transcription via the estrogen receptor, *Reg. Toxicol. Pharmacol.* 34: 182–187.

Soto, M.A., Justicia, H., Wray, J.W. and Sonnenschein, C. (1991) p-Nonyl-phenol: An estrogenic xenobiotic released from 'modified' polystyrene, *Environ. Health Perspect.* 92: 167–173.

AR-mediated toxicity

Keller, E.T., Ershler, W.B. and Chang, C. (1996) The androgen receptor: A mediator of diverse responses, *Frontiers Biosci.* 1: d59–d71.

Tomura, A., Goto, K., Morinaga, H., Nomura, M., Okabe, T., Yanase, T., Takayanagi, R. and Nawata, H. (2001) The subnuclear three-dimensional image analysis of androgen receptor fused to green fluorescence protein, *J. Biol. Chem.* 276: 28395–28401.

p,p′-DDE-induced endocrine-disrupting effects

Kelce, W.R., Lambright, C.R., Gray, L.E. and Roberts, K.P. (1997) Vinclozolin and p,p′-DDE alter androgen-dependent gene expression: *In vivo* confirmation of an androgen receptor-mediated mechanism, *Toxicol. Appl. Pharmacol.* 142: 192–200.

You, L., Casanova, M., Archibeque-Engle, S., Sar, M., Fan, L.Q. and Heck, H.D.A. (1998) Impaired male sexual development in perinatal Sprague-Dawley and Long-Evans Hooded rats exposed *in utero* and lactationally to p,p′-DDE, *Toxicol. Sci.* 45: 162–173.

You, L., Sar, M., Bartolucci, E., Ploch, S. and Whitt, M. (2001) Induction of hepatic aromatase by p,p′-DDE in adult male rats, *Mol. Cell. Endocrinol.* 178: 207–214.

PPARs

Kersten, S., Desvergne, B. and Wahli, W. (2000) Roles of PPARs in health and disease, *Nature* 405: 421–424.

Schoonjans, K., Staels, B. and Auwerx, J. (1996) Role of the peroxisome proliferator-activated receptor (PPAR) in mediating the effects of fibrates and fatty acids on gene expression, *J. Lipid Res.* 37: 907–925.

Vamecq, J. and Latruffe, N. (1999) Medical significance of peroxisome proliferator-activated receptors, *Lancet* 354: 141–148.

Peroxisome proliferators

Bentley, P., Calder, I., Elcombe, C., Grasso, P., Stringer, D. and Wiegand, H.J. (1993) Hepatic peroxisome proliferation in rodents and its significance for humans, *Food Chem. Toxicol.* 31: 857–907.

Lee, S.J., Pineau, T., Drago, J., Lee, J.O., Owens, D.L., Kroetz, P.M., Fernandez-Salguero, P.M., Westphal, H. and Gonzalez, F.J. (1995) Targeted disruption of the alpha isoform of the peroxisome proliferator-activated receptor gene in mice results in abolishment of the pleiotropic effecs of peroxisome proliferators, *Mol. Cell. Biol.* 15: 3012–3022.

PPARα ligand/activator-mediated hepatocarcinogenesis

Corton, J.C., Anderson, S.P. and Stauber, A. (2000) Central role of peroxisome proliferator-activated receptors in the actions of peroxisome proliferators, *Annu. Rev. Pharmacol. Toxicol.* 40: 491–518.

Cosulich, S., James, N. and Roberts, R. (2000) Role of MAP kinase signalling pathways in the mode of action of peroxisome proliferators, *Carcinogenesis* 21: 579–583.

Hasmal, S.C., James, N.H., Macdonald, N., Gonzalez, F.J., Peters, J.M. and Roberts, R.A. (2000) Suppression of mouse hepatocyte apoptosis by peroxisome proliferators: Role of PPARα and TNFα, *Mut. Res. Fund. Mol. Mech. Mutagenesis* 448: 193–200.

Clofibrate-mediated cytoprotection against hepatotoxicants

Chen, C., Hennig, G.E., Whiteley, H.E., Corton, J.C. and Manautou, J.E. (2000) Peroxisome proliferator-activated receptor alpha-null mice lack resistance to acetaminophen hepatotoxicity following clofibrate exposure, *Toxicol. Sci.* 57: 338–344.

Manautou, J.E., Hart, S.G.E., Khairallah, E.A. and Cohen, S.D. (1996) Protection against acetaminophen hepatotoxicity by a single dose of clofibrate: effects on selective protein arylation and glutathione depletion, *Fund. Appl. Toxicol.* 29: 229–237.

Manautou, J.E., Hoivik, D.J., Tveit, A., Hart, S.G.E., Khairallah, E.A. and Cohen, S.D. (1994) Clofibrate pretreatment diminishes acetaminophen's selective covalent binding and hepatotoxicity, *Toxicol. Appl. Pharmacol.* 129: 252–263.

Mehendale, H.M. (2000) PPAR-α: A key to the mechanism of hepatoprotection by clofibrate, *Toxicol. Sci.* 57: 187–190.

PPARγ

Fajas, L., Auboeuf, D., Raspé, E., Schoonjans, K., Lefebvre, A.M., Saladin, R., Najib, J., Laville, M., Fruchart, J.C., Deeb, S., Vidal-Puig, A., Flier, J., Briggs, M.R., Staels, B., Vidal, H. and Auwerx, J. (1997) The organization, promoter analysis, and expression of the human PPARγ gene, *J. Biol. Chem.* 272: 18779–18789.

Spiegelman, B.M. (1998) PPAR-γ: Adipogenic regulator and thiazolidinedione receptor, *Diabetes* 47: 507–514.

Uppenberg, J., Svensson, C., Jaki, M., Bertilsson, G., Jendeberg, L. and Berkenstam, A. (1998) Crystal structure of the ligand binding domain of the human nuclear receptor PPAR-γ, *J. Biol. Chem.* 273: 31108–31112.

PPARγ and TZD-mediated bone marrow adipogenesis and hepatic steatosis

Bedoucha, M., Atzpodien, E. and Boelsterli, U.A. (2001) Diabetic KKA[y] mice exhibit increased hepatic PPARγ1 gene expression and develop hepatic steatosis upon chronic treatment with antidiabetic thiazolidinediones, *J. Hepatol.* 35: 17–23.

Boelsterli, U.A. and Bedoucha, M. (2002) Toxicological consequences of altered peroxisome proliferator-activated receptor-γ (PPARγ) expression in the liver: Insights from models of obesity and type 2 diabetes, *Biochem. Pharmacol.* 62: 1–10.

Camp, H.S., Li, O., Wise, S.C., Hong, Y.H., Frankowski, C.L., Shen, X., Vanbogelen, R. and Leff, T. (2000) Differential activation of peroxisome proliferator-activated receptor-gamma by troglitazone and rosiglitazone, *Diabetes* 49: 539–547.

Gimble, J.M., Robinson, C.E., Wu, X.Y., Kelly, K.A., Rodriguez, B.R., Kliewer, S.A., Lehmann, J.M. and Morris, D.C. (1996) Peroxisome proliferator-activated receptor-gamma activation by thiazolidinediones induces adipogenesis in bone marrow stromal cells, *Mol. Pharmacol.* 50: 1087–1094.

Tolman, K.G. (2000) Thiazolidinedione hepatotoxicity: A class effect?, *Int. J. Clin. Pract.* 113: 29–34.

Weinstock, R.S., Murray, F.T., Diani, A., Sangani, G.A., Wachowski, M.B. and Messina, J.L. (1997) Pioglitazone: *In vitro* effects on rat hepatoma cells and *in vivo* liver hypertrophy in KKAy mice, *Pharmacology* 54: 169–178.

Chapter 14

Interactions of xenobiotics with ion transporters

Contents

Certain xenobiotics can specifically interfere with ion transporters through specific interactions at the transporter's binding site(s). Depending on the concentration of the xenobiotic, the overall function of the ion transporter will be impaired, and toxicity may ensue. Because ion transporters are crucial for many biological functions, inhibition of these transporters is likely to result in disruption of ion homeostasis and loss of cell function.

Ion transporters are membrane proteins that either undergo conformational changes upon binding of a substrate (they are then called ion carriers), or water-filled pores, featuring ion-selective transport of substrates through open-closed function (they are then called ion channels). Both forms of ion transporting proteins can theoretically transport ions in both directions of the membrane. In general, the vectorial transport is largely governed by the electrochemical gradient of the substrate.

As in many other cases, such a highly specific affinity of a xenobiotic for a crucial biomolecule is often seen with naturally occurring compounds. Indeed, the examples below are all highly effective plant or animal toxins. Because of these properties, some of these compounds have been applied as biochemical tools or even efficaceous pharmaceutical drugs.

14.1. Interactions with neuronal Na⁺ channels

Sodium channels are essential for the function of excitable cells. When certain toxins, such as tetrodotoxin, specifically block the Na⁺ channel, then this may result in severe neurotoxicity.

Tetrodotoxin (TTX) is a potent neurotoxin found in the ovary, intestine and liver of the puffer fish. Interestingly, the fish are not able to synthesize TTX by themselves; instead, they accumulate TTX which is produced by marine bacteria. Puffer fish themselves are resistant to the bacterial toxin because they feature a mutation in the biomolecule to which TTX normally binds with high affinity (the Na⁺ channels); TTX is unable to bind to the mutated form of the Na⁺ channel.

Accidental poisoning with TTX is frequent in Japan, where the fish is eaten in Fugu restaurants after careful removal of the toxic organs. About one-third of the poisonings end fatally. Initial symptoms include numbness of the lips and tongue, followed by paresthesia of extremities. The next more serious stage includes muscle fatigue, dizziness, followed by bradycardia, hypotonic blood pressure, and finally respiratory failure and muscle paralysis develop.

Mechanisms of tetrodotoxin toxicity: TTX selectively blocks the voltage-dependent Na⁺ channels of excitable tissues including nerve cells. As a result, no action potential can be built up, while the resting potential of the cell remains unaffected.

TTX is effective in blocking the Na⁺ channel only when it is applied to the external surface of the nerve membrane. This implies that TTX acts from the outside, 'plugging' the Na⁺ channel at its external mouth. Indeed, molecular structure elucidation and models have revealed that TTX, a bulky and hydrophilic compound containing a cationic group and a guanidine moiety, enters the cell in part via the Na⁺ channel, whereby the other part of the molecule blocks its outer mouth, irrespective of whether the channel is open or closed (see Figure 14.1).

Na⁺ channels are large monomeric proteins forming a voltage-gated ion channel. The Na⁺ transporter has been cloned and its three-dimensional structure elucidated. The channel is formed by four homologous repeats that form hairpin-like structures partially traversing the cell membrane, and creating a hydrophilic environment inside the pore. The ion selectivity is given, in part, by the sequence-aligned residues at the inside of the pore.

In neurons, the axonal membrane is highly polarized under resting conditions, featuring a positive charge at the extracellular side and a negative charge

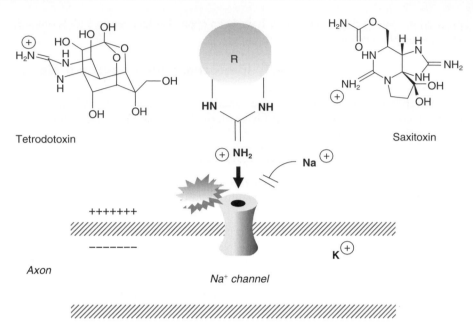

Figure 14.1. Tetrodotoxin plugs and blocks the voltage-dependent Na⁺ channel in neurons.

at the cytoplasmic side of the cell membrane. This inside-out negative membrane potential (−60 to −90 mV) is maintained by the Na⁺, K⁺-pump, an ATP-dependent transporter that pumps in one catalytic step three Na⁺ ions out of the cell and two K⁺ ions into the cell. Upon a stimulus, the membrane rapidly depolarizes; this is achieved by rapid opening of the Na⁺ channels. The rapid Na⁺ influx causes an inside-positive potential (+30 mV). This is followed by a slower efflux of K⁺, and finally the resting potential is restored. This so-called action potential is the key event in the propagation of the signal along the neuronal axon.

A very similar mode of action is the underlying cause of the toxicity of a related biomolecule, saxitoxin ('paralytic shellfish poison'). Saxitoxin is produced by marine dinoflagellates and can accumulate in shellfish. Similarly to TTX, saxitoxin binds to the Na⁺ channel with high affinity and plugs the channel, so that sodium influx and formation of the action potential is prevented.

Other xenobiotics are able to disrupt Na⁺ channel function by a different mechanism. For example, the pyrethroids, a group of insecticides, as well as the organochlorine pesticide DDT, bind to the open Na⁺ channel and prevent the channel from closing again. By it being kept in the open state, a complete repolarization of the neuronal membrane cannot be attained. This results in a prolonging effect on the depolarization phase and repetitive after-firing and hyperexcitation.

14.2. Interactions with the Na⁺, K⁺-pump

Some xenobiotics can exert their toxicity by selectively interfering and blocking the sodium–potassium pump, a ubiquitous and crucial ion transporter. Such compounds include cardiac glycosides and their derivatives.

> **Cardiac glycosides** are naturally occurring compounds derived from *Digitalis* species. These compounds have been therapeutically used to treat cardiac insufficiency (however, due to their narrow therapeutic window and high potential toxicity, alternative treatment is sought). The active compounds are **digitoxin** and **digoxin**, which have an aglycone moiety (digitoxigenin) coupled to a deoxysugar via a glycosidic bond.
>
> The manifestations of digitoxin-induced toxicity include disruption of cardiac function, but also gastrointestinal and neuronal toxicity. In the healthy person, the cardiac symptoms are extreme bradycardia (slowing down of the heart frequency) and atrial fibrillation, while in the cardiac patient the symptoms are arrhythmia, extrasystoles, and ventricular fibrillation, which can be fatal.

Mechanisms of digitoxin-induced cardiac toxicity: Cardiac glycosides specifically inhibit the Na⁺, K⁺-pump. They do so by binding to specific amino acid residues of the protein, immobilizing the critical domains of the transporter, and thus inhibiting cation transport. Because the Na⁺, K⁺-pump is an ATP-dependent transporter that mediates the efflux of 3 Na⁺ ions (in exchange for an influx of 2 K⁺ ions) and builds up an outside–inside Na⁺ gradient, inhibition of this transporter results in a collapse of the Na⁺ gradient. Normally, high extracellular Na⁺ concentrations are required to drive sodium-dependent secondary transporters. In cardiomyocytes, one such transporter is the Na⁺, Ca²⁺ exchanger (i.e. Na⁺ influx is the driving force for Ca²⁺ efflux from the cell). Hence, cardiac glycosides cause an increase of the intracellular Ca²⁺ levels. Influx of calcium ions into these excitable cells, however, is the signal for the activation of myosin/actin. Hence, inhibition of Na⁺, K⁺-ATPase will ultimately result in an overstimulation of the cell, causing cardiac arrhythmia and fibrillation (see Figure 14.2).

> The **Na⁺, K⁺-ATPase** translocates sodium and potassium ions across the cell membrane against concentration gradients utilizing ATP as the driving force. It is an integral membrane protein found in the cells of all higher eukaryotes. The protein is composed of α- and β-subunits and forms several transmembrane helices that form 'hairpin' loops. Upon binding of Na⁺ and K⁺, the protein undergoes a conformational change.
>
> The three-dimensional organization and the structural basis of the mechanism of ATPase inhibition by cardiac glycosides have long remained unknown. However, recent random mutation analyses have identified a number of specific amino acid residues in the extracellular and transmembrane domains that are determinants of the cardiac glycoside sensitivity.

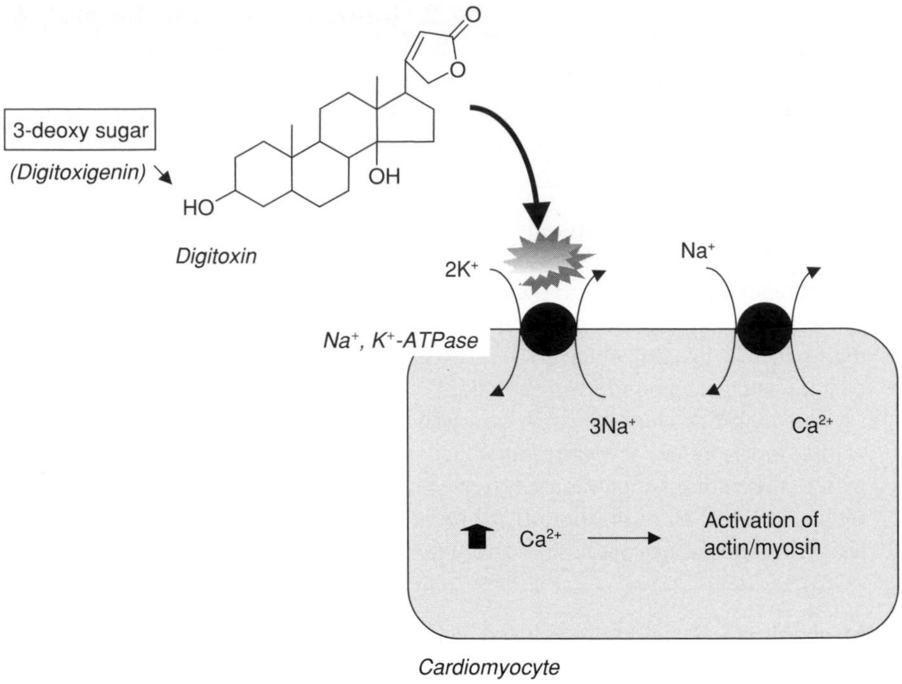

Figure 14.2. Inhibition of Na⁺, K⁺ pump by cardiac glycosides indirectly causes accumulation of intracellular Ca²⁺ in cardiac cells.

Learning points

- Certain xenobiotics can bind with high selectivity and affinity to ion channels. For example, tetrodotoxin or saxitoxin, both of which are bulky hydrophilic molecules with a spacious cationic guanidine moiety, specifically bind to and inhibit the Na⁺ channel on excitable cells. These compounds plug the ion channel, thus inhibiting rapid Na⁺ influx and preventing the initiation of an action potential.
- Digitoxin and other cardiac glycosides specifically bind to critical domains of the Na⁺, K⁺-ATPase and thus inhibit conformational changes that are associated with cation transport. This results in a collapse of the Na⁺ gradient and inhibition of other sodium-driven ion transporters. Inhibition of the Na⁺, Ca²⁺ exchanger in cardiomyocytes causes intracellular Ca²⁺ accumulation and overstimulation by actin/myosin activation.

Further reading

TTX toxicity
Narahashi, T. (2000) Neuroreceptors and ion channels as the basis for drug action: Past, present, and future, *J. Pharmacol. Exp. Ther.* 294: 1–26.

Na⁺ channels

Sato, C., Ueno, Y., Asai, K., Takahashi, K., Sato, M., Engel, A. and Fujiyoshi, Y. (2001) The voltage-sensitive sodium channel is a bell-shaped molecule with several cavities, *Nature* 409: 1047–1051.

Yamagishi, T., Li, R.A., Hsu, K., Marban, E. and Tomaselli, G.F. (2001) Molecular architecture of the voltage-dependent Na channel: Functional evidence for α helices in the pore, *J. Gen. Physiol.* 118: 171–181.

Na⁺, K⁺-ATPase

Palasis, M., Kuntzweiler, T.A., Arguello, J.M. and Lingrel, J.B. (1996) Ouabain interactions with the H5–H6 hairpin of the Na, K-ATPase reveal a possible inhibition mechanism via the cation binding domain, *J. Biol. Chem.* 271: 14176–14182.

Chapter 15

Disruption of cellular energy production by xenobiotics

Contents

Mitochondria are key to the maintenance of many cellular functions and are the powerplants of cellular energy production. In addition, mitochondria mediate physiological processes and are involved in signal transduction and regulation of cell proliferation, differentiation, apoptosis (see section 7.2), and other processes. Because of their pivotal function, however, mitochondria are vulnerable and are crucial targets of many adverse activities of xenobiotics. Indeed, the role of mitochondrial toxicity has been recognized for an increasing number of xenobiotics.

A variety of molecular mechanisms are involved in the disruption of mitochondrial function, the most important of which are highlighted in the following sections.

15.1. Mitochondrial targets and xenobiotic-induced bioenergy crisis

The production of ATP plays an important role for the biosynthesis of endogenous compounds, transport processes, generation of kinetic energy, and other functions,

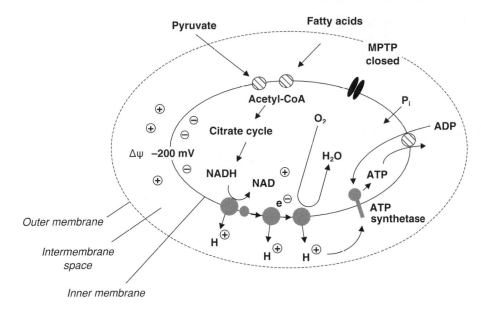

Figure 15.1. Pivotal steps in normal mitochondrial energy production
(see text for explanation).

and the maintenance of adequate ATP levels is crucial for most cells. Because
energy production, i.e. the ATP synthetase-mediated synthesis of ATP from ADP
and inorganic phosphate (P_i), is the ultimate step in a complex reaction network,
any process that disturbs or blocks this reaction network will ultimately result in
an inhibition of ATP synthesis, which is the common endpoint of toxicity.

Normal mitochondrial function: Let us recall that a number of interrelated
mechanisms have to remain operative in mitochondria to guarantee proper function
(see Figure 15.1).

1 Uptake of the substrates, pyruvate (from glucose degradation) and fatty acids,
   that will ultimately be oxidized. These substrates cannot simply diffuse into the
   mitochondrial matrix where they will be oxidized, but have to be transported
   across the mitochondrial membranes. The outer mitochondrial membrane is
   quite permeable for compounds smaller than approximately 14 kD and does not
   represent a barrier for most xenobiotics. The inner mitochondrial membrane, in
   contrast, is not freely permeable to ions and metabolites. Instead, specific proteins have to transport the substrates into the matrix. For example, long-chain
   fatty acids are first 'activated' by binding to CoA, and these activated fatty acids
   are coupled to a shuttle compound, carnitine. The resulting acylcarnitine is then
   transported across the inner membrane, and the fatty acid moiety is released into
   the mitochondrial matrix.
2 In the matrix, both pyruvate and fatty acids are converted or broken down to
   acetyl-CoA, the major substrate that enters and drives the citrate cycle. Fatty acids
   are cleaved to C2-moieties by the process of β-oxidation. The major function of
   the citrate cycle is to produce reducing equivalents, i.e. reduced NADH.

3 Electrons produced from NADH oxidation are transported via a downhill multi-step reaction cascade (the electron transport chain) to finally reduce molecular oxygen to water. Naturally, molecular oxygen is another driving force for the electron transport chain and must be available. The electron transport chain is composed of four protein complexes, assembled from a number of peptide subunits (but only three of them span the entire inner membrane). For example, the first complex (complex I) oxidizes NADH and in turn reduces the mobile electron carrier, ubiquinone (which is embedded in the lipid membrane).

4 The energy released from NADH oxidation (and further downhill from the oxidation of other intermediates) is used to pump protons outwards and expel them across the inner mitochondrial membrane into the intermembraneous space. Proton pump activity is present at three distinct sites in the electron transport chain. Due to this process, an inside-out negative membrane potential (Δ_Ψ) is generated, making the intermembrane space an acidic compartment.

5 The energy of this proton gradient is used to drive the ATP synthetase; during the influx of protons from the intermembrane space into the matrix, a portion of the ATP synthetase complex rotates, and ATP is assembled from ADP and P_i.

Interference with mitochondrial function by xenobiotics: Chemicals can interfere at any of these steps that participate in mitochondrial energy production. For example, one of the most important targets is the inner mitochondrial membrane. If the permeability of the inner membrane is increased by a toxic action of a xenobiotic, then the Δ_Ψ will collapse, because there will be a rapid influx of protons across the membrane. Alternatively, if the electron transport chain is directly inhibited, the energy supply for driving the proton pumps is impaired. Because ultimately the proton gradient is the driving force for ATP synthetase activity, net ATP production will be inhibited.

Three important features of the inner mitochondrial membrane are toxicologically relevant. First, its lipid composition; it is a peculiarity of the inner membrane that it does not contain cholesterol but is rich in cardiolipin. A number of xenobiotics have a high affinity for cardiolipin and accumulate therefore at the inner mitochondrial membrane. Second, the high inside negative transmembrane potential; because of this electochemical gradient, a number of small cationic xenobiotics may accumulate and thus reach high intramitochondrial concentrations. Finally, the mitochondrial permeability transition pore (MPTP) (see section 7.2). This megachannel that spans across the inner and outer membrane and which is composed of a number of protein complexes is normally closed, thus making the membrane impermeable for large compounds and allowing the proton gradient to be maintained. However, xenobiotics can cause the MPTP to open, which will not only result in a collapse of the Δ_Ψ but also in the release of signaling molecules from mitochondria into the cytosol, e.g., cytochrome *c*. These mediators have been implicated in triggering apoptosis (see section 7.2).

Other possible sites of xenobiotic attack involve blocking of the citrate cycle (no NADH will be produced), inhibition of substrate uptake (no fuel available), inhibition of fatty acyl β-oxidation (no acetyl-CoA will be produced and fatty

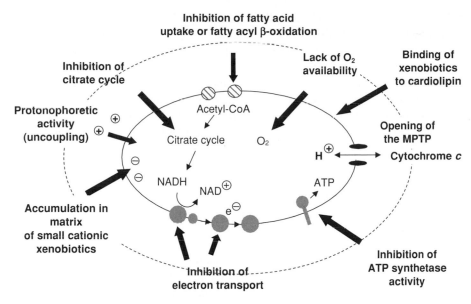

Figure 15.2. Possible sites of xenobiotic interference with mitochondrial function, resulting in mitochondrial toxicity.

acids will accumulate), blocking of the electron transport chain, or finally specific inhibition of the ATP synthetase activity, all of which will ultimately result in loss of energy production (see Figure 15.2).

Some organs are particularly sensitive towards xenobiotic-induced energy depletion. For example, tissues that are known to be highly oxygen-dependent are the cardiac muscle and skeletal and smooth muscle tissue, as well as the CNS and the peripheral nervous system. These organs will be among the first to be affected when xenobiotics cause a general depletion of ATP. Other tissues that are highly susceptible to mitochondrial injury are the kidney and the β-cells of the pancreas. In other cases, toxicokinetic or toxicodynamic factors may determine a more localized tissue- or organ-selective mitochondrial damage.

Many cells can react to sustained mitochondrial functional impairment by compensatory stimulation of *de novo* synthesis of mitochondria, but this effect is limited.

A well-known phenomenon is uncoupling of the oxidative phosphorylation, induced by a variety of xenobiotics. This implies that the electron transport and, hence, the pumping of protons into the intermembrane space are dissociated (uncoupled) from their major function, i.e. driving ATP synthetase. This is brought about by a futile cycling of protons back to the matrix, due to the protonophoretic activity of certain xenobiotics.

15.2. Protonophoretic and uncoupling activity of xenobiotics

Many small xenobiotics which are lipophilic and weakly acidic can act as protonophores. One example is pentachlorophenol.

Pentachlorophenol (PCP) is a widely used fungicide and wood impregnating agent. Its health hazard in the workplace has been known for a long time. Exposure to high concentrations has led to increase in body temperature, perspiration, thirst, and in extreme cases muscle fatigue, respiration problems, and dizziness. These symptoms are compatible with a lack of energy supply.

A different problem is a possible connection between low PCP exposure, as may occur inside houses, and possible (non-specific) health problems. Traces of PCP have been found in the urine, as PCP occurs ubiquitously, but there is no scientifically-based evidence for a health hazard after this low exposure to PCP. One possible explanation for the observed potential toxicity is contamination of PCP with other chlorinated agents, including polychlorinated dibenzodioxins.

Molecular mechanisms of pentachlorophenol toxicity: PCP is a weak acid (pK$_a$ ~5) and is therefore dissociated at physiological pH. It can easily penetrate the permeable outer mitochondrial membrane and reach the intermembrane space, where it is protonated, due to the high proton density. The uncharged lipophilic molecule can cross the inner mitochondrial membrane where it is readily dissociated, due to the inside negative potential and the inside–out pH difference of approximately 0.6 pH units. The negatively charged PCP anion is then expelled back to the intermembrane space, and the cycle is repeated. Importantly, this mechanism shuttles back the protons into the matrix and thus results in a futile cycling, preventing the protons from accumulating in the intermembrane space and from driving the ATP synthetase. Thus, PCP is a 'protonophore' (it transports protons). The result is uncoupling of the oxidative phosphorylation (see Figure 15.3).

The consequences of uncoupling (besides insufficient ATP production) are increased oxygen consumption and increased loss of energy in the form of heat. In other words, under these conditions the mitochondrion has turned from a cellular powerplant into a heat-producing organelle.

Many drugs and other xenobiotics cause uncoupling of oxidative phosphorylation *in vitro*. However, it is only for a few of them that the concentrations attained *in vivo* are high enough to become relevant. This mechanism of burning fat without producing energy has previously been thought to be useful for the development of drugs against obesity. However, the further development of such drugs, including the powerful uncoupler dinitrophenol and other lipophilic phenols, had to be discontinued from further development due to severe adverse effects and deaths.

Interestingly, uncoupling of oxidative phosphorylation is physiologically used by some hibernating animals and newborn animals (and humans) to produce heat in the absence of ATP production. This effect is brought about by several specific mitochondrial proteins, called uncoupling proteins (UCP), present in brown adipose tissue.

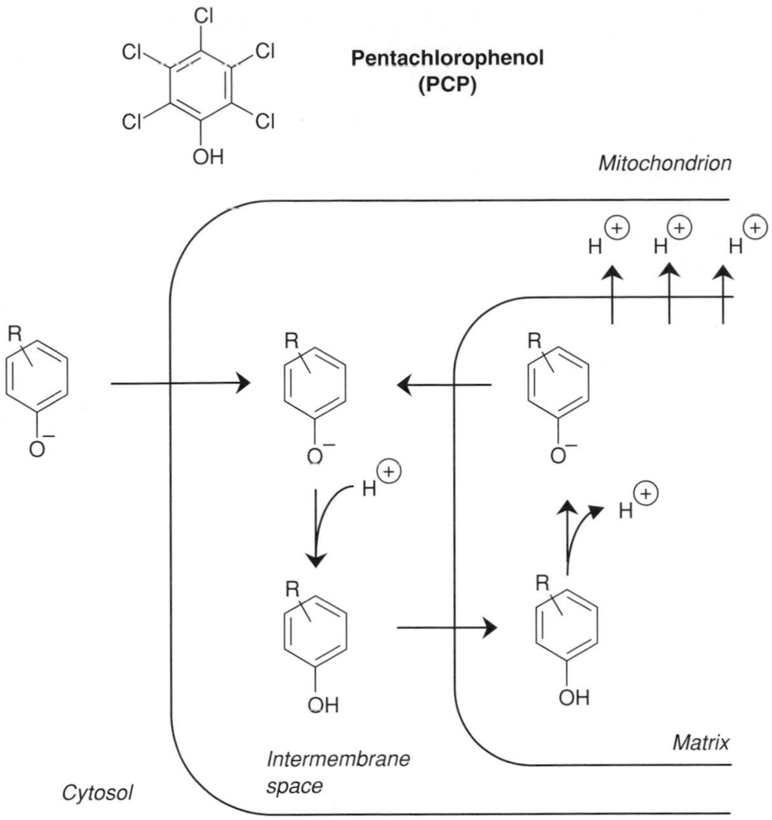

Figure 15.3. Pentachlorophenol is an uncoupler because it transports protons back into the matrix, thus dissipating the mitochondrial membrane potential.

15.3. Inhibition of NADH production

NADH is the major reducing equivalent in the mitochondrion and is used to provide electrons for maintaining the proton pumps, reducing oxygen to water, and finally to synthesize ATP from ADP and P_i. Hence, inhibition of the production of NADH by xenobiotics must invariably lead to impaired energy production and toxicity.

This disruption can occur at several distinct sites including the β-oxidation pathway, a major energy (NADH)-generating process, and the citrate cycle.

15.3.1. Inhibition of mitochondrial fatty acyl β-oxidation

Fatty acids are progressively shortened into acetyl-CoA products by a process called β-oxidation. Either these acetyl-CoA units are then condensed to ketone bodies and exported or they enter the citrate cycle for further oxidation and NADH production.

Because the enzymes involved in the β-oxidation process are located in the mitochondrial matrix, fatty acids must first cross the inner (impermeable) mitochondrial membrane. While short-chain and medium-chain fatty acids can easily cross the membrane, long-chain fatty acids (i.e. C_{14}–C_{18}) require a specific transport system. In a first step, they are activated by coenzyme A to the CoA thioester, which allows for a subsequent coupling to carnitine, a shuttle molecule that transports the long-chain fatty acids across the membrane and reactivates them by binding again to CoA. In the matrix, the fatty acyl-CoA is then enzymatically shortened by two carbons via a multistep process by which acetyl-CoA, the substrate for the citrate cycle, is generated. During this oxidative process, NADH is generated.

Xenobiotics can interfere with any of these enzymatic steps of the β-oxidation process. For example, if xenobiotics interfere with the availability of the cofactor, coenzyme A, then fatty acyl activation and transmembrane transport are severely impaired. This can happen if a carboxylic acid-containing xenobiotic is coupled to CoA, a process by which the available co-factor is sequestered by the formation of acyl derivatives. An example is the drug valproic acid.

Valproic acid (VPA) is a widely-used anti-epileptic drug. It is a relatively safe drug but nevertheless has been associated with adverse reactions including hepatotoxicity. Two clinical forms of liver injury have been described; a mild form, characterized by transient increases in serum aminotransferase activities, and a more severe form, typically associated with jaundice and necrosis. This latter adverse drug reaction is a rare event (incidence in children approx. 1/5,000, in adults 1/20,000–40,000). Interestingly, VPA-induced liver injury also presents as microvesicular steatosis. Ultrastructural analysis reveals the presence of swollen mitochondria with degenerated structures.

Mechanisms of valproate toxicity: Valproic acid is a branched-chain fatty acid. Like natural fatty acids, VPA forms valproyl-CoA-thioesters, carnitine esters, and subsequently undergoes mitochondrial β-oxidation. Besides mitochondrial metabolism, VPA is also metabolized by CYP to Δ^4-VPA (4-ene VPA). Once formed, this oxidative metabolite can undergo mitochondrial β-oxidation, and the first step (dehydrogenation) of this pathway results in the formation of $\Delta^{2,4}$-VPA (2,4-diene VPA) (see Figure 15.4).

At least two mechanisms have been implicated in VPA mitochondrial toxicity. First, because VPA and VPA metabolites decrease the cellular levels of free CoA (and of carnitine), it is generally believed that this sequestration is the major cause of the inhibition of mitochondrial β-oxidation and its consequences. As it is the medium-chain acyl CoA synthetase (which is located in the matrix of mitochondria) that most probably couples VPA to CoA, it is the intramitochondrial pool of CoA that is depleted. This explains why the β-oxidation of short- and medium- as well as long-chain fatty acids is inhibited.

Second, another possible mechanism of injury is a direct inhibition of the enzymes involved in the β-oxidation process. This is brought about by the metabolite of VPA, Δ^4-VPA, which is activated by CoA inside the mitochondria and which itself undergoes the first step of β-oxidation (dehydrogenation) to the $\Delta^{2,4}$-VPA. This would provide a likely explanation of why CYP inducers potentiate the liver toxicity of VPA.

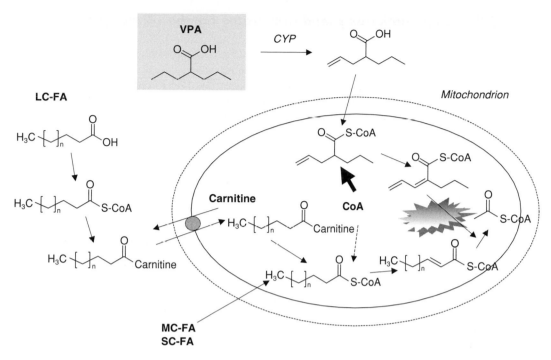

Figure 15.4. Mitochondrial fatty acid β-oxidation and mechanisms of valproic acid (VPA)-induced inhibition of β-oxidation. VPA sequesters intramitochondrial CoA (thick arrow) and therefore prevents fatty acid activation. In addition, its oxidative metabolite, Δ^4-VPA, undergoes the first step of β-oxidation to $\Delta^{2,4}$-VPA. The latter is an electrophilic metabolite that directly reacts with and inhibits enzymes involved in β-oxidation. LC-FA, long-chain fatty acid; MC-FA, medium-chain fatty acid; SC-FA, short-chain fatty acid.

Because mitochondrial β-oxidation of fatty acids is the primary source of energy in some organs (liver, heart) in the fasting state, sustained inhibition of β-oxidation can lead to a severe energy crisis. Indeed, in patients with preexisting mitochondrial diseases (e.g. decreased activities of complex I and IV), the risk for VPA-induced fulminant liver failure is increased.

Another side-effect of the inhibition of β-oxidation is accumulation of fatty acids. This can take extreme forms and lead to the development of microvesicular steatosis.

Microvesicular steatosis is phenotypically characterized by the accumulation of many small to mid-size lipid droplets in hepatocytes, distending the cells. This fatty change is distinct from the macrovesicular type of steatosis (large fat droplets, often associated with a disturbance in the secretion of lipids as very-low-density lipoproteins). Microvesicular steatosis is typical for drugs inhibiting β-oxidation including valproate. The consequences can be severe; for example, this condition, irrespective of the etiology, often leads to fulminant liver failure. The accumulation of these lipids also invariably causes increased rates of lipid peroxidation (see section 5.2.3) and oxidative stress.

15.3.2. Xenobiotics as pseudosubstrates for the citrate cycle

Xenobiotics which interrupt the citrate cycle cause a block in the production of NADH. NADH is the major reducing equivalent, providing electrons that drive the electron transport chain and are ultimately used to reduce molecular oxygen to water. Such an interrruption of the cycle can occur when a xenobiotic mimics a natural substrate that is part of the citrate cycle. One example is fluoroacetate, which mimics acetate but cannot be fully metabolized like acetate.

Fluoroacetate is a natural substance occurring in certain plants in Southern Africa (*Dichapetalum*), South America (*Palicourea*), and Australia (*Gastrolobium*, *Acacia*), and the compound is toxic to animals that consume these plants. Due to its acute toxicity, fluoroacetate was developed as a rodenticide ('compound 1080') during the Second World War. Toxic effects in humans have occurred; the symptoms of intoxication with fluoroacetate are convulsions (reflecting CNS toxicity), cardiac arrhythmias and fibrillation. These symptoms are ultimately due to a lack of ATP supply, and the organ selectivity of the effects mirrors the high sensitivity of the brain and heart to be among the first organs that succumb to energy deprivation.

It was found that citrate accumulates in tissues of fluoroacetate-exposed organisms. Because citrate is one of the intermediates in the citrate cycle, it was concluded and later confirmed that the subsequent reaction in the cycle, i.e. isomerization of citrate to isocitrate, was inhibited by fluoroacetate.

Mechanisms of fluoroacetate toxicity: Fluoroacetate is an analog of acetate. Normally, acetate is coupled to CoA (and thereby activated) and subsequently combined with oxaloacetate (C4 body) to form citrate (C6). In a next step, citrate undergoes isomerization to isocitrate, which is further oxidized to α-ketoglutarate, thereby reducing NAD^+ and forming NADH and H^+.

The crucial step during the isomerization of citrate to isocitrate is catalyzed by aconitase, an enzyme containing a [4Fe–4S] cluster. In a first step, the negatively charged oxygen atoms of citrate bind to a specific iron of the cluster of aconitase.

Fluoroacetate mimics the first few steps of acetate metabolism, i.e. it couples to CoA to form fluoroacetyl-CoA. Condensation with oxaloacetate yields fluorocitrate. However, the following isomerization step is not possible, because fluorocitrate inhibits aconitase. The strongly electronegative fluorine atom interacts with the iron center of aconitase, making an isomerization impossible. The entire citrate cycle comes to a stop, and NADH production is inhibited. This process is called a 'lethal synthesis', because the organism synthesizes substrate analogs which in a later step block the metabolism and irreversibly damage the organism (see Figure 15.5).

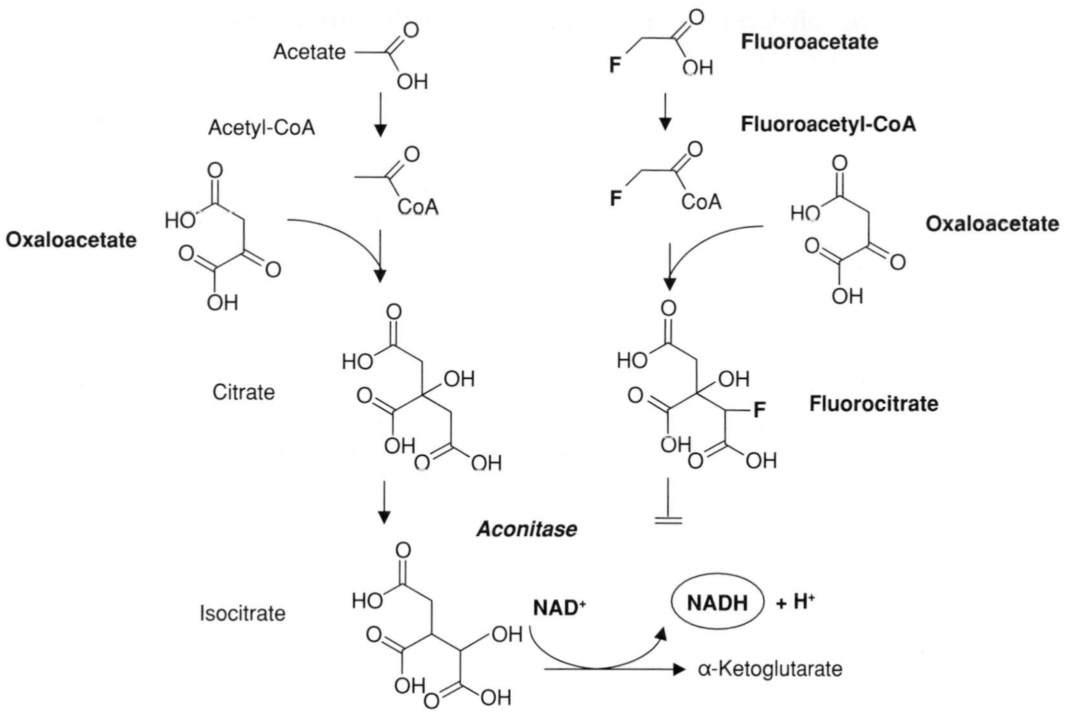

Figure 15.5. Fluoroacetate is an analog of acetate and is gated into the citrate cycle and processed to fluorocitrate. Fluorocitrate, however, inhibits the enzyme aconitase and, hence, blocks the entire citrate cycle, resulting in a an inhibition of NADH production.

15.4. Inhibition of the electron transport chain and increased generation of ROS

Xenobiotics can inhibit the electron flow at several points of the electron transfer cascade. Wherever it may occur, the result will be a decreased proton pump function and, ultimately, inhibition of ATP synthetase.

There are two types of electron transport chain inhibitors. The first type of compounds block the electron transport by binding to one of the components of the electron transport chain. Examples include rotenone (a naturally occurring compound and widely used experimental tool) and cyanide (see below). The second type are compounds that actually stimulate electron flow through the initial parts of the transport chain, but which at one site or another divert the electron flow from their normal path by accepting the electrons themselves. Examples are redox cycling agents such as doxorubicin.

One of the most frequent sites of interference is complex I (NADH:ubiquinone oxidoreductase, an enzyme complex in the inner mitochondrial membrane). This can be brought about by a xenobiotic which diverts electrons from their normal flow and which acts as an electron acceptor. Thus, in addition to causing decreased energy production, such partially reduced xenobiotics can pose a 'reductive stress', which can entail a host of secondary reactions. A typical example is doxorubicin.

Doxorubicin (Adriamycin®) is an anti-neoplastic agent belonging to the anthracycline class and used for the treatment of various solid cancers and lymphomas. Its use has, however, been limited because of the risk of cumulative and dose-dependent irreversible cardiomyopathy that leads to congestive heart failure. During the first years on the market, this organ-selective toxicity became evident in a relatively large number of patients, especially in children, where the incidence of arrhythmias was relatively high and degeneration of the cardiac muscle tissue was often seen. Despite this increased risk, doxorubicin has remained in use due to its high antitumor efficacy. However, newer anthracycline derivatives have meanwhile been developed, clearly featuring a substantially reduced cardiotoxic potential.

Mechanisms of doxorubicin toxicity to mitochondria: One of the mechanisms that might explain the mitochondria-selective toxicity is that doxorubicin has a high affinity for cardiolipin at the inner mitochondrial membrane and therefore accumulates at that subcellular location.

A look at the chemical structure of doxorubicin (a tetracyclic aglycone to which an amino sugar is attached via a glycosidic bond) reveals that it possesses a quinone moiety. Doxorubicin is an excellent electron acceptor and diverts electrons exclusively from complex I of the respiratory chain, thereby reducing the quinone to its semiquinone radical. This latter is unstable and rapidly autoxidizes to the parent quinone. Due to its high redox potential (approximately −320 mV), it reduces molecular oxygen to the superoxide anion radical and thus undergoes redox cycling (see section 5.1.1). Possible consequences, which can all be explained by this redox cycling activity and production of oxidative stress, include oxidation of mitochondrial glutathione, induction of the MPTP, and cardioselective oxidation of mitochondrial DNA.

While there is sufficient evidence to support the concept that doxorubicin toxicity is based on the production of ROS and inhibition of ATP production, the question arises as to why doxorubicin selectively damages the myocardium and exerts a cardiospecific toxicity. It produces ROS in many other cell types, too!

Several hypotheses, which are not mutually exclusive, have been established and all contribute to the tissue selectivity of toxicity. First, the heart simply needs a high and continuous supply of ATP for its uninterrupted function and is thus extremely vulnerable. Second, the heart has a very low antioxidant capacity and is prone to succumb to the consequences of oxidative stress. For example, GS-peroxidase and catalase activity in heart muscle are very low. Third, doxorubicin can alter cardiac-specific transcription. Indeed, oxidative stress alters the structure and function of lipid components that act as second messengers. For example, doxorubicin can indirectly alter the protein kinase C-mediated regulation of intracellular Ca^{2+} and down-regulate the expression of several nuclear genes encoding enzymes that play a central role in normal energy production. These include the heart- and muscle-specific isoform of ADP/ATP translocase, and also of components of the electron transport chain. The ADP/ATP translocase transports newly synthesized ATP from the inner side of mitochondria into the cytosol, and ADP from the cytosol into mitochondria. This protein is abundant in the inner mitochondrial membrane, and also constitutes part of the MPTP.

Another question is why the effect of doxorubicin is persistent for many weeks after cessation of treatment, and why oxidative stress continues long after discontinuation of the drug. An attractive hypothesis and key mechanism explaining these observations is the fact that doxorubicin directly oxidizes and damages mitochondrial DNA. This effect of doxorubicin could explain why the toxic effects on the heart are irreversible. According to this concept, the accumulation of oxidized DNA bases could be causally linked with the irreversible cardiomyopathy in patients, since expression of the mitochondrial genome is crucial to the integrity of the respiratory chain. It is therefore possible that newly synthesized dysfunctional mitochondria may continue to produce high levels of ROS, even after cessation of doxorubicin administration, and thus would provide a continuous source of oxidative damage to the mitochondrial DNA.

Mitochondrial DNA (mtDNA) is highly susceptible to oxidation by ROS. The reasons are manifold.

1 mtDNA in the matrix is in close proximity to the site where relatively large amounts of ROS are generated constantly, even under basal conditions of respiration and in the absence of xenobiotics.
2 Unlike nuclear DNA, mtDNA does not encode RNA and proteins with nonsense sequences, except for a small sequence. Therefore, any mtDNA oxidation is likely to result in a biologically significant effect.
3 mtDNA does not possess any protective histones, and the DNA repair mechanisms for mtDNA are much less effective than those for the nuclear DNA. Therefore, oxidative injury in the mitochondria leads to accumulation of oxidative base damage. In fact, mtDNA exhibits a more than ten-fold higher basal incidence of oxidized deoxyguanosine than nuclear DNA.

Thus, the initial redox cycling event of doxorubicin, fueled by NADH and driven by diverting electrons from complex I, and the subsequent production of ROS are coupled to a redox-sensitive regulation of heart-specific genes and oxidative mtDNA damage that ultimately lead to a depletion of ATP and to the precipitation of irreversible cardiomyopathy (see Figure 15.6).

Xenobiotics can also bind to other sites of the electron transport chain and block electron flow. For example, cyanide and azide are well-known compounds that bind to the terminal protein complex, the cytochrome c oxidase (complex IV).

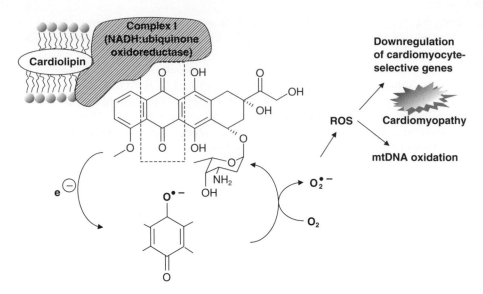

Figure 15.6. Redox cycling of the quinone–semiquonone moiety of doxorubicin leads to the generation of oxidative stress which affects the mitochondrial DNA as well as altering cardiomyocyte-specific gene expression.

Cyanide is a well-known and potent toxin. It is used as KCN or NaCN in the metal industry. Cyanide also occurs naturally as glycosides (amygdalin) in bitter almonds, where the cyanide content can be up to 0.1 percent. In the gut, intestinal bacteria can enzymatically cleave the glycoside and release glucose, benzaldehyde, and cyanide. HCN is volatile and has been used as a disinfectant, but importantly, it is also generated during combustion of polyurethane polymers, as used for furniture. Cyanide toxicity is a great problem in fires in houses or airplanes, where it is produced rapidly and in great amounts.

At physiological pH, HCN is not dissociated and rapidly diffuses across cell membranes. The symptoms of cyanide poisoning are hyperpnea and red coloration of the skin (oxygen-saturated blood). Toxicity is manifested by general malaise, vomiting, and ultimately respiratory block. The neurons of the respiratory center are particularly sensitive to energy deprivation.

Mechanisms of cyanide toxicity: Cyanide avidly binds to Fe^{3+} (but not Fe^{2+}), which is abundant in heme-containing proteins that undergo redox cycling. Because the cytochrome a_3 moiety of the complex IV, which is the terminal protein complex of the electron transport chain, is a redox-active heme protein, cyanide binds to this site. However, binding is not specific nor selective, and cyanide also binds to other heme-containing enzymes (CYPs, peroxidases, cytochrome c, oxidized hemoglobin or myoglobin). In view of the rapid onset of the potent toxic effects on mitochondria, an inhibition of the other enzymes seems, however, less relevant.

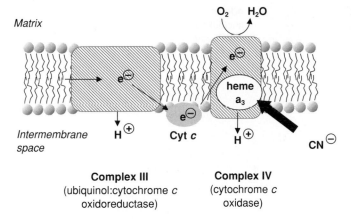

Figure 15.7. Cyanide binds to the heme a_3 subunit and inhibits the terminal cytochrome c oxidase (complex IV) of the electron transport chain.

Block of complex IV by cyanide causes a rapid and severe depletion of cellular ATP content that results in cell death due to energy impairment (see Figure 15.7).

Understanding the molecular mechanisms of cyanide toxicity has greatly helped in developing an antidote against acute cyanide intoxication. Because binding of cyanide to ferric iron-containing heme proteins is not specific for cytochrome c oxidase, an efficient therapy could aim at offering to the body abundant amounts of other ferric iron-containing heme that would absorb the cyanide from the vital mitochondrial heme proteins. A large potential pool of heme, of course, is contained in the circulating hemoglobin, but $Hb–Fe^{2+}$ is not redox-active. $Hb–Fe^{2+}$ can, however, be rapidly converted to $Hb–Fe^{3+}$ by methemoglobin-forming xenobiotics (e.g. nitrite or dimethylaminophenol) (see section 5.2.2). In fact, cyanide has an even greater affinity for $Hb–Fe^{3+}$ than for complex IV! For example, 30 percent met-Hb can bind approximately five lethal doses of cyanide. The resulting CN–methemoglobin complex is converted by thiosulfate ($Na_2S_2O_3$) to SCN, which is less toxic and is subsequently excreted in the urine.

15.5. Opening of the mitochondrial membrane permeability transition pore (MPTP)

Recently, the phenomenon of 'membrane permeability transition' has been increasingly recognized as an important mechanism of cell death (see section 7.2), and it is more than just a biochemical curiosity (as it was considered a number of years ago). Indeed, many xenobiotics are able to cause an opening of a physiological pore in the mitochondrial membrane and thus rapidly increase the permeability for solutes of the otherwise largely impermeable inner mitochondrial membrane. This has dramatic consequences.

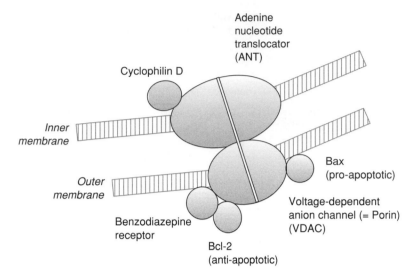

Figure 15.8. Model of the membrane permeability transition pore (MPTP) and its components.

The membrane permeability transition pore (MPTP) is a membrane-bound protein complex in mitochondria. It is composed of a number of proteins including the voltage-dependent anion channel (VDAC), located in the outer membrane; the ADP/ATP exchanger, located in the inner membrane; and cyclophilin-D, located in the matrix, at the contact sites between the mitochondrial inner and outer membranes. This complex is associated with a number of other proteins including Bax and Bcl-2 which play a role in apoptosis (see section 7.2). This complex forms a pore which under normal conditions is closed (see Figure 15.8).

The pore's physiological function has been suggested to regulate mitochondrial Ca^{2+} by periodically and transiently ridding mitochondria of excess metabolites and ions including Ca^{2+}. Therefore, it seems logical that addition of calcium ionophores to cultured cells (which results in a rapid rise in mitochondrial Ca^{2+} and overloading) abruptly leads to an opening of the MPTP.

Upon opening of the pore, a channel of approximately 2.0–2.6 nm is generated, allowing molecules with an M_r of ~1500 to pass across the channel. This is probably brought about by a cooperative behaviour of pairs of the involved proteins. The accessory protein, Bax, binds to the pore proteins and further increases the permeability. Interestingly, cyclosporin A (which binds to cyclophilin) can very efficiently block this pore, an effect which is often used experimentally to prove that a certain toxicity is mediated via opening of the MPTP.

The consequences of this rapid opening of the pore are obvious and dramatic. The inner membrane is depolarized and the mitochondrial membrane potential (proton gradient) collapses because protons rapidly stream back into the matrix. Hence, the oxidative phosphorylation is uncoupled. In addition, intramitochondrial solutes are released. Finally, because the osmolarity of the matrix is higher than that of the cytosol, the mitochondria swell due to rapid water influx (from this observation, i.e. that mitochondria swell due to a sudden altered state of increased permeability, the term 'permeability transition' was derived). The inner membrane can compensate the increase in volume because of the folded cristae, but the outer membrane ruptures. Altogether, an energy crisis is initiated and, if the effect is rapidly propagated, the cell eventually dies of apoptosis or necrosis.

As oxidative stress is a major inducer of MPTP opening, many chemicals that are prooxidants can also induce the MPT. This can occur directly (by producing ROS) or indirectly (by increasing concentrations of $NAD(P)^+$, GSSG, or other disulfides). One important group of compounds that are known to produce oxidative stress and, hence, induce MPTP opening are the toxic hydrophobic bile acids which accumulate in cholestasis.

Toxic hydrophobic bile acids are primary or secondary (i.e. produced from metabolism by the intestinal flora) bile acids that can accumulate in the liver under conditions of cholestasis. This occurs also by xenobiotics which have the potential to induce cholestasis (see section 3.3.1). For example, the glycine conjugate of chenodeoxycholic acid (one of the most abundant primary bile acids in humans) becomes toxic when it accumulates and reaches high cellular concentrations. In fact, under conditions of cholestasis, chenodeoxycholic acid concentrations can be increased up to 20-fold in the liver.

Hydrophobic bile acids can readily induce cell death in hepatocytes. For example, low micromolar concentrations (as typically present in cholestasis) of toxic bile acids induce apoptosis in cultured hepatocytes. These hydrophobic bile acids exhibit detergent-like properties, but the concentrations used to induce cell death are far lower than those which would induce membrane disruption by detergent activity. Therefore, other mechanisms are likely to be involved.

Glycochenodeoxycholate-induced cell death is accompanied by activation of mitogen-activated protein (MAP) kinases, typical for compounds producing oxidative stress. Indeed, hydrophobic bile acids induce oxidative stress in hepatocytes, probably by interfering with the electron transport chain and thereby diverting electrons to molecular oxygen, resulting in the generation of ROS. Furthermore, the feeding of hydrophobic bile acids recruits the pro-apoptotic protein Bax, which associates with mitochondria and assists in inducing the MPTP opening (see Figure 15.9).

Oral administration of another bile acid, ursodeoxycholic acid (UDCA) can protect against cholestasis-induced liver damage (UDCA is a secondary bile acid and structural isomer of chenodeoxycholic acid, which is generated by intestinal bacteria). The cytoprotective mechanisms are severalfold and not yet fully understood, but evidence indicates that UDCA can inhibit the opening of the MPTP. For example, it prevents the recruiting of Bax from the cytosol and inhibits Bax from being associated with the megapore. In fact, UDCA has been therapeutically used with success.

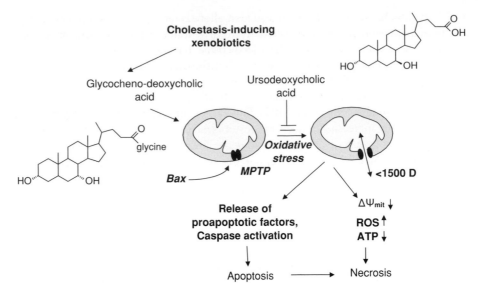

Figure 15.9. Toxic hydrophobic bile acids can induce opening of the MPTP through oxidative stress, leading to both apoptosis and necrosis. The hydrophilic bile acid, ursodeoxycholate, is protective because it inhibits the opening of the pore and blocks cell death.

Learning points

- Mitochondrial toxicity induced by xenobiotics is based on a variety of mechanisms all of which result in a decrease in cellular ATP production and an ensuing energy crisis. Sites of interference with normal mitochondrial function include substrate and oxygen availability, citrate cycle and NADH production, electron transport and proton pump function, and ATP synthetase-driven ATP production.
- Uncoupling of the oxidative phosphorylation can be induced by protonophores which shuttle the protons from the intermembrane space back into the matrix in a futile manner.
- Inhibition of mitochondrial fatty acid β-oxidation can be caused by sequestration of carnitine or CoA or by direct inhibition of the enzymes involved. The resulting accumulation of fatty acids can culminate in the development of microvesicular steatosis, a dangerous condition.
- Inhibition of the electron transport chain at complex I can divert electrons and result in the production of ROS. This can potentially cause oxidative damage to the sensitive mitochondrial DNA.
- Doxorubicin can injure cardiac muscle because it has a high affinity to the mitochondrial cardiolipin, because it is a redox cycling agent, and because it alters kinase-mediated regulation of intracellular calcium and down-regulates the expression of genes involved in normal energy production.

- Oxidative stress and other forms of chemically-induced stress induced by xenobiotics can cause the opening of the mitochondrial permeability transition pore. This not only causes a collapse of the mitochondrial membrane potential which leads to ATP deprivation but also facilitates the release of proapoptotic factors.

Further reading

Interference with mitochondrial function

Saraste, M. (1999) Oxidative phosphorylation at the *fin de siècle*, *Science* 283: 1488–1493.

Wallace, K.B. and Starkov, A.A. (2000) Mitochondrial targets of drug toxicity, *Annu. Rev. Pharmacol. Toxicol.* 40: 353–388.

Microvesicular steatosis and valproate toxicity

Berson, A., DeBeco, V., Lettéron, P., Robin, M.A., Moreau, C., ElKahwaji, J., Verthier, N., Feldmann, G., Fromenty, B. and Pessayre, D. (1998) Steatohepatitis-inducing drugs cause mitochondrial dysfunction and lipid peroxidation in rat hepatocytes, *Gastroenterology* 114: 764–774.

Fromenty, B. and Pessayre, D. (1995) Inhibition of mitochondrial beta-oxidation as a mechanism of hepatotoxicity, *Pharmacol. Ther.* 67: 101–154.

Fromenty, B. and Pessayre, D. (1997) Impaired mitochondrial function in microvesicular steatosis, *J. Hepatol.* 26: 43–53.

Grillo, M.P., Chiellini, G., Tonelli, M. and Benet, L.Z. (2001) Effect of α-fluorination of valproic acid on valproyl-S-acyl-CoA formation *in vivo* in rats, *Drug Metab. Dispos.* 29: 1210–1215.

Krähenbühl, S., Brandner, S., Kleinle, S., Liechti, S. and Straumann, D. (2000) Mitochondrial diseases represent a risk factor for valproate-induced fulminant liver failure, *Liver* 20: 346–348.

McLaughlin, D.B., Eadie, M.J., Parker-Scott, S.L., Addison, R.S., Henderson, R.D., Hooper, W.D. and Dickinson, R.G. (2000) Valproate metabolism during valproate-associated hepatotoxicity in a surviving adult patient, *Epilepsy Res.* 41: 259–268.

Fluoroacetate toxicity

Lauble, H., Kennedy, M.C., Emptage, M.H., Beinert, H. and Stout, C.D. (1996) The reaction of fluorocitrate with aconitase and the crystal structure of the enzyme-inhibitor complex, *Proc. Natl Acad. Sci. USA* 93: 13699–13703.

Doxorubicin toxicity to mitochondria

Jeyaseelan, R., Poizat, C., Wu, H.Y. and Kedes, L. (1997) Molecular mechanisms of doxorubicin-induced cardiomyopathy – Selective suppression of Reiske iron-sulfur protein, ADP/ATP translocase, and phosphofructokinase genes is associated with ATP depletion in rat cardiomyocytes, *J. Biol. Chem.* 272: 5828–5832.

Scheulen, M.E. and Kappus, H. (1992) Anthracyclines as model compounds for cardiac toxicity, *Tissue-specific Toxicity. Biochem. Mech.* 221–253.

Singal, P.K., Iliskovic, N., Li, T.M. and Kumar, D. (1997) Adriamycin cardiomyopathy: Pathophysiology and prevention, *FASEB J.* 11: 931–936.

Zhou, S., Palmeria, C.M. and Wallace, K.B. (2001) Doxorubicin-induced persistent oxidative stress to cardiac myocytes, *Toxicol. Lett.* 121: 151–157.

Cyanide toxicity

Fosslien, E. (2001) Review: Mitochondrial medicine – Molecular pathology of defective oxidative phosphorylation, *Ann. Clin. Lab. Sci.* 31: 25–67.

Zhang, J.G., Tirmenstein, M.A., Nicholls-Grzemski, F.A. and Fariss, M.W. (2001) Mitochondrial electron transport inhibitors cause lipid peroxidation-dependent and -independent cell death: Protective role of antioxidants, *Arch. Biochem. Biophys.* 393: 87–96.

The MPTP

Bernardi, P. (1999) Mitochondrial transport of cations: Channels, exchangers, and permeability transition, *Physiol. Rev.* 79: 1127–1155.

Crompton, M. (1999) The mitochondrial permeability transition pore and its role in cell death, *Biochem. J.* 341: 233–249.

Lemasters, J.J. (1998) The mitochondrial permeability transition: From biochemical curiosity to pathophysiological mechanism, *Gastroenterology* 115: 783–786.

Toxic hydrophobic bile acids

Gores, G.J. (2000) Mechanisms of cell injury and death in cholestasis and hepatoprotection by ursodeoxycholic acid, *J. Hepatol.* 32 (Suppl. 2): 11–13.

Rodrigues, C.M.P. and Steer, C.J. (2000) Mitochondrial membrane perturbations in cholestasis, *J. Hepatol.* 32: 135–141.

Rolo, A.P., Oliveira, P.J., Moreno, A.J.M. and Palmeira, C.M. (2001) Chenodeoxycholate is a potent inducer of the permeability transition pore in rat liver mitochondria, *Biosci. Rep.* 21: 73–80.

Yerushalmi, B., Dahl, R., Devereaux, M.W., Gumpricht, E. and Sokol, R.J. (2001) Bile acid-induced rat hepatocyte apoptosis is inhibited by antioxidants and blockers of the mitochondrial permeability transition, *Hepatology* 33: 616–626.

Chapter 16

Outlook: from mechanisms to individual expression of genes

The past years have seen an unprecedented increase in the knowledge and understanding of the molecular mechanisms that underlie the toxicity of xenobiotics. These include novel pathways of bioactivation or inactivation, mechanisms of macromolecular binding, receptor binding and activation, and, importantly, novel signaling pathways and specific gene activation mechanisms. Yet many questions are still unresolved and there is a long way to go before we elucidate some of the complexities and interactions of these mechanisms.

Two major factors have been contributing to this accelerated increase in our knowledge. The first factor is related to the recent elucidation of the DNA sequence of the human genome and the identification of hitherto unknown genes, which have revolutionized science. This major achievement has primarily yielded a large amount of new information. The great challenge nowadays, however, is not so much obtaining the information but rather its interpretation. The human genome has approximately 97 percent of 'junk' DNA, and the rest consists of genes. A current British project uses the genome of the puffer fish (Fugu) to bring more clarity into the distinction between relevant gene-related DNA and irrelevant information. This fish has only ~400 million base pairs, and not ~3 billion as humans, and one can surmise that it is primarily the 'junk' DNA that has been eliminated during evolution rather than the indispensable genes. But even if we are left with 'only' approximately 30,000 genes for humans, the puzzling question is how such a small number of genes can act in a concerted manner to fulfill all the necessary functions of life. It has become clear that we must get away from the 'one-gene' concept for one function. It is the interplay and crosstalk between many genes, their time- and situation-dependent multifunctionality, and the equilibrium between many simultaneous pathways that determines the outcome. Probably the same holds true if we specifically address some unresolved questions related to mechanisms of toxicity.

The second factor is the galloping advances in molecular technology. With the recent advent of refined analytics, but primarily of the possibilities to analyze thousands of genes and proteins with the new genomics, transcriptomics, and proteomics techniques, it has become possible to analyze in a short time the time- and concentration-dependent effects of xenobiotics on gene expression at both the transcript and the protein level. DNA microarrays allow one to monitor the activation or inactivation of specific genes as a response to exposure to a xenobiotic. Again, things have turned out to be more complex than anticipated, and the real difficulty is in the handling and interpretation of all these data rather than in actually obtaining the information. We have long realized that the search for a 'tox gene' (e.g. one that would explain the pathways leading to the toxicity of TCDD) has become obsolete, and that it is again the interplay and network of many different pathways that determine such toxicities. In addition, novel techniques in genetics will disclose many new SNPs (single nucleotide polymorphisms), in addition to the well-known genetic polymorphisms for enzmyes, receptors, etc. This, it is hoped, will help in the future to explain some of the rare idiosyncratic reactions to a certain chemical.

In addition to 'toxicogenetics' (genetic analysis by which one might be able to identify susceptible population or patient subsets) and 'toxicogenomics' and 'proteomics' (the technology applications by which one might be able to identify hazardous compounds), another technique has recently gained much attention. With the advent of 'metabonomics', which is based on multivariate statistical analysis of NMR spectroscopic data on small molecules in biofluids, cells, and tissues, it has become possible to analyze and quantify the dynamic metabolic response of living systems to xenobiotics. Together with the other '-omics', metabonomics will undoubtedly provide novel information on mechanisms underlying adaptive and toxic responses to toxicants, as well as identifying biomarkers of exposure.

Thus, molecular toxicology has come a long way. After the intense research activities in the past decades (still ongoing) that have centered around defining the hazard for old and new xenobiotics, the focus of the research activities has more recently moved to the elucidation of molecular mechanisms (still ongoing). Increased emphasis, however, will undoubtedly be put on the analysis of individual expression of genes that will modulate these mechanistic pathways. In addition, the molecular mediators and downstream effector mechanisms and their finely tuned regulation will be better analyzed and, it is hoped, better understood.

However, in spite of the ever-deeper complexities in mechanistic toxicology and the clear focusing on gene expression pathways, it is easy to lose sight of the general picture. The molecular details reveal a new dimension to our understanding of how cells and organisms respond to a challenge by a potentially harmful chemical, but there remains the urgent need to understand the basic chemical, biochemical and physiological links. One purpose of this textbook was to remind the reader of these general links, and not to get lost in the molecular details.

Further reading

Bartosiewicz, M.J., Jenkins, D., Penn, S., Emery, J. and Buckpitt, A. (2001) Unique gene expression patterns in liver and kidney associated with exposure to chemical toxicants, *J. Pharmacol. Exp. Ther.* 297: 895–905.

Ingelman-Sundberg, M. (2001) Genetic variability in susceptibility and response to toxicants, *Toxicol. Lett.* 120: 259–268.

Nicholson, J.K., Lindon, J.C. and Holmes, E. (1999) Metabonomics: Understanding the metabolic responses of living systems to pathophysiological stimuli via multivariate statistical analysis of biological NMR spectroscopic data, *Xenobiotica* 29: 1181–1189.

Robertson, D.G., Reily, M.D., Sigler, R.E., Wells, D.F., Paterson, D.A., and Braden, T.K. (2000) Metabonomics: Evaluation of nuclear magnetic resonance (NMR) and pattern recognition technology for rapid *in vivo* screening of liver and kidney toxicants, *Toxicol. Appl. Pharmacol.* 57: 326–337.

Stevens, J.L. and Marnett, L.J. (1999) Defining molecular toxicology: A perspective, *Chem. Res. Toxicol.* 12: 747–748.

Waring, J.F., Jolly, R.A., Ciurlionis, R., Lum, P.Y., Praestgard, J.T., Morfitt, D.C., Buratto, B., Roberts, C., Schadt, E. and Ulrich, R.G. (2001) Clustering of hepatotoxins based on mechanisms of toxicity using gene expression profiles, *Toxicol. Appl. Pharmacol.* 175: 28–42.

Zbinden, G. (1992) The three eras of research in experimental toxicology, *Trends Pharmacol. Sci.* 13: 221–223.

Review Q&A

Introduction

Q: Two compounds may induce toxicity via the same mechanism, yet cause different toxic effects. Alternatively, two other compounds may cause the same toxic effects, but by different mechanisms. Can you give plausible explanations for these possibilities?

A: pp. 2, 4–5

Q: Give practical reasons why the elucidation of mechanisms underlying the toxicity of xenobiotics is important.

A: p. 3

Q: What is the underlying mechanism that explains why thalidomide embryotoxicity is enantiospecific?

A: pp. 10–12

Organ-selective toxicity

Q: Which molecular mechanisms can plausibly explain possible neurotropic or cardiotropic toxicity of xenobiotics?

A: pp. 16, 45–47, 123, 292

Q: How can cysteinyl–Hg complexes get inside a cell?

A: pp. 17–18

Q: Why do certain cephalosporins accumulate inside proximal tubular cells while others do not?

A: pp. 26–28

Q: What is the biological basis for the liver-selective organotropic toxicity of many xenobiotics?

A: p. 24

Cellular transport and selective accumulation of potentially toxic xenobiotics

Q: What are possible molecular mechanisms which cause xenobiotics to accumulate in a specific cell type and exert cell- or tissue-specific toxic effects, and how are these pathways regulated?

A: pp. 17, 32

Q: Why does paraquat accumulate in alveolar cells while diquat does not?

A: pp. 35–36

Q: What are the underlying mechanisms for MPP$^+$-induced neuronal injury?

A: pp. 38–39

Q: Why does benoxaprofen (or similar compounds) readily precipate in bile canaliculi?

A: pp. 41–43

Q: What is the molecular basis of the blood–brain barrier?

A: pp. 45–46

Bioactivation of xenobiotics to reactive metabolites

Q: Can you name possible evolutionary advantages of the development of a wide array of (often highly preserved) drug-metabolizing enzyme systems?

A: pp. 52–53

Q: How does phenobarbital regulate the expression of CYPs? What are the differences from CYP3A4 regulation by other compounds?

A: pp. 56, 58–59

Q: Why can grapefruit juice augment the pharmacological action of nifedipine?

A: pp. 60–61

Q: What is the molecular basis for the protein-reactivity of acyl glucuronides?

A: pp. 66–67, 201–202

Q: Why can the polymorphic genotype of NAT be important in benzidine toxicity?

A: pp. 71–72

Q: What are the sequential mechanistic steps that cause benzohydroquinone glutathione-S-conjugate nephrotoxicity?

A: pp. 77–79

Q: By what mechanisms can a xenobiotic become phototoxic?

A: p. 81

Q: What are the possible consequences of heat shock protein damage by a reactive metabolite?

A: pp. 86–87

Xenobiotic-induced oxidative stress: cell injury, signaling, and gene regulation

Q: How can a quinone induce oxidoreductive stress in a cell?

A: p. 97

Q: What are the molecular mechanisms contributing to bleomycin-induced lung injury?

A: pp. 106–107

Q: Delineate the molecular mechanisms of initiation and progression of asbestos-induced pulmonary injury.

A: pp. 108–109

Q: What are the molecular and toxicological consequences of DNA base oxidation?

A: pp. 113–116

Q: Name at least three major functions of GSH and thioredoxin.

A: pp. 124, 130

Q: What is the ARE and how can stress genes become activated?

A: pp. 137–138

Q: What are the major signaling pathways activated by ROS?

A: pp. 139–141

Disruption of cellular calcium homeostasis

Q: What is the role(s) of calcium in tri-*n*-butyltin-induced cell injury?

A: p. 150

Mechanisms of necrotic and apoptotic cell death

Q: Where is the 'point of no return' in xenobiotic-induced apoptosis or necrosis?

A: pp. 157, 159, 161

Q: What is the causal relationship between oxidative stress and apoptosis?

A: pp. 160, 166–167

Q: By what mechanisms can caspases become activated?

A: pp. 154, 164–165

Q: What is the role of Fas in xenobiotic-induced apoptosis?

A: pp. 162–163

Q: What is the mechanistic basis for Bcl-2-mediated anti-apoptotic effects (and for Bax-mediated pro-apoptotic effects)?

A: pp. 168–169

Q: What are the consequences of sustained inhibition of apoptosis in a tissue?

A: pp. 170–172

Impairment of cell proliferation and tissue repair

Q: At what points of the cell cycle can xenobiotics interfere with normal function, and what are the downstream biological consequences?

A: p. 176

Q: What is the mechanistic role of p53?

A: pp. 178–179

Q: What is the underlying mechanism of paclitaxel-mediated cell killing?

A: pp. 180–181

Q: Why can certain organochlorine pesticides potentiate the hepatotoxicity of CCl$_4$?

A: p. 184

Covalent binding of reactive metabolites to cellular macromolecules

Q: Both the hepatotoxic drug acetaminophen (APAP) and its non-hepatotoxic structural analog (AMAP, having the phenolic group in the *meta*-position) are bioactivated in the liver and form covalent adducts (although targeting different proteins). What are the possible reasons for the differential toxicity of these congeners, and how could a possible causal involvement of covalent protein modification in the hepatic toxicity of APAP be proved?

A: pp. 190–192

Q: Define an electrophile.

A: pp. 187–188

Q: What are major possible consequences of protein adduct formation?

A: pp. 193–194

Q: What is the molecular mechanism contributing to microcystin toxicity?

A: pp. 195–197

Q: Why is 2,6-heptanedione not neurotoxic while 2,5-hexanedione is?

A: p. 199

Q: Why are hepatic canalicular proteins preferentially acylated by the reactive diclofenac acyl glucuronides and their positional isomers?

A: pp. 202–204

Q: What are the molecular mechanisms of benzo[*a*]pyrene alkylation of guanine?

A: pp. 206–207

Immune mechanisms

Q: Why does everybody exposed to a pro-hapten not develop an immune-mediated toxic reaction in the particular organ or tissue where the protein modification occurs?

A: pp. 229, 231–232

Q: What is the role of Kupffer cells in mediating toxicity?

A: pp. 213–216

Q: How does TCDD impair thymus function and what are the consequences?

A: pp. 218–219

Q: What is the causal relationship between the Toxic Oil Syndrome and autoimmune disease?

A: pp. 221–223

Q: Why can penicillins elicit immunoallergic reactions?

A: pp. 225–226

Q: Why does isoflurane less frequently cause drug-induced hepatitis than halothane?

A: p. 227

Q: What is an idiosyncratic drug reaction?

A: pp. 231–232

Cytokine-mediated toxicity

Q: What is the role of the TNF receptor in xenobiotic-induced toxicity?

A: pp. 164–165, 239–240

Specific inactivation of enzymes and other proteins

Q: Real-case scenario, Switzerland, 1998: To reduce the populations in small lakes of a rapidly proliferating predator crayfish species, imported from Louisiana and which does not belong to the normal European ecofauna, the authorities had considered the use of fenthion. Fenthion is a phosphorothionate pesticide. Environmentalists raised concerns about a health hazard for humans and animals. Based on mechanistic considerations – false alarm or legitimate concerns?

A: pp. 248–249

Q: What is the molecular basis for thyroid function disruption by PCBs, and why are *meta*-substituted PCBs more toxic than *ortho*-substituted PCBs?

A: p. 250

Nuclear receptor-mediated toxicity

Q: List at least three pieces of evidence that the AHR is causally involved in TCDD toxicity.

A: p. 257

Q: What is the molecular mechanism underlying *p*-nonylphenol-associated estrogenic activity?

A: pp. 20, 258–260

Q: Try to convince somebody with sound arguments (based on mechanisms) that (a) most xenoestrogens do not pose a hazard to human health, (b) some xenoestrogens are indeed hazardous to human health.

A: pp. 260, 263

Q: What are the downstream consequences of PPARα activation by xenobiotics (clofibrate)?

A: pp. 264–266

Q: What is the role of PPARγ in normal and pathophysiological conditions and how can a PPARγ ligand and activator (a thiazolidinedione) disrupt the normal function?

A: pp. 264, 269–271

Interactions of xenobiotics with ion transporters

Q: What is the molecular basis for tetrodotoxin neurotoxicity?

A: p. 277

Q: Describe the molecular pathways underlying the cardiotoxicity of digitoxin.

A: p. 279

Disruption of cellular energy production by xenobiotics

Q: What are possible molecular targets for xenobiotics that can compromise mitochondrial function and cause toxicity?

A: pp. 284–285

Q: Explain valproic acid-induced toxicity – molecular mechanisms and consequences?

A: pp. 288–289

Q: What are the molecular mechanisms contributing to doxorubicin-induced cardiotoxicity?

A: pp. 292–294

Q: Give causes and consequences of the opening of the MPTP in mitochondria.

A: pp. 166, 295–297

Index